Identity Revisited and Reimagined

Sangeeta Bagga-Gupta · Aase Lyngvær Hansen
Julie Feilberg
Editors

Identity Revisited and Reimagined

Empirical and Theoretical Contributions on Embodied Communication Across Time and Space

Springer

Editors
Sangeeta Bagga-Gupta
School of Education and Communication
Jönköping University
Jönköping
Sweden

Aase Lyngvær Hansen
Department of Research and Development
Statped
Trondheim
Norway

Julie Feilberg
Language and Communication Studies
Norwegian University of Science and Technology
Trondheim
Norway

ISBN 978-3-319-58055-5 ISBN 978-3-319-58056-2 (eBook)
DOI 10.1007/978-3-319-58056-2

Library of Congress Control Number: 2017941467

Printed on acid-free paper

This Springer imprint is published by Springer Nature
The registered company is Springer International Publishing AG
The registered company address is: Gewerbestrasse 11, 6330 Cham, Switzerland

On being, becoming and belonging
and
other positionings in the 21st century

"The Sanskrit word dharma *is the nearest synonym [...] for the word civilisation... The specific meaning of* dharma *is that principle which holds us firm together and leads us to our best welfare. The radical meaning of this word is the essential quality of a thing"*

—Nobel laureate Rabindranath Tagore 1861–1941, Crisis in Civilisation & Other Essays, 18–19

Foreword

Identity is a heavily researched field, studied from multiple angles and through diverse lenses and in different settings, whether those of different institutions within, or sectors of, society. Some approaches look at the predictable configurations of identity, or the factors that contribute to formation, display and components of identity. Others try to work out the structure or shape to the diverse manifestations of identity, and still others study identity according to categories and traditions of different academic disciplines, or inform analysis of identity through examination of incidents taken to illustrate or instantiate the psychological, linguistic, philosophical, sociological or embodied character of identity. This volume breaks new ground in approach and content, summed up in its title of a*revisiting* of the approaches to identity scholarship to*reimagine* the object of analysis. The volume is extremely well edited by Sangeeta Bagga-Gupta, Aase Lyngvær Hansen and Julie Feilberg so that despite the wide range of studies, approaches, settings and problems discussed they are held together by a common emphasis of combining empirical documentation with refined thinking. The revisiting takes the reader across the global North and global South, to and in virtual worlds, as well as settings of immediate physical and spatial contact between actors and in an array of kinds of identity, including the various ways that ability, physical and otherwise, is marked and constructed in social life.

This book aims to transcend limitations of identity scholarship so much of which has been framed by static concepts and non-dynamic understandings of the individual self, relations between individual and group, and the dynamic interplay of the multiple groups and identities that individuals negotiate and affirm/deny in various interactions. For this reason, the chapters make complexity and diversity a central element of analysis. Many contributors stress intersectional stances and most report empirically driven studies of local work, often taking a micro-level analysis. Inevitably, perhaps, communication is always involved, internal communication of an identity forming or identity displaying group, and external communication between that group and various interlocutors beyond it. Communication involves a fusion of structure and purpose, the structure comes to us from the past, such as the words and forms of expression that our languages bequeath us, and our application of those in original meaning making in the present for our specific purposes. The form that communication takes combines the inherited and validated patterns of the past with pragmatic needs in the here and now. Between these planes, but structuring them too, is a space where identities are played out as interlocutors seek not only to send messages but to be present and identified with these messages in the context of actually occurring interaction. In this way, communication patterns we inherit are also changed to make room for how new identity formations name the world and seek to change it in their image.

All chapters represent a challenge to analyses of identity that make use of demarcated fields of study, with their bounded high abstractions, whether of gender, race, or language grouping, and instead turn the spotlight to identity as a social practice, negotiated and enacted in encounters, always interactional though often framed by inherited (historical) formations.

In my own work on language policy in conflict zones in Southeast Asia, I read this volume with an eye to what it can teach us about struggle in the social and public life of communities. The struggle I have in mind is that in which national institutions are confronted with demands for recognition of difference, and how this difference or these multiple differences are represented, displayed, negotiated, accommodated or repudiated. The social identity formations, the "new" identities that demand inclusion, are themselves, sometimes if not often, struggling for internal self-definition even as they demand the institutions of their society acknowledge their presence. What we need to learn from researchers of identity is a response to the new kinds of conflict, struggle and demands in today's world, between citizens and states and their autonomous institutions, networks and discourses. These new kinds of conflict are widespread, after all, despite proclamations that the world is getting more peaceable (cf Steven Pinker 2011, *The Better Angels of Our Nature: Why Violence has Declined*) there is immense conflict at the sub-national level all across the world in which something like identity is present, prominent, and problematical. In a review of the Pinker book, philosopher John Gray described it as an "attempt to ground the hope of peace in science", and while science in the sense intended is unlikely to produce peace, research, knowledge accumulation and reflection and dialogue must play their proper roles.

The contemporary science of conflict analysis is in any case muddled, even at the most basic level of quantification. Some claim that overall levels of violence and conflict are at historically low levels and declining, contested by research that shows multiplying forms and intensifying levels of violence, tension, and dislocation globally.

Conflict today is most often intra- and sub-national, some of it intergenerational, rather than the more conventionally identified international and sharp-focused wars that flare and end and that make up the bulk of what is taught in history curriculums in schools. There are innumerable instances of conflict today that is chronic in nature, and within polities rather than between them, and within many polities that are secure and unlikely to dissipate. The boundaries of conflict are less and less about nation and territory, though there are too many conventional conflicts as well, and more and more conflicts within nations and networked across them. This new geography of conflict is not itself completely new, but certainly more pronounced, more spread, and perhaps more intractable than before, and infused with disputes characterized by rival and seemingly irreconcilable differences of identity.

These problems give rise to the critical importance of research on identity and have given rise to new thinking about conflict and conflict types. One clear example is the work of "new war" scholars emerging in the last decades, who aim to open up understanding of the new shape and form of violent conflict. Silent or absent in much of this literature are questions of language and culture grievance even though language and culture grievance are often present, but also silenced or absent is any "re-visiting" or "re-imagining" of identity, such as is undertaken in this book.

Some conflicts are network based. Network conflicts involve a struggle for power beyond state actors alone, such as in Syria today, where global non-state armed groups, religiously defined, nationality defined and ideologically defined actors, some aspiring to statehood, others wanting to preserve current statehood or to dismantle existing states, are all involved. Ethno-linguistic grievance, and demands for restitution and recognition of past injustice also serve to surface new kinds of conflict or new dimensions to existing conflict. It would be incorrect to imagine that these are new in any totally original unprecedented sense. Their newness resides in the hybrid forms they take and the globalization of the identity formations that instantaneous communications and the multicultural realities of most nation states make possible. It is in much more complex polities that new conflicts occur and in which new kinds of identity offer us entrée to understanding and to the possibility of mitigation of tension and problems. In this context, new research evidence and considered reflections on the problematic of identity are welcome and those reported in this fine book are an important instalment in this wider task of helping us, as citizens and as scholars, to contribute to forging new kinds of social relations that are collaborative, inclusive and peaceable. Another practical need is to better inform dialogue and facilitation methods used in post-conflict negotiations so that these are more grounded in the reality of new formations of identity.

It has long been apparent that the gulf that predictably and profoundly stalks academic life, between reflection and action, and that gives rise to popular characterizing of ivory towers and unworldly academics, is not only regrettable but also dangerous. It is often deeply untrue. This is partly because the academy itself is a real part of the real world, whose inhabitants (scholars, researchers and teachers) engage continuously with the practical and the everyday, perhaps not always with their research, but at least in their "other life" as citizens. For this reason, the extreme version of the stereotype of unworldly ivory tower academics is often plain wrong. In any case, not all scholarship needs to engage with the everyday and the practical. Yet there remains much to lament about separation between "the academy" and "the world" in many areas where knowledge generated through research and reflection can improve social and community life.

When scholarship reflects on issues so critical to the conduct of social and political life divisions between "theory" and "practice" worlds must be overcome. The reflected, reflexive and nuanced considerations of phenomena in the academy, on topics such as identity, and the daily practical tasks of tackling identity conflicts and problems in civil life, work, and education, need to be brought into interaction with each other. Identity is a topic of today, for the world of today, with consequences for aspirations of equality, participation and intercultural communication that motivate many of us in our work as both scholars and citizens. The innovative work of scholars who might offer hope for new ways to work with problematical concepts needs to be connected quickly and substantively to the work of practitioners in a range of fields where identity problems pose serious challenges to institutional or civic life.

Politicians frequently describe social cohesion as reliant on the vehicles of shared language, common citizenship, sense of belonging and democratic expression. All these remain important instruments and practices for coherence and resilience, but the proliferation of ways in which groups identify and their desires for identity recognition impose on us a need to expand, extend and deepen our understanding of how socially cohesive public life can be imagined.

Identity is a predictable and profound component of the roiling tensions of our contemporary world yet its treatment in journalistic coverage and political debate is superficial and outdated. We need the kind of steady, sobering, historically attuned and globally oriented scholarship the chapter authors in this book offer us, on identity and its complexities, to take into our classrooms, research projects and civic life. But we also need to adapt, communicate and exchange identity research work with policy makers, conflict analysts, social planners and a host of others, who also do "identity work" as they manage relations between people within nations or institutions, delivering services and distributing goods, making economies function, promoting welfare and equality and supporting civil peaceful civil co-existence.

The stable identity formations of ethnic culture, official language, national state and organized religion of the past are today multiplied and supplemented by new formations and new elements of identity. Lobby groups, promotional interests and other forms of political representation give voice to these mixed, diverse and mobile configurations of the ways in which the social spaces we inhabit are proliferating with social groupings to which we are attached and which interact with each other. At the beginning of 2017, there can hardly be a more urgent task than for researchers to revisit and reimagine identity, and to then engage with policy makers about the new formations that constitute our social selves, and participate in the design of the practices and understandings of an improved civil life for all.

Joseph Lo Bianco
Professor of Language and Literacy Education
Melbourne Graduate School of Education
The University of Melbourne
Melbourne
Australia

Preface

While there is no dearth of scientific literature in the area of identity, a common point of departure in dealing with it is from philosophical, policy studies and/or political science points of view. Another routine manner in which identity gets approached in research is through sector framed domains that build upon identity categories such as gender, ethnicity, class, functional dis/abilities, nation state. Disciplinary framed fields such as education, special education, health sciences, including the multidisciplinary fields of language and communication studies, disability studies, gender studies, have focused the concept of identity in a range of ways. Such an interest often tends to be discussed in terms of what can be called "identity sectors".

The majority of institutional settings such as K-12 education, higher education, care services, including special interest groups, provide enclaves that encompass people of *all* ages, gender, class, race, functional abilities, etc. While this is also the case in everyday life contexts inside and outside institutional settings, certain institutions (for instance, governments, company boardrooms) tend to be homogenous as far as identity markers such as gender, ethnicity and functional ability are concerned.

The empirically framed theoretical contributions in this book explore dimensions of life inside and outside institutional settings that allow for dynamic viewings of human identity processes. Going beyond traditional identity sectors explicitly, the contributions both revisit and reimagine identity positions in settings across the global North and the global South. They also traverse across face-to-face and digital sites, bringing with it dialoguing in the current age of ubiquitous virtual communication and globalization. Highlighting the need to recognize decolonial perspectives, the use of concepts such as the "global North" and "global South" attempts to frame all geopolitical spaces, including Nordic nation states like those of Norway and Sweden, in terms of contexts where marginalization and colonial power hierarchies have existed and continue to exist. This then goes beyond understandings of nation states in terms of historical coloniality and opens up for the recognition of current ways in which marginalization processes get played out across the globe.

In addition to going beyond bounded identity fields and challenging static and demarcated descriptions of identity, the chapters in this book present theoretical and/or empirical explorations of the ways in which human beings position themselves and get positioned across sites in different practices. Taking a social practice perspective, the chapters in this book build upon the premise that both institutions and individuals are shaped by the "living and daily doings" of members of institutions in different settings. Each contribution takes as its point of departure the complexities that characterize and shape both individuals and communities—past and present, engaging with the increasing pace of change and diversification that interfaces at global, geopolitical and local scales. In other words, the contributions take a social practice perspective as a point of departure for exploring the performance, living and doing of identity positions across time and space. Many of the contributions take an intersectional stance and the majority report upon empirically driven studies that explore the ways in which micro- as well as multi-scalar analyses of naturally occurring human communication and behaviours contribute to our understanding of identification processes; the ways in which more recent dialogical and social theoretical-analytical frameworks allow for attending to the complexity and dynamics of identity processes; the ways in which institutional settings, media settings, community of practices and affinity spaces provide affordances and obstacles for different types of identity positions; and the ways in which shifts in identity positions can be traced across time and space (in for instance, interactional and/or historical data).

In other words, this book explicitly focuses ongoing or recently completed research that discusses results specifically from a social practice perspective, representing different domains and disciplines that build upon interactional and/or historical studies where identity positions and processes are centre-staged. Secondly, the book's contribution lies in the fact that it explicitly discusses methodological and conceptual issues of relevance in the light of present-day diversification, including virtual and physical mobility across time and space. The chapters challenge demarcated fields of study and conceptions of identity *as* gender, identity*as* functional disability, identity*as* race, identity*as* or based upon language groupings, etc. Furthermore, the book offers theoretical and methodological discussions by contributors whose empirical work illustrates global North–South perspectives. Finally, an important and unique contribution of the book is mainstreaming not only marginalized areas of study (for instance, the area of disability and differently abled studies, gender studies) but also bringing into the mainstream voices of marginalized authors and reviewers (including authors and reviewers with diverse experiences within scholarship).

The vast majority of the individual contributions in the book "Identity Revisited and Reimagined" have developed from further reviewed and revised versions of selected peer-reviewed drafts presented and discussed at the international conference–workshop "Revisiting Identities, REID" organized by the CCD, Communication, Culture and Diversity research environment in Sweden (www.ju.se/ccd). The conference was awarded a grant by the Swedish Research Council. In addition to this grant, we would like to acknowledge support grants awarded to the

REID project by (i) the Faculty of Humanities and Social Sciences at Örebro University, Sweden, (ii) NTNU, Trondheim, Norway, and (iii) the Center for Rehabilitation Research, Örebro County Council, Sweden. Resources from the CCD research environment and the hospitality offered by the Statped Midt at Trondheim, Norway, have made possible editorial meetings during 2015 and 2016. We also gratefully acknowledge the unflinching administrative support of Ms. Kicki Ekberg for the CCD activities that lead up to REID and this volume. Finally, the support of the Springer publication team headed by Hendrikje Tuerlings and including Esther Otten and Cynthia Kroonen is gratefully acknowledged.

In particular, we are thankful to each of the following external reviewers for their participation in the REID project during 2015–2016: Arnfinn Vonen, Norway; Ernst Thoutenhoofd, Sweden; Giulia Messina Dahlberg, Sweden; Gunnar Grepperud, Norway; Guy Karnung, Sweden; Hilde Haualand, Norway; Ingela Holmström, Sweden; Jonathan White; Sweden; Lazaro Moreno Herrera, Sweden; Mathew Martin, India; Mats Tegmark, Sweden; Mila Vulchanova, Norway; Patrick Stefan Kermit, Norway; Rolf Piene Halvorsen, Norway; Synnøve Matre, Norway; Sylvia Vigmo, Sweden; Tone Pernille Østern, Norway. We are also indebted to the publishers' external reviewers who remain anonymous and whose two rounds of feedback during 2016 have been appreciated.

The book "Identity Revisited and Reimagined. Empirical and Theoretical Contributions Across Time and Space" is divided into four parts. Part I consists of four chapters that contribute to the theme "Conceptual Framings of Identity in a Multifaceted World". Part II, "Making, Undoing and Remaking: Performing Identities", presents work in three chapters. The next three chapters in the book come together in Part III: "Politically Framed Identities in Embodied Interaction". The final part in this book, "Identity Work in Institutional and Technology Mediated Environments", presents studies in four chapters. A short editorial introduction opens each of the four sections that make up this book. A Foreword by Prof. Joseph Lo Bianco, chair of Language and Literacy Education, Melbourne Graduate School of Education, University of Melbourne, Australia, presents an introductory commentary related to identity, peace and conflict mediation and situates the book against current geopolitical issues across planet earth. An Afterword presents reflections on the volume by senior professor Roger Säljö from Gothenburg University, Sweden.

Jönköping, Sweden/AMU, Aligarh, India
Trondheim, Norway/Khao Lak, Thailand
Trondheim, Norway/London, England
January 2017

Sangeeta Bagga-Gupta
Aase Lyngvær Hansen
Julie Feilberg

The original version of the book frontmatter was revised: Editor affiliation in copyright page has been updated and abstracts for all chapters in online version have been included. The erratum to the chapter is available at 10.1007/978-3-319-58056-2_15

Contents

Editors and Contributors

About the Editors

Sangeeta Bagga-Gupta is Full Professor of Education since 2016 at Jönköping University, Sweden. She has been full professor at Örebro University, Sweden since 2007. She is also adjunct professor 2016–2017 at Aligarh University, India. Her multidisciplinary, multi-scalar ethnographically framed research focuses communication, learning and identity from sociocultural and decolonial framings. She publishes extensively and in a number of different research domains. She is the Principle Investigator of the new Swedish Research Council project*Participation for all? School and post-school pathways of young people* (2016–2020) and has been the leader of the research group CCD, *Communication, Culture and Diversity* since the end of the 1990s.

Aase Lyngvær Hansen is Assistant Professor (emerita) of Language and Communication at the Norwegian University of Science and Technology, Trondheim, Norway. Her multidisciplinary research focuses on interaction and learning in visually oriented classrooms. She has also worked for many years as a teacher of the deaf and as a developer of teaching material for the deaf on video, DVD and Internet.

Julie Feilberg is Assistant Professor of Language and Communication at the Norwegian University of Science and Technology, Trondheim, Norway. Her research focuses child language development and professional and institutional discourse. She has also served for many years as pro-rector with responsibility for education and quality learning at the Norwegian University of Science and Technology.

Contributors

Ellen Andenæs Norwegian University of Science and Technology, Trondheim, Norway

Sangeeta Bagga-Gupta School of Education and Communication, Jönköping University, Jönköping, Sweden

David Block ICREA/University of Lleida, Lleida, Spain

Marina Everri Department of Psychological and Behavioural Science, London School of Economics, London, UK

Julie Feilberg Norwegian University of Science and Technology, Trondheim, Norway

Annaliina Gynne School of Education, Culture and Communication, Mälardalen University, Västerås, Sweden

Aase Lyngvær Hansen Norwegian University of Science and Technology, Trondheim, Norway

Johan Hjulstad Department of Language and Literature, Norwegian University of Science and Technology, Trondheim, Norway

Elizabeth Keating University of Texas, Austin, USA

Irene W. Leigh Department of Psychology, Gallaudet University, Washington, DC, USA

Paul McIlvenny Department of Culture and Global Studies, Aalborg University, Aalborg, Denmark

Sigrun Marie Moss Department of Psychology, University of Oslo, Oslo, Norway

Jenny Rosén Department of Language Education, Stockholm University, Stockholm, Sweden; Dalarna University, Falun, Sweden

Julia Sacher University of Cologne, Cologne, Germany

Laura Sterponi Language Literacy and Culture at the Graduate School of Education, University of California, Berkeley, USA

Elina Tapio Humak University of Applied Sciences, Helsinki, Finland

Abbreviations

CCM	Chama cha Mapinduzi (The party of the Revolution) (political party)
CDA	Critical Discourse Analysis
cf.	*confer*, see also
CIC	Categorization of Identities and Communication
CIRCA	Clandestine Insurgent Radical Clown Army
COP 15	Fifteenth session of the Conference of the Parties
CORE	Congress of Racial Equality
CUF	Civic United Front (political party)
DAS	Deaf Acculturation Scale
DIMuL	"Doing Identity in and through Multilingual Literacy Practices", project name
e.g.	*example given*, for example
ECTS-credit	European Credit Transfer and Accumulation System credit
EMCA	Ethnomethodological Conversation Analysis
f.	following (page, line)
ff.	following (pages, lines)
FinSL	Finnish Sign Language
GNU	Government of National Unity
i.e.	*id est*, that means
IAEA	International Atomic Energy Agency
ibid.	*ibidem*, in the same place
IOC	International Olympic committee
LGBT	Lesbian, Gay, Bisexual, Transgender/Transsexual
LGBTQ	Lesbian, gay, bisexual, transgendered and queer
LIMCUL	The Swedish National Research School "Young People's Literacies, Multilingualism and Cultural Practice in Everyday Society". The research school is supported by the Swedish Research Council
MCA	Membership Categorization Analysis

MDA	Mediated Discourse Analysis
NSL	Norwegian sign language
SFI	Swedish for Immigrants
SLA	Second-Language Acquisition
SLL	Second-Language Learning
UN	United Nations
UNMOVIC	United Nations Monitoring, Verification and Inspection Commission
USA	United States of America
VME	Video Mediated Environment, or video-*only* mediated environment
WMD	Weapons of Mass Destruction

List of Figures

List of Tables

List of Transcripts

Part I
Conceptual Framings of Identity in a Multifaceted World

Theorizing issues related to identity from a range of ways, the four chapters that constitute the first part of the volume "*Identity Revisited and Reimagined. Empirical and Theoretical Contributions Across Time and Space*" present conceptual framings related to identity in and across spaces, interactions, methodologies, and mobilities. Going beyond essentialistic bounded understandings of identity, or the novelty ascribed to human diversity across spaces in the twenty-first century, the individual chapters in this part highlight the many-ways-of-being (particularly Chaps. 1 and 4), the embodiment and resistance or counter-positionings (particularly Chaps. 2 and 3), and the contextualization of performances of identity (all four chapters) in and across time and space. They contribute to furthering our understandings of "normal diversity" (compare with super/hyper-diversity) and theorize identity in a multifaceted world.

In Chap. 1, "Many Ways-of-Being Across Sites. Identity as (Inter)action," Sangeeta Bagga-Gupta, Julie Feilberg, and Aase Lyngvær Hansen call attention to how identity gets framed in both everyday media contexts and research contexts across time and space. Their chapter challenges specific ways-of-being that get fossilized in traditional identification categories across contexts. Bagga-Gupta, Feilberg, and Hansen focus identity positions and research on aspects of identity, by taking a point of departure in the geopolitical spaces of Norway and Sweden, including virtual spaces and academic global spaces. Focusing identity discussions by representatives of "Generation Z" (among other sources), the chapter aims to illustrate key conceptual dimensions prevalent in contemporary human and social science theories of identity. The work presented in this chapter builds upon an understanding of identity as interaction and multiple ways-of-being, where diversity is a cornerstone concept. The chapter aims to tweeze out commonsensical understandings as they are represented in mass-media texts; trace a brief historical development and focus of research on identity in some Scandinavian contexts; and finally, highlight the ways decolonial perspectives can (potentially) shape academic work on identity.

David Block in Chap. 2 "Positioning Theory and Life-Story Interviews: Discursive Fields, Gaze and Resistance" offers a working model for making sense of life-story interviews, including embodied interactions that transpire during them. This model extends positioning theory and makes use of the concept of discursive fields as a backdrop. Block argues that we need to take an approach to life-story interviews which moves beyond an exclusively microlevel analysis (examining, e.g., the minutest of features of spoken language, such as pronoun use or accent) or an exclusively content-based analysis (which, in essence, plays the story told in the interview back to the reader). Instead, he proposes that we take seriously that interviews are social events, sociohistorically embedded in multiple phenomenological layers. His point of departure is that while this view of interviews is by now fairly well accepted in principle, many narrative researchers continue to fail to take it fully into account. The chapter does not aim to make available concrete recommendations about how to incorporate this more socially sensitive view of interviews into narrative research; rather, it aims to further discussion in a debate opened long ago by scholars such as Jerome Bruner, who wrote about interviews as social events, sociohistorically embedded in multiple phenomenological layers.

The chapter builds upon a life-story interview excerpt, which Block argues is interpretable only if we take an expansive approach in the analysis. Block discusses positioning theory as a means through which we can make sense of interactions that get played out during interviews. He develops an extension of positioning theory with the aim of understanding interviews as social phenomena, drawing on authors such as Judith Butler, Mikhail Bakhtin, James Paul Gee, Karl Marx, and Michel Foucault. The interview excerpt data used functions as a tool to which the author adds layers in order to substantiate his emergent model of analysis. The chapter presents salient issues that arise in all research where life-story interviews are used.

In Chap. 3, "Refusing What We Are: Communicating Counter-Identities and Prefiguring Social Change in New Social Movements," Paul McIlvenny points to the need (i) for revisiting and challenging how we conceptualize identity and (ii) for rethinking studies of discourse and identity. In this chapter, he uses Ethnomethodological Conversation Analysis (EMCA) to examine how "counter-identities" are achieved and made accountable in interactional practices of a mock protest event. McIlvenny highlights that protests by a range of new social movements have been studied extensively, but that few studies have focused on the communicative practices and mediated actions in which new identities and forms of subjectivity are discursively produced. In this chapter, he deploys and investigates what Michel Foucault called "counter-conducts," practices in which alternative modes of being governed are performed. By questioning the conduct of their conduct, participants simultaneously question the relationship of the self to itself, playing with and risking identity in the process. The case study presented in the chapter analyzes video recordings of a "United Nathans weapons inspectors" protest theater event that took place in 2003. Using EMCA, McIlvenny examines how counter-identities get played out in the interactional practices of the prefigurative protest event. McIlvenny argues that such an approach helps document the ways in which fields of visibility and modes of rationality are sequentially and categorically organized in the contingent accomplishment of counter-identities.

In Chap. 4, "Center-Staging Language and Identity Research from Earthrise Perspectives. Contextualizing Performances in Open Spaces," Sangeeta Bagga-Gupta uses the phenomenon of moonrise–sunrise metaphorically to explicate two perspectives that highlight the ways in which communication and identity are commonly approached and/or understood. Represented by moonrises, the first position highlights a relatively less "visible" norm that nevertheless potently shapes these understandings. Bagga-Gupta highlights that this dominant default norm is marked by a monolingual–monocultural or monoethnic perspective. It is "naturalized" in Eurocentric global North discourses and is often not made visible in either mundane discourses or the academic literature. In contrast, the more visible second position, represented by sunrises, highlights the common human condition vis-à-vis communication and identity. Bagga-Gupta argues that the latter position paradoxically gets marked as the deviant, marginalized, not-normal in global North discourses. Position 2 gets framed in academic discourses and commonsensical thinking through concepts such as bi-/multi-/pluri-/translingualism, bi-/multiculturalism, and multiethnicities. Recent terminology that has emerged within European literature on globalization, framed by migration flows into European geopolitical spaces (and digitalization), includes concepts such as super/hyperdiversity. Bagga-Gupta argues that the more common human condition of diversity gets deviantly framed, marking and making visible (albeit as the not-normal) multiple language varieties and membership in multiple cultures and ethnicities. The chapter illustrates how these two positions represent normative global North discourses where communication and identity, including culture, are approached through, as well as reduced to, technicalities and essentialistically framed epistemologies. Such understandings are critically relevant for the organizing of institutionalized learning for children and adults across geopolitical spaces, in general, and in global North contexts like those of Sweden more especially.

Going beyond these two hegemonic positions and informed by decolonial alternative epistemologies, Bagga-Gupta center-stages a third perspective wherein language-use or languaging and identiting or identity-positionings, including culturing, represent dynamically different ways of approaching and/or understanding human behavior and the human condition. Drawing upon the iconic images taken by the crew of Apollo 8 in December 1968, the phenomenon of "Earthrise" is deployed to substantiate such an alternative position. Bagga-Gupta illustrates how the phenomena of earthrise contrasts in significant ways with moonrise and sunrise conceptualizations of language and identity.

Chapter 1
Many Ways-of-Being Across Sites. Identity *as* (Inter)action

Sangeeta Bagga-Gupta, Julie Feilberg and Aase Lyngvær Hansen

1.1 Introduction

With its origin in the latin *idem*, meaning "the same", identity refers to aspects that pertain to a person, group or a phenomenon that is stable in some sense over time (Gleason 1983; Wetherell 2010; Wetherell and Mohanty 2010). Taylor (1989) suggests that a concept such as identity was unthinkable before the 16th century. Its usage, nevertheless, has a long history. It was identified in the 16th century in the English language, where it resembles the concept of identic similarity (likeness) used in mathematics. One currently finds the word identity in the natural sciences, for instance in the disciplines of medicine, biology, chemistry, physics etc. (see below). Identity was used by philosophers like Leibniz and Locke in discussions on the relationship between mind and matter, from the 18th century onwards. This usage was further developed by philosophers like Friedrich von Schelling in what he termed identity philosophy (Craig 1998). At the beginning of the 20th century, the work of the psychoanalyst Erik H. Erikson incorporated the concept of identity into social psychology (Erikson 1968). Since the 1950s it has become a core concept both in the social sciences and in the humanities (Gleason 1983). More recently, Wetherell calls for the need to see "identity as an open problematic—a site gathering together a wide range of concerns, tropes, curiosities, patterns of thoughts, debates around certain binaries and particular kinds of conversations" (2010:1). The concept, one can say, is heavily theorized in contemporary academic

S. Bagga-Gupta (✉)
School of Education and Communication, Jönköping University, Jönköping, Sweden
e-mail: Sangeeta.bagga-gupta@ju.se

J. Feilberg · A.L. Hansen
Norwegian University of Science and Technology, Trondheim, Norway
e-mail: julie.feilberg@ntnu.no

A.L. Hansen
e-mail: aaselyngvarhansen@gmail.com

S. Bagga-Gupta et al. (eds.), *Identity Revisited and Reimagined*,
DOI 10.1007/978-3-319-58056-2_1

discussions (at least in the global North; for some discussions on the situation in the global South see Hasnain et al. 2013; Bagga-Gupta et al. 2013). It is a concept that is a paradigmatic product of its historical conditions, formulated and reformulated in strategic ways by the period or movement under which it emerged and the preoccupations of its theorists (Benwell and Stokoe 2006).

The idea of a stable, bounded identity, "the real self", more or less seen as a psychological phenomenon or "a stable structure located primarily in the individual psyche or in fixed social categories" (Bucholtz and Hall 2005: 586), represents the core in many theories of identity that have emerged from global North settings. Such an "essentialist view" continues to dominate scholarship despite having been challenged in numerous ways over time. This hegemonic view differs substantially from conceptions of identity as a fluid, malleable product that is discursively produced as people position themselves and get positioned in social interaction across a range of contexts, including textual settings. This latter view of identity is often referred to as a "social constructionist" perspective (Benwell and Stokoe 2006).

The work presented in this chapter takes a social constructionist point of departure on identity. It furthermore presents some empirically framed analysis of different data-sets from some global North contexts, and brings to bear the relevance of decolonial perspectives in these contexts. We here call for a return to an understanding of identity in terms of performance, *as* action. This means that we call for center-staging the sites of identity formation both analytically *and* methodologically. This perspective is not being offered as something novel per se since such a position has existed in one way or another for a long time within academic disciplines such as (certain branches of) anthropology, sociology, psychology, as well as multidisciplinary areas of scholarship. However, in addition to re-emphasizing the need to attend to identity as performance, as action in scholarship, what this chapter attempts to do is to highlight the myriad ways in which such a position gets articulated within and across contemporary sites such as mass-media settings and in academic genres, *and* furthermore calls for augmenting these from decolonial perspectives.

More specifically, the work presented in this chapter focuses upon identity positions and research on aspects of identity, by taking a point of departure in the geopolitical spaces of Norway and Sweden, including virtual spaces and academic global spaces. Scandinavian geopolitical spaces are traditionally not associated with 19th and 20th century European colonization. Our focus upon these geopolitical spaces builds upon a conviction that there exists a need to address issues of decolonialism across sites in contemporary discussions of globalization. Recent decolonially framed scholarship gives recognition to issues of power hegemony, marginalization, including colonialism in both global North *spaces* and global South *spaces*, including the global South in global North *places* (and vice versa; see Sect. 1.4 below and Bagga-Gupta, Chap. 4 this volume). In addition to highlighting the hegemonies of the global North and the marginalization of global South thinking and knowledge regimes, such work is re-emerging and is becoming re-configured in "Southern" epistemologies, ontologies and cosmologies. This work no longer emerges only from southern places. More significantly, it is scholarship from across south-north geographical places and from global South spaces that contributes to such theorizing. Our previous and ongoing work, including our argumentation in this chapter, highlights the significance of, as well as contributes to, such thinking. Thus, it is the very decolonialization of knowledge structures that are at stake here and our work attempts to contribute to a small, growing body of literature that calls for the *reconfigurations of centers and margins* (Appadurai 1996; Bagga-Gupta 2013; Hasnain et al. 2013; Omoniyi 2015; Maldonado-Torres 2011).

Section 1.2 presents an analytical teaser of some slices of data from the domain of contemporary mass-media sites. More specifically, we present some reflections first on a data-set from a recent portrayal of a teenager across physical and virtual in-flight magazine texts as well as the teenagers' own blog texts (Sect. 1.2.1). Thereafter, Sect. 1.2.2 presents analysis of another mass-media data-set that is more traditional and currently has a material and digital presence, i.e. newspapers. These sets of analysis illuminate aspects of identity work and some of the current social mass-media landscapes and conditions under which identity processes circulate and are negotiated.

Taking these analyses as a point of departure for understanding identity empirically, Sect. 1.3 moves on to focus upon research on identity in some Scandinavian contexts. More specifically, we turn our gaze at the body of Ph.D. theses presented in Norway and Sweden during the last 25 years. Doctoral theses in these settings (where we are ourselves situated), constitute a specific academic genre that are publically defended and digitally catalogued. Access to them across time and space is thus possible. Furthermore, this genre constitutes a substantial piece of work that a junior scholar produces during the course of his/her socialization trajectory into mainstream academics (in these and many other geopolitical spaces). The final section of this chapter—Sect. 1.4—brings together the issues that emerge in the analysis of the different data-sets (the mass-media materials and the academic texts) and current attempts to re-emphasize the need to see the layers of identity issues embedded in "diversity", a cornerstone concept in current scholarship, political discourses, policies, etc. Going beyond current popular nomenclature of "hyper-diversity", "super-diversity" (Vertovec 2006; see also Blommaert 2010) and "complex diversity" (Kraus 2012), we highlight the need for engaging with decolonial perspectives and critiques that are re-emerging in Southern scholarship, with the intent of shaping research work on identity in the Scandinavian contexts. Furthermore, we argue for the need to re-vitalize understandings of diversity from an action and a multiple viewing of identity positions. The issues that we raise in this chapter, thus contribute towards nuancing contemporary (largely Eurocentric) discourses of diversity and call for identity to be understood in discussions of diversity as an emergent dimension of interaction across time and space and in terms of multiple ways-of-being.

1.2 Identity and Identity-Positions in Global North Mass-Media Sites

1.2.1 A Contemporary Mass-Media Example Across Physical-Digital Sites: Elise By Olsen

The youth culture and style magazine Recence Paper, started by Elise By Olsen, a 14-year old from the geopolitical spaces of Norway, is showcased in a recent article in a British daily newspaper, the Guardian, as follows: the Recence Paper is a,

> youth culture magazine exposing the lifestyle of youth and its subculture. A youth generation that is tired of a society that ruins collective self-confidence with an expectation of perfection that is forced upon them. These youth are part of a generation that will not be limited to gender binaries. They will not accept the obligations of commercialism (Ferrier 2015, http://recenspaper.com/about/).

Prior to starting the Recence Paper, Elise By Olsen had begun blogging (when she was eight years old) and had established a global blog network by the time she turned 13. Featured in the in-flight magazine of the airline Norwegian, Elise By Olsen is quoted as saying: "We are generation Z. We are fed up with all the commercials that are dumped on us, the impossible beauty standards which ruin our self-confidence, and the gender stereotypes that put us in a box" (Olsson 2015: 25).

> For By Olsen, it's a cri du coeur against Scandinavian norms. 'A lot of the time here', she says, 'people look the same, dress the same, and all the magazines have this clean aesthetic. At school there's a uniform: preppy shirt, Canada Goose jacket, Uggs, make-up. We want to say that you don't have to be girly, you don't have to be understated—you can be loud and colourful, and be yourself' (Olsson 2015: 25).

Commenting on By Olsen's Instagram account, the journalist Olsson writes that it, "reveals a lot of selfies, and lot of attitude" (Olsson 2015: 25; see Fig. 1.1).

> 'I wear short crop tops and have pink hair—I'm used to being stared at, online and offline'. If it all seems slightly solipsistic to anyone who grew up pre-internet (when teenagers didn't generally have public profiles), to her 'it's just the way it is, it's natural to us. Most of us grow up with a public persona, and we create this curated little world' (By Olsen cited in Olsson 2015: 25).

The articles and interviews with a representative of "Generation Z", directly and indirectly serve to illustrate several dimensions of identity that are salient in contemporary theories of identity and identity research (as we will also see in Sect. 1.3 below). First of all, By Olsen implicitly draws a distinction between an inner or hidden "self" that we as readers can understand is different from the same person's "public personae" and "public profile" ("you don't have to be understated, can be loud and colourful, and be yourself"). She furthermore highlights that the public persona is part of a "curated little world". In other words, the young blogger sees at least this latter type of identity, the public personae, as a social phenomenon that is staged and cultivated in socio-cultural discursive contexts, here specific digital media sites.

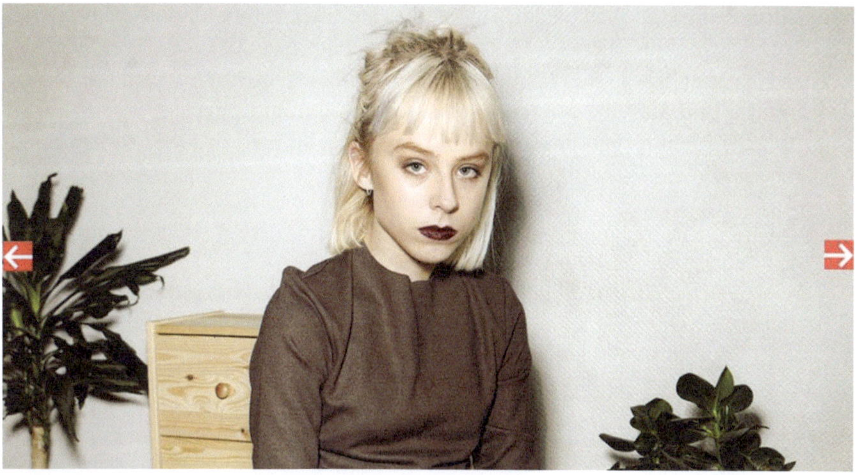

Fig. 1.1 Elise By Olsen: Is this girl the future? (Screen grab from the Norwegian magazine; http://www.norwegian.com/magazine/features/2015/07/is-this-girl-the-future, May 2016)

Secondly the interviews with the young blogger serve to illustrate discursive processes where positioning of the self via ones clothes, attitudes, language use and style is explicitly articulated: “I wear short crop tops and have pink hair—I’m used to being stared at, online and offline”. Such articulations are juxtaposed against the backdrop of others who do not follow similar conventions: “people look the same, dress the same, and all the magazines have this clean aesthetic. At school there’s a uniform: preppy shirt, Canada Goose jacket, Uggs, make-up”. This identity positioning, or what we call “identit*ing*” (Bagga-Gupta 2017; Bagga-Gupta et al. 2016), by the blogger is accomplished across different contexts and media; through talk and text: instagram, interviews, blogs, a blogging network, a digital magazine and a printed and digital newspaper.

A third point of relevance relates to the explicit categories of identity that By Olsen refers to. Her talk illustrates that one identity category can contain several layers of subcategories. Generation Z in the in-flight magazine text thus refers to an identity category where ‘age’, a particular ‘point in time’ in ‘global North’ spaces are significant dimensions, and include ‘feminism’, ‘gender’, and ‘Scandinavian norms’.

A fourth, central theme related to the concept of identity that gets highlighted in the interview excerpts, blog texts, etc., is that identity can be conceived of as emerging at both local and global discursive levels. The global level is here represented by commercial powers and the cultural values vis-à-vis the right expression related to “beauty” (for instance, “a society that ruins collective self-confidence with an expectation of perfection”) and the gender binaries that serve to categorize and constrict individuals and groups. A final topic that can be noted for present purposes, in this data-set, is the reference to the “riot” on behalf of one identity category (Generation Z). The riot counters the voices that serve to suppress

Generation Z through the categorizations that are forced upon them by commercial forces and society at large.

At an overall level, the narratives and discourses in how a teenage blogger writes, talks, and thereby *does* identity across digital and physical spaces are relevant to how identity gets implicitly and explicitly framed in other contemporary mass-media sites.

1.2.2 Identifications Across Physical-Digital Mass-Media Sites

The citations on and by Elise By Olsen presented and discussed above, are somewhat different but also, echo the ways in which identity is used and understood in other mass-media sites. These relate to both essentialist and constructionist perspectives on identity. A concordance-search[1] for the word identity in a corpus of newspaper articles for the period 1998–2015 in the geopolitical spaces of Norway, reveals that this basic meaning of identity—identity understood as name or identification—is routinely used in everyday languag*ing* (Bagga-Gupta 2014; Garcia 2009; Linell 2009). For instance: "The publisher knows the identity of the author" and "coming to Berlin without a passport and a clear identity"; or in phrases that contain "false identity" and "wrong identity". This fundamental meaning of identity is also encapsulated in daily life artifacts that have the explicit purpose of identifying who an individual "really is": a passport, a bank ID card, a driving license, a national ID number etc. The phrase "creating identity" receives 991229 hits in the corpus of newspaper texts searched for the period 1998–2015. Judging by the number of times it is deployed in this genre of mass-media (i.e. Norwegian newspapers during the last circa 20 years), the word identity is obviously an important concept in Norwegian society. This resembles the popularity of the concept in scholarship, at least since the 1950s, as well.

The concept of identity in a broader sense comes into use in different areas in everyday life and crops up in quite distinct clusters of meaning in our concordance-search data-set. At one level, personal identity is understood as being different from collective identities. Thus for instance, "Indigenous peoples are inflicted with a romanticizing collective culture". A large number of formulations in this data-set furthermore connect identity to a group of people or sector framed domains. Thus for instance, the newspaper texts highlight *ethnic* identity, *professional* identity, *linguistic* identity, *minority* identity, *Sami* identity, *homosexual* identity, *racial* identity, *deaf* identity, etc. In addition to referring to *individuals* and *collectives*, the word identity also refers to *institutions*, *organizations* and *places* in this data-set; the latter are referred to as having identities. Thus for instance, identity

[1]The key word (here identity) and a specified number of words that surround every instance where the key word is used are noted in a concordance-search.

of the state, the school system, the labor party, football teams, the identity of cities. etc. A particular urban architecture, for instance, gets framed as endorsing the uniqueness of a west-coast city in Norway: "the wharfs carry the identity of Bergen".

Another (very frequent) cluster of meanings relates to the more abstract issue of *belonging* somewhere in time and space. Thus, expressions like European identity, national identity, regional identity, local identity, geographical identity, inter-municipal identity, cultural- and historic identity highlight belongingness in this specific data-set.

The word identity is, furthermore, positioned as *nouns*, *adjectives* and *verbs* in the concordance-corpus analysis. Thus for instance, in phrases like: social understanding and identity, language and identity, pronounced identity, rigid identity, inferiority feeling and identity, friendship and identity, economically motivated identity, known identity, visual identity, need for identity, longed-for identity, etc. The commonsensical notion of identity appears in these types of examples to be something that is at times fixed, and at other instances fluid and boundary-less. In the latter, it is rather a status that is positioned, claimed, refused, negotiated and established. This is reminiscent of a constructionist analytical perspective on identity. Furthermore such verb-like examples are constituted by *words of action*. As the examples presented above illustrate, the verbs connected to identity in the newspaper data-set display a wide variety of actions and emotions. In this data-set identity can be lacking, given, felt, developed, created, built, secured, carried, strengthened, fought for, looked for, marked, hidden, refreshed, mirrored, shifted, swapped and stolen, just to mention a few descriptors.

The two specific tangible and digital mass-media data-sets focused upon in this section highlight some interesting patterns and issues. Given that identity is something that is constantly in creation and therefore is understood *as action* (Bagga-Gupta 2013, 2017), there exists a need for studying identity construction in a wide range of spoken, written, signed talk and text frameworks, and across different contexts (Benwell and Stokoe 2006). It can be explored in everyday conversation, in institutional settings, in narratives and stories, in commodified contexts, across spatial locations and in the research enterprise itself (as we have done in this section and will do in the next one). By focusing social interactions inside, outside and across institutional settings, attention can be drawn to how identities are constructed and revealed, and how they are shaped by the organizational structure and distinctive characteristics of institutions (Mäkitalo and Säljö 2000).

Narratives or accountings constitute another pathway to illuminate identiting or identity processes. Narratives are powerful sites in themselves for understanding the fluid nature of identity formation. Here transfer or the sharing of knowledge bound to cognitive issues of constructed and perceived memory are often made relevant (Bruner 1990). Using the "now situation" and contrasting it to the "then-situation" can here be a valuable lens for scrutinizing identity. In both situations, interactionally framed research and research that takes a narrative or accounting point of departure, people can be seen to commodify and market themselves in a range of social media and in-real-life sites. Self-branding is part of a trend that Davis (2003) suggests we all experience, given that many aspects of the consumer society contribute to a redefinition of the self in commodity terms.

The narratives and discourses in interviews and texts and the picture of a teenage blogger that emerges, as well as the narratives and discourses that have been identified in newspaper texts across two decades, highlight the heterogeneity of ways in which identity gets conceptualized. These multiple ways-of-being illustrate how identity gets implicitly and explicitly framed in contemporary mass-media sites. This resembles in many ways, as the next analytical section highlights, how identity is being conceptualized in scholarship currently. Such a plurality is in line with how theories of identity are being discussed in the literature today (Benwell and Stokoe 2006; Wetherell 2010; Wetherell and Mohanty 2010).

1.3 A Selective Overview of Research into Identity

As highlighted in the introduction above, there is growing recognition regarding the multiple layered dimensions of identity within scholarship and the many ways in which identity is (and has been) discussed in the literature. This recognition opens the way to go beyond the binary division between essentialist and constructionist positions that have framed research on identity across time. In addition to this issue, there continues to exist a frustration within scholarship with regards to what identity is. Giving recognition to the difficulties related to creating a common framework within scholarship on what identity is or can be, Wetherell (2010) highlights that,

> Very few concepts have been as generative [as identity]. In many ways, though, this success and spread are quite astonishing. Nearly every scholar who works on identity complains about its slippery, blurred and confusing nature. Identity is notoriously elusive and difficult to define and nearly every generation of scholars since the 1950s has included some keen to dismiss it as a consequence concluding it has no analytic value or purchase. Yet the study of identity persists and prospers, and the territory traced out and retraced by identity continues to be indispensable (2010: 1).

The sentiment illustrated in Wetherell's quote relates to and reflects what has emerged in the analysis of the contemporary digital-textual mass-media world example of Elise By Olsen and the newspaper data analyzed and discussed in Sect. 1.2 above. Interestingly, and going beyond the binary divisions of essentialist and constructionist positions, scholars currently also highlight the heterogeneous dimensions related to identity. Thus for instance, Bucholtz and Hall (2005) discuss the following key points related to identity:

(1) identity is the product rather than the source of linguistic and other semiotic practices and therefore a cultural rather than a primarily psychological phenomenon;
(2) identities encompass macro-level demographic categories, temporary and interactionally specific stances and participant roles, and local, ethnographically emergent cultural positions;

(3) identities may be indexed through labels, implicatures, stances, styles or linguistic structures and systems;
(4) identities are relationally constructed through several, often overlapping, aspects of the relationship between self and other, including similarity/difference, genuineness/artifice and authority/delegitimacy; and
(5) identity may be in part intentional, in part habitual, and less than fully conscious, in part an outcome of interactional negotiation, in part an outcome of larger ideological processes and structures (2005: 585).

With this as a brief introduction to more recent and emerging shifts related to voices about the complexities of identity, and continuing our quest for throwing light on identity by focusing upon how it gets played out in different empirical sites, this section looks at research on identity across two and a half decades that is emerging in two Scandinavian contexts. In other words, this section presents a meta-view of identity in identity scholarship.

The research genre represented by doctoral thesis (in geopolitical spaces like Norway and Sweden), constitute an interesting data-set for present purposes. Doctoral thesis in these settings (and also elsewhere), are the result of the highest formal education that a student-scholar participates in within academia. Produced within the frameworks of established research, they (not infrequently) represent both mainstream scholarship as well as openings towards new(er) scholarship. Doctoral theses in Norway and Sweden are publically defended and digitally catalogued. This means that they can be conveniently accessed for analytical purposes. An absence of overviews on the state of research on identity from Scandinavian geopolitical spaces is one rationale for studying the types and directions of research efforts that frame this domain. The following types of questions have been posed in order to understand how identity gets conceptualized in this specific body of literature across 25 years: What is the focus vis-à-vis identity, and how (if at all) has the research focus on identity developed across time? What settings are explored? What are the theoretical and methodological points of departure in the doctoral dissertations that have been identified? What themes do the studies conducted during the last 25 years focus upon? What kinds of data do they explore?

The following search engines were scrutinized: BIBSYS Ask/Oria (search conducted on 31-08-2015), DiVA (search conducted on 13-10-2015), and UiO-DUO (search conducted on 31-08-2015). Tabel 1.1 lists some of the parameters and areas of interest vis-à-vis identity that emerged in these searches.

1. DuO is a search motor for the University of Oslo. Here two search words were used, *identitet* (Norwegian) and the English word *identity*. The search was conducted for doctoral theses published during the last 25 years (1990–2015). 1305 titles emerged.

Table 1.1 Parameters related to Ph.D. theses identified in three database searches for the period 1990–2015

Database	Duo	Bibsys/Ask	Diva
Years covered	1990–2015	1990–2015	2004–2015
Number of titles	1305	1086	162
Disciplines	Humanities, Social Sciences and Natural Sciences[a]	Humanities and Social Sciences	Humanities and Social Sciences
Identity research related to…	Medicine Biology Physics Chemistry Psychotherapy Mental Health Nationalism Religion Education Culture Disability Teacher Language Deaf Migration Psychology	Gender Nationalism Citizenship Religion Professionalism Teacher Contractor Language Culture Education Language Sociology Music Youth Deaf Politics Ethnicity Sport Health Politics	Gender Education Pedagogics Psychology Religion Politics Digital gaming Nationality Parent Migration Health care worker Political Digital Dementia Language Deaf

[a]This search engine did not allow for the elimination of the natural sciences

2. Bibsys Ask/Oria is the main search motor for both Norwegian and international publications in Norway.[2] Here the search words used were *identit** which expands to both Nordic and English versions of the word identity. The search covered doctoral theses published within the humanities and the social sciences in Norway and Sweden during the last 25 years (1990–2015). 1086 titles were identified, highlighting a large variation in the area of identity research.
3. DiVA—Academic Archive On-line, is a search tool for research publications and student thesis written at 40 universities and research institutions in Sweden and Norway. DiVA began its development in 2000 at the Electronic Publishing Centre at Uppsala University Library in Sweden. Our search in DiVA covered the period 2004–2015 and 162 titles were identified.

The shortlisting of relevant doctoral theses was conducted by scrutinizing if the term identity (or its specific Scandinavian permutations; see above) was up-fronted in the title or within the key-words or thesis abstract. This curiosity driven process revealed a large variety of topics within identity research in this data-set. Most of

[2]It was replaced by the search motor Oria in November 2015.

the registered theses thus identified were published during the last part of the search period.[3] The topics explored in the identified scholarship can be broadly categorized as falling under the realm of traditional domains such as *ethnicity*, *nationality*, *gender*, *religion*, *language*, *politics*, *professionalism* and *culture*. These doctoral theses can also be grouped in terms of *personal* identity, *self*-identity, *musical* identity, *deaf* identity, *immigrant* identity, *sport* identity and *social* identity. Interestingly, changes in societal dimensions during the last quarter of a century in some ways reflect shifts in identity research topics noted in this analysis. Thus for instance, the growth of technology and internet development has given rise to new areas of identity research. Table 1.1 presents specific dimensions and the areas of foci in the area of identity in this data-set across the three databases.

The largest number of identified doctoral studies fall within the domains of the humanities and the social sciences, while a smaller number of theses related to identity issues lie within the domains of medicine, health science and architecture. The educational sciences theses fall within the humanities and social sciences domains. The majority of the identified doctoral studies focus on *particular identity categories*. In this data-set we thus find studies of *national* identity development in conflict areas: Moss (2015), for instance, has studied political, ethnic and religious identity strategies in conflict settings in African states, and Felberg (2008) presents a discourse analysis of the construction of Serbian and Montenegrin identities and relations during the Nato bombing of Yugoslavia in 1999. Other examples of works in this category are studies of *professional* identity in the case of adult learners (for instance Tønseth 2011), in medical institutions (for instance Sebrant 2000; Bovim 2010); in the instance of cleaners (for instance Aurell 2001); personnel working in ICT-organizations (for instance Haugseth 2012); and the case of artists (for instance Sandve 2014).

Other types of identity categories represented in this data-set include studies of *minorities* like people with a diagnosis such as hard-of-hearing, deaf or disabled (for instance Breivik 2001, 2007; Olaussen 2010); of immigrants, and of indigenous groups like the Sami and Kven people (for instance Blix 2013). Some of the doctoral studies that have been identified focus issues connected to particular *age groups*, like for instance pupils between 9 and 13 years (Schreiner 2006), tweens (Eriksen 2013), young parents and retired people; and finally studies of identity, *gender* and *sexuality* (Aurell 2001; Ohnstad 2009; Bergdahl 2010; Mellingen 2013). Some other salient themes that emerge in this literature include *language* and identity (see for instance Straszer 2011; Ahlgren 2014), *food*, *body* and identity (e.g. Stjerna 2007); identity positioning in *digital contexts* (e.g. Bjørgen 2014), *political* identity staged in *rap music* (e.g. Sandve 2014), identity and *therapeutic development* (for instance Skatvedt 2009), *youth* identity and *science teaching* (e.g. Schreiner 2006). The studies examine identity constructions across *discourse contexts*. As can be surmised, the identified theses cover a diverse body of themes,

[3]Doctoral theses in these contexts are published in a limited non-commercial edition by the doctoral students' university.

from novels (Bergdhal 2010) to therapeutic interactions (Andersson 2008). They represent a large body of contexts like informal interactions in a range of institutions, multiethnic settings in schools and interaction in geriatric wards. Other contexts that are salient include a focus upon novels, film, rap music, mass-media, official documents, virtual environments and spaces like geographical regions, city neighborhoods and homes.

The vast majority of the identified theses, especially the more recent ones, highlight that they build upon a constructionist or discursive understanding of identity. A wide range of *theoretical approaches* within this perspective have been identified. Postcolonial theory, Performative Theory, Positioning theory, Narrative theory, Critical discourse theory, Queer theory and Literature theories are some of the primary areas that are up-fronted. The *types of data* that are represented include for the most part interviews, questionnaires, texts, field notes from participant observations, and (a few) focus everyday interactions (for instance Eriksen 2013). Embodiment in the form of non-verbal communicative elements that constitute part of the analysis is more or less non-existent in this data-set.

The analysis of scholarship represented by doctoral students' theses across a quarter of a century highlights recent shifts in analytical foci and the multiple and heterogeneous nature of the domain of identity research in the two geopolitical Scandinavian contexts that have been focused upon here. The identified studies seem to uncommonly privilege methodological approaches where the focus is upon everyday social interactions. Some theses do focus upon discourses or languaging in textual sites. However the issue that is relevant for present purposes is that while the sites of identity formation are highlighted analytically (i.e. a constructionist perspective is payed homage to), the methodological framings of the majority of the studies identified tend to make use of units-of-analysis where texts (literary materials, policy, etc.), and, peoples' or institutions' accountings of identity are privileged. This lends support to our call for re-emphasizing the need to attend to identity *as* action in the domain of identity scholarship. While postcolonialism does emerge as a theme (or rather a perspective), it does so only in a couple of theses that have been identified. As is the case with most postcolonial scholarship (see below), these too build upon a philosophically oriented theoretical view, rather than a theoretically framed, empirical focus. The final section in this chapter highlights the relevance of decolonial perspectives and critiques in an attempt to highlight their relevance for scholarship on diversity and identity across time and space, and particularly in global North spaces like Scandinavian contexts.

1.4 Many-ways-of-Being. Identity, Decoloniality

We have made the case for the relevance of studying geopolitical spaces of Scandinavia from decolonial perspectives, not only because of the substantial shifts in demography in the region in the new millennium, but because decolonial perspectives have relevance for highlighting and attending to marginalization processes in global North spaces in more general terms as well. There is growing awareness that we need to recognize global North hegemonies and also augment these with "alternative voices" from global South spaces (Hasnain et al. 2013; Bagga-Gupta 2013) in a number of research domains, not least those related to the human condition. We have, in this chapter, drawn upon a range of different sources primarily from northern places. Our aim has been to highlight how identity gets framed currently in specific mass-media sites and in a research genre with the intent of center-staging the webs-of-understandings that are indexed in the concept identity. This concept is recognized as being notoriously slippery. A related and equally slippery concept, diversity is a corner-stone concept related to domains of scholarship like multiculturalism, interculturalism and bi/multilingualism, at least, since the turn of the century. Diversity is also significantly related to the concept identity and is more clearly being (re)recognized as a simple term for a complex phenomenon (see https://southernmultilingualisms.org/). This concept is commonly and broadly understood in terms of "an instance of being composed of differing elements or qualities" and "the inclusion of different types of people in a group or organization" (http://www.merriam-webster.com/dictionary/diversity, 15 Dec 2015). For present purposes, what these mainstream understandings of diversity and their relationship to multi/inter/pluri-culturalism and bi/multilingualism have in common is their stratifying functions; the latter—multi/inter/pluri-culturalism and bi/multilingualism—all index (and thereby maintain) *boundaries between bounded separate identity-positions*. Here power hegemonies are salient and specific identity-positions, both inside and outside scholarship, become relevant sites for illuminating the playing out and negotiation of the human condition. Postcolonial and decolonial scholarship has special relevance with regards to these issues, not least for re-vitalizing and contributing to the recent (primarily European) nomenclature related to globalization and recent migrations (for instance, "super-diversity", "hyper-diversity", "complex diversity").

A decolonial perspective can be understood in terms of a humanistically framed socially oriented position (Maldonado-Torres 2011; Mignolo 2000, 2009). This perspective constitutes an emerging domain that has key relevance in the current scholarship that attends to issues of power hegemonies at different scales across time and space. In comparison to *post*-colonial framings, *de*-colonial perspectives represent a turn that acknowledge that coloniality is well and thriving in the midst of contemporary communities and nation-states across the globe—in the east, west, north, south (Bagga-Gupta 2004, 2015, 2017; Maldonado-Torres 2011; Mignolo 2000, 2009; Omoniyi 2015). Making visible coloniality within all *spaces* and *places*, such a perspective takes issue with temporal framings in the "post" of post-colonialism and the spatial framings of coloniality as belonging to the 19th and 20th century power structures of specific European nation-states over geopolitical places in Third World continents. In other words, decoloniality encompasses geopolitical spaces across the inhabited continents, including nation-states like Norway and Sweden that are not commonly associated with colonial 19th and 20th century empires. They thus attempt to make visible global North hegemonies—inside European, Asian, African, etc. spaces where *alternative epistemologies* are marginalized or made invisible across time and space (Bagga-Gupta 2013, 2015, 2017; Bhabha 1994; Hasnain et al. 2013; Wiley 2006).

We furthermore call attention to the need for *going beyond* discussions about marginalization and power hegemonies in the post—as well as decolonial body of scholarship. Taking the case of a constructionist perspective on identity thus implies, we argue, that there is need for recognizing the methodological implications of the fact that social interaction including languaging or the doing of language and communication constitutes a fundamental dimension of socialization and the doing of identity across the life trajectory. In other words, such a position highlights that languag*ing* (or language-use) and identit*ing* (or identity work) entail an orientation towards (methodological) approaches where the study of time and space and a focus upon human beings in interaction across different sites and modalities (for instance modalities like oral, written, signed) are salient. The significant issue here is that a socioculturally framed decolonial position focuses on the interrelated nature of identiting, languaging and learning and at the same time sees these as actively constituted in life across institutions, communities and policies (Bagga-Gupta et al. 2016; Holland et al. 1998). The analysis presented in Sects. 1.2 and 1.3 in this chapter highlight some methodological ways of attending to identiting in different data-sets. Other types of data-sets which incorporate everyday life in terms of interactional recorded data also allow for focusing upon identity as action.

Going beyond essentialist understandings of identity, present day performatory or action related formulations of identity in terms of identiting, make salient the multiple ways-of-being as well as identity as (inter)action. Taking an action and a performativity methodological analytical approach, identiting is understood as being staged in everyday languaging and interaction inside, outside and across institutional settings. In everyday life, at home and at work, individuals display, perform and ascribe aspects of identity intentionally, as a dimension of habit and mundane social practice (Bucholtz and Hall 2005).

The movement of people and information across spatial boundaries in contemporary times, furthermore challenges the mythical harmonious link between geographical regions and people at all spatial scales (Paasi 2002). The International Olympic Committee's unique action in June 2016 wherein a nation-*less* team called the "Refugee team" for the 2016 summer Olympics was constituted, immediately made headlines across the globe. Ten athletes displaced from conflict regions of the world were chosen to become members of this nation-less Refugee team that does not have access to a national-flag or a national anthem at the Rio Olympics. Such an action is unprecedented in the history of the Olympics or the post-World War II global setting. The commentary that followed the IOC's action in social-media spaces highlighted, among other issues, that the idea of the nation-state has become so naturalized in our collective global imagination that such an action is seen as revolutionary (which in one sense it is).

Having said this, and as we have shown and argued for, there also exists a need to recognize the more "local" effect of spatial identity work within the immediate scale of human beings surroundings, including coloniality within and across spaces and places. At another scale, migration patterns across the globe, in addition to the recent IOC stance and action, call attention to the fallacy of taking nation-states and nationhood as static entities which can be the basis of saying meaningful things about the people who are its citizens or who pass into them or through them, or who are displaced within them. In other words, nation-states as a unit-of-analysis—a relatively recent construction—continues in the current historical period to destruct, collate and emerge on the global stage. Thus, nation-states constitute a poor unit-of-analysis when it comes to characterizing human identity (Bagga-Gupta 2012, 2013, 2015; Gal and Irvine 1995; Rosén and Bagga-Gupta 2013) and a decolonial perspective is central here. Decoloniality both encompasses an interest in language, identity and hegemony as well as the fallacy of essentializing identity—irrespective of whether the focus is at the individual or collective (like the nation-state) scale.

Our point is that in addition to conceptual issues vis-à-vis identity and hegemony, significant issues related to a screwed methodological focus has shaped the scholarship that focuses upon identity (and diversity) and the scholarship that takes a decolonial point of departure. Traditionally, decolonial literature draws upon rich experiences of scholars who have moved from the east/south to the west/north or on literature that emerges from the east/south or individuals who can claim a birth relationship to specific nation-states. This scholarship and/or authorship is poorly represented by studies that build upon empirical data where the focus is upon social practices of peoples' lives across the globe–the north, south, east, west. Drawing upon a socio-culturally oriented framework, we argue for the need to understand the methodological foci in research that potentially contributes to a decolonial perspective.

In other words, this discussion takes cognizance of the static problematic nature of scholarship that

- takes singular identity-positions at the individual scale (such as gender, ethnicity, functionality, age, class etc. in terms of identity and diversity) or the collective scale (such as nation-states) as given neutral units-of-analysis, and
- builds upon a unit-of-analysis marked by boundaries (Bagga-Gupta 2013).[4]

Moving beyond a focus on particularities and divisions that mark individuals, collectives but also activities or places or specific scales, a boundary-turn perspective recognizes the irreducibility of social action and narratives across time and space (and across the use of material and intellectual tools). Thus, taking socio-culturally framed conceptual discussions on the irreducible nature of individuals interacting with one another and cultural tools across time and space as a fundamental unit-of-analysis (Linell 2009; Säljö 2005), we argue for the need to have empirical data inform discussions on identity. This is significant given that it is often pre-theorized static demarcated concepts like ethnicity, gender, dis/abilities

[4]Here attention can be drawn to the Boundary Turn (Bagga-Gupta 2013) other associated turns like the Colonial Turn and the Mobility Turn (Landri and Neuman 2014; Sheller and Urry 2006) in the literature on language, culture and identity since the 1990 s (see also Clifford 1997; Hasnain et al. 2013; Scollan and Scollan 2004).

pertaining to identity and diversity that inform policy, but also academic discussions related to globalization.

Taking a social constructionist view of identity and pushing for empirical data-based scholarship, the analysis of a range of data-sets presented in this chapter has attempted to make visible the multiple ways-of-being where identity is understood as action or what we call identit*ing* (Bagga-Gupta 2017; Bagga-Gupta et al. 2016). Furthermore, our analysis illustrates the case for going beyond discussions that emerge from single data-sets in addition to a focus upon separate a priori identity positions in analysis work.

We also take issue with data-sets that primarily privilege people and institutions' accountings of their own or others' identities or analysis of literary accounts only. The conceptually framed methodological issues pushed in this chapter are important, not least since they go beyond accountings, policies, activism with regards to power hegemonies and instead center-stage the webs-of-understandings that are indexed in the very doing of identity across sites.

References

Ahlgren, K. (2014). *Narrativa identiteter och levande metaforer i ett andraspråksperspektiv* (Narrative identities and living metaphors from a second language perspective). Ph.D. thesis, University of Stocholm, Stockholm.

Andersson, K. (2008). *Talking Violence, Constructing Identity, Young Men in Institutional Care*. Ph.D. thesis, University of Linköping, Linkøping.

Appadurai, A. (1996). *Modernity at large: Cultural dimensions of globalization*. Minneapolis, MN: University of Minnesota Press.

Aurell, M. (2001). *Arbete och identitet: Om hur städare blir städare* (Work and identity: On how cleaners become cleaners). Ph.D. thesis, University of Linköping, Linkøping.

Bagga-Gupta, S. (2004). Challenging understandings in pluralistic societies–language and culture *loose* in school *sites* and *losing sight* of democratic agendas in education? *Utbildning och Demokrati. Tidskrift för didaktik och utbildignspolitik/Education and Democracy. Journal of didactics and politics of education*, *13*(3), 11–36.

Bagga-Gupta, S. (2012). Privileging identity positions and multimodal communication in textual practices: Intersectionality and the (re)negotiation of boundaries. In A. Pitkänen-Huhta & L. Holm (Eds.), *Literacy practices in transition: Perspectives from the Nordic countries* (pp. 75–100). Bristol: Multilingual Matters.

Bagga-Gupta, S. (2013). The Boundary-Turn. (Re)locating culture, identity and language through the epistemological lenses of time, space and social interactions. In I. Hasnain, S. Bagga-Gupta & S. Mohan (Eds.), *Alternative voices*: *(Re)searching language, culture, identity*... (pp. 28–49). Newcastle-upon-Tyne: Cambridge Scholars Publishing.

Bagga-Gupta, S. (2014). Languaging: Ways-of-being-with-words across disciplinary boundaries and empirical sites. In H. Paulasto, H. Riionheimo, L. Meriläinen, & M. Kok (Eds.), *Language contacts at the crossroads of disciplines* (pp. 89–130). Newcastle-upon-Tyne: Cambridge Scholars Publishing.

Bagga-Gupta, S. (2015) *Language learners* and *learning language*. Webs-of-understandings in the era of reinforced boundaries. Paper at the invited symposium The boundary turn. Challenges in researching and theorizing learning and diversity from decolonial perspectives, 16 biennial EARLI 2015 conference: Towards a reflective society. Synergies between learning, teaching and research, Cyprus, August 25–29 2015.

Bagga-Gupta, S. (2017). Going beyond oral-written-signed-virtual divides: Theorizing languaging from social practice perspectives. *Writing & Pedagogy*, 9(1).

Bagga-Gupta, S., Hasnain, I., & Mohan, S. (2013). Introduction: (re)searching language, culture and identity. In I. Husnain, S. Bagga-Gupta, & S. Mohan (Eds.), *Alternative Voices: (re) searching language, culture and identity* (pp. 1–27). Newcastle upon Tyne: Cambridge Scholars Publishing.

Bagga-Gupta, S., Messina Dahlberg, G., & Winther, Y. (2016). Disabling and enabling technologies for learning in higher education-for-all. Issues and challenges for whom? *Informatics 3*,(21), 1–19. doi:10.3390/informatics3040021

Benwell, B., & Stokoe, E. (2006). *Discourse and identity*. Edinburgh: Edinburg University Press.

Bergdahl, I. L. S. (2010). *Kärleken utan namn Identitet och (o)synlighet i svenska lesbiska romaner* (Love without name and (in)visibility in Swedish novels). Ph.D. thesis, University of Umeå, Umeå.

Bhabha, H. (1994). *The location of culture*. London: Routledge.

Bjørgen, A. M. (2014). *Digitale praksiser i samspill mellom kontekster. En undersøkelse av 9–13 åringers bruk, opplevelser og fortolkninger av digital teknologi i overganger mellom skole og fritid* (Digital practices in interplay between contexts. A survey of 9-13 years olds use, experiences and interpretations of digital technology in transition between school and leisure time). Ph.D. thesis, University of Oslo, Oslo.

Blommaert, J. (2010). *The sociolinguistics of globalization*. Cambridge: Cambridge University Press.

Blix, B. H. (2013). *The construction of Sami identity, health, and old age in policy documents and life stories. A discourse analysis and a narrative study*. Ph.D. thesis, University of Tromsø, Tromsø.

Bovim, R. V. (2010). *Arbeidsskapte identiteter: En studie av forutsetninger for identitet og tilhørighet i en organisatorisk kontekst* (Work shaped identities. A study of prerequisites for identity and belonging in an organizational context). Ph.D. thesis, The Norwegian University of Science and Tehnology, Trondheim.

Breivik, J. K. (2001). *Deaf identities in the making: Methaphores and narrations in translocal lives*. Ph.D thesis, University of Oslo, Oslo.

Breivik, J. K. (2007). *Døv identitet i endring. Lokale liv–globale bevegelser*. Deaf identity in change. Local lives–global movements. Oslo: Universitetsforlaget.

Bruner, J. (1990). Culture and human development: A new look. *Human Development 33*, 344–355. https://doi.org/10.1159/000276535.

Bucholtz, M., & Hall, K. (2005). Identity and interaction: A sociocultural linguistic approach. *Discourse Studies, 7*(4–5), 585–614.

Craig, E. (Ed.). (1998). *Routledge encyclopedia of philosophy*. London and New York: Routledge.

Davis, J. E. (2003). The commodification of self. *The Hedgehog Review, 5*(2), 41–49.

Erikson, E. H. (1968). *Identity: youth and crisis*. London: Faber & Faber

Eriksen, I. M. (2013). *Young norwegians: Belonging and becoming in a multiethnic high school*. Ph.D. thesis, University of Oslo, Oslo.

Felberg, T. (2008). *Brothers in arms? Discourse analysis of Serbian and Montenegrin identities and relations as constructed in Politika and Pobjeda front page articles during the NATO bombing of Yugoslavia in 1999*. Ph.D. thesis, University of Oslo, Oslo.

Ferrier, M. (2015). Rising star: meet Oslo's 15-year-old answer to Tavi Gevinson. *The Guardian*. Retrieved from http://www.theguardian.com/fashion/2015/may/20/rising-star-meet-oslos-15-year-old-answer-to-tavi-gevinson

Gal, S., & Irvine, J. T. (1995). The boundaries of languages and disciplines: How ideologies construct difference. *Social Research, 62*(4), 967–1001.

Garcia, O. (2009). *Bilingual education in the 21st century. A global perspective*. Malden, MA: Blackwell.

Gleason, P. (1983). Identifying identity: A semantic history. *The Journal of American History, 69* (4), 910–931.

Hasnain, I., Bagga-Gupta, S., & Mohan, S. (Eds.). (2013). *Alternative voices: (Re)searching language, culture, identity*. Newcastle-upon-Tyne: Cambridge Scholars Publishing.

Haugseth, J. F. (2012). *Forenklingens logikk: En studie av reproduksjonen av profesjonell identitet i IKT-organisasjoner* (The logic of simplification. A study of reproduction of professional identity in ICT-organisations). Ph.D. thesis, Norwegian University of Science and Technology, Trondheim.

Holland, D., Lachicotte, W., Jr., Skinner, D., & Cain, C. (1998). *Identity and Agency in Cultural Worlds*. Cambridge, Massachusetts: Harvard University Press.

Kraus, P. A. (2012). The politics of complex diversity: A European Perspective. *Ethnicities 12*(1), 3–25.

Landri, P., & Neuman, E. (2014). Introduction. Mobile Sociologies of Education. *European Educational Research Journal, 13*(1), 1–8.

Linell, P. (2009) *Rethinking Language, Mind, and World Dialogically. Interactional and Contextual Theories of Human Sense-making*. Charlotte, NC: Information Age Publishing.

Mäkitalo, Å., & Säljö, R. (2000). Talk in institutional context and institutional context in talk. *Categories and situated practices. Text, 22*(1), 57–82.

Maldonado-Torres, N. (2011). Thinking through the decolonial turn: Post-continental Interventions in theory, philosophy, and critique—An introduction. *Transmodernity: Journal of Peripheral Cultural Production of the Luso-Hispanic World, 1*(2), 1–15.

Mellingen, H. I. (2013). *Fra smertespråk til lykkenormativitet. Kjønn, seksualitet og religiøs identitet i et performativitetsperspektiv* (From the language of pain to the normativity of happiness. Gender, sexuality and religious identity in a performativity perspective). Ph.D. thesis, University of Agder, Kristiansand.

Mignolo, W. (2000). (Post) Occidentalism, (Post) Coloniality, and (Post) Subaltern Rationality. In F. Afzal-Khan & K. Seshadri-Crooks (Eds.), *The Pre-Occupation of postcolonial studies* (pp. 86–118). Durham: Duke UP.

Mignolo, W. (2009). Epistemic disobedience, independent thought and decolonial freedom. *Theory, Culture and Society, 26*(7–8), 159–181.

Moss, S.M. (2015). *Negotiations of identities in Rwqanda, Zanzibar and Sudan*. Ph.D. thesis, Norwegian University of science and Technology, Trondheim.

Ohnstad, A. (2009). *Lesbiske identiteter: skeive bevegelser* (Lesbian identities: quer movements). Ph.D. thesis, University of Oslo, Oslo.

Olaussen I. (2010). *Disability, technology & politics: the etangled experience of being hard of hearing*. Ph.D. thesis,University of Oslo, Oslo.

Olsson, A. (2015). Is this girl the future. *Norwegian.com*. Retrieved from http://www.norwegian.com/magazine/features/2015/07/is-this-girl-the-future

Omoniyi, T. (2015). *Illusions and delusions of the centre within the framework of globalization*. Invited symposium at conference The Sociolinguistics of Globalisation: (De)centering and (de)standerdization. The University of Hong Kong. June 3–6 2015.

Paasi, A. (2002). The problem with spatial identity: revisiting the “sense of place”. *Tijdschrift voor economische en sociale geografie., 93*(2), 37–148.

Rosén, J. K., & Bagga-Gupta, S. (2013). Shifting identity positions in the development of language education for immigrants: An analysis of discourses associated with ‘Swedish for immigrants’. *Language, Culture and Curriculum, 26*(1), 68–88.

Säljö, R. (2005) *Lärande och kulturella redskap: Om lärprocessser och det kollektiva minnet*. [Learning and Cultural Artefacts: On Learning Processes and Collective Memory]. Stockholm: Prisma.

Sandve, B. (2014). *Staging the real: Identity politics and urban space in mainstream Norwegian rap music*. Ph.D. thesis, University of Oslo, Oslo.

Schreiner, C. (2006). *EXPLORING A ROSE-GARDEN Norwegian youth's orientations towards science–seen as signs of late modern identities Based on ROSE (The Relevance of Science Education), a comparative study of 15 year old students' perceptions of science and science education*. Ph.D. thesis, University of Oslo, Oslo.

Scollan, R., & Scollan, S. W. (2004). *Nexus analysis. Discourse and the emerging internet*. London: Routledge.

Sebrant, U. (2000). *Organiserande och identitet: om arbetsorganisation i geriatrisk vård* (Organising and identity: about work organisation in geriatric health care). Ph.D. thesis. Stockholms University, Stockholm.

Sheller, M., & Urry, J. (2006). The new mobilities paradigm. *Environment and Planning A, 38*(2), 207–226. doi:10.1068/a37268

Skatvedt, A.H. (2009). *Alminnelighetens potensial: en sosiologisk studie av følelser, identitet og terapeutisk endring* (The potential of commonality: a socological study of emotions, identity and therapeutic change). Ph.D. thesis, University of Oslo, Oslo.

Stjerna, M.L. (2007). *Föreställningar om mat och ätande. Risk, kropp, identitet och den "frågasatta" maten i vår tid* (Notions of food and eating. Risk, identity, the body and 'contested' food in contemporary society). Ph.D. thesis,University of Stockholm, Stockholm.

Straszer, B. (2011). *"Ungerska för rötternas skull": Språkval och identitet bland andragenerationens ungrare i Sverige och Finland* (Language choice and identity among second-generation Hungarians in Sweden and Finland). Ph.D. thesis, Uppsala University, Acta Universitatis Upsaliensis. Studia Uralica Upsalienisa, Uppsala.

Taylor, C. (1989). *Sources of the self: The making of a modern identity*. Cambridge, MA: Harvard University Press.

Tønseth, C. (2011). *Voksne i læring: Identitetskonstruksjon i lys av Kompetansereformen* (Learning adults. Identity constructions in light of the Reform of Competency). Ph.D. thesis, Norwegian University of Science and Technology, Trondheim.

Vertovec, S. (2006). *The emergence of super-diversity in Britain*. Centre of Migration, Policy and Society. University of Oxford.

Wetherell, M. (2010). The field of identity research. In M. Wetherell & C. T. M. Mohanty (Eds.), *The sage handbook of identities* (pp. 3–26). London: Sage Publications.

Wetherell, M., & Mohanty, C. T. M. (Eds.). (2010). *The SAGE handbook of identities*. London: SAGE Publications.

Willey, T. (2006). The lessons of historical investigation: Investigations for the study of language policy and planning. In T. Ricento (Ed.), *An introduction to language policy: Theory and method* (pp. 13–152). Oxford: Blackwell Publishing.

Ref Elise By Olsen http://www.ink-live.com/emagazines/norwegian-magazine/1978/july-2015/#1/z

Searches on identity (English), identitet (Norwegian) and identit* (loaded 31.08.15)

Bibsys Ask Oria: http://ask.bibsys.no/ask/action/result?cmd=&kilde=biblio&fid=alle&term=identit%3F&op=and&fid=alle&term=&bibliografi=&materiale=doktoravh&arstall=&sortering=sortdate-&treffPrSide=50

UiO-DuO: https://www.duo.uio.no/discover?filtertype=type&filter_relational_operator=equals&filter=Doktoravhandling

Identity: https://www.duo.uio.no/discover?scope=%2F&query=identity&submit=&filtertype_0=type&filter_0=Doktoravhandling&filter_relational_operator_0=equals

Identitet: https://www.duo.uio.no/discover?query=identitet&scope=/&filtertype=type&filter_relational_operator=equals&filter=Doktoravhandling

DiVA: (loaded 13.10.15): http://www.diva-portal.org/smash/resultList.jsf?dswid=-7276&p=51&fs=false&language=en&searchType=RESEARCH&query=&af=%5B%5D&aq=%5B%5B%7B%22freetext%22%3A%22identity%22%7D%5D%5D&aq2=%5B%5B%7B%22dateIssued%22%3A%7B%22from%22%3A%221990%22%2C%22to%22%3A%222015%22%7D%7D%2C%7B%22language%22%3A%22eng%22%7D%2C%7B%22publicationTypeCode%22%3A%5B%22comprehensiveDoctoralThesis%22%5D%7D%5D%5D&aqe=%5B%5D&noOfRows=50&sortOrder=author_sort_asc&onlyFullText=true&sf=all

Author Biographies

Sangeeta Bagga-Gupta is Full Professor of Education since 2016 at Jönköping University, Sweden. She has been full professor at Örebro University, Sweden since 2007. She is also adjunct professor 2016–2017 at Aligarh University, India. Her multidisciplinary, multi-scalar ethnographically framed research focuses communication, learning and identity from sociocultural and decolonial framings. She publishes extensively and in a number of different research domains. She is the Principle Investigator of the new Swedish Research Council project *Participation for all? School and post-school pathways of young people* (2016–2020) and has been the leader of the research group CCD, *Communication, Culture and Diversity* since the end of the 1990s.

Julie Feilberg is Assistant Professor of Language and Communication at the Norwegian University of Science and Technology, Trondheim, Norway. Her research focuses child language development and professional and institutional discourse. She has also served for many years as pro-rector with responsibility for education and quality learning at the Norwegian University of Science and Technology.

Aase Lyngvær Hansen is Assistant Professor (emerita) of Language and Communication at the Norwegian University of Science and Technology, Trondheim, Norway. Her multidisciplinary research focuses on interaction and learning in visually oriented classrooms. She has also worked for many years as a teacher of the deaf and as a developer of teaching material for the deaf on video, DVD and Internet.

Chapter 2
Positioning Theory and Life-Story Interviews: Discursive Fields, Gaze and Resistance

David Block

2.1 Introduction

in the faculty / I already knew really nice German people / besides like all Germans / they walked around with this completely false idea / that we Spanish women are an inexhaustible well of bodily joy >laughing< / which meant I had a lot of friends / so in this sense / on the one hand I felt accepted / not only by the foreign students / but by the Germans in the faculty / and at the same time tremendously rejected by officialdom / only one professor took me seriously during the entire year / I wasn't used to that / and the others made it clear that they thought I was (.5) a total airhead / and that was the hardest part (.5) seeing that / I don't know / for the first time / this had never happened to me before / that they didn't take me seriously / for being a woman / for being a foreigner / all of which meant / ehrm / that since then I have had a pretty appalling impression of Germany / I don't have any / I haven't gone back / I haven't read any German since / nothing in German since then / some kind of total rejection / (Elena 27/09/01)

en la facultad / ya conocía a gente alemana muy maja / además como todos los alemanes / iban con esta idea totalmente falsa / de que las españolas somos un pozo inagotable de alegría para el cuerpo >laughing> / pues tenía muchísimas amistades / entonces en este sentido / por un lado me sentía muy integrada / tanto con los otros extranjeros / como con los alemanes de la facultad / y al mismo tiempo tremendamente rechazada por las instancias oficiales / solo un profesor me tomó en serio en todo el año / yo no estaba acostumbrada a eso / y los demás me habían claramente hecho ver que pensaba que yo tenía (.5) un vacío total en el cerebro / y eso fue lo más duro (.5) ver que / no sé / por primera vez / que no me había pasado nunca / que no me tomaban en serio / por ser mujer / y por ser extranjera / con lo cual / pues / tengo una impresión de Alemania desde entonces bastante horrorosa / no tengo ningún / no he vuelto / no he vuelto a leer alemán / nada en alemán desde entonces/ una especie de rechazo total / (Elena 27/09/01)

D. Block (✉)
ICREA/University of Lleida, Lleida, Spain
e-mail: dblock@dal.udl.cat

S. Bagga-Gupta et al. (eds.), *Identity Revisited and Reimagined*,
DOI 10.1007/978-3-319-58056-2_2

This excerpt is taken from a life-story interview which I carried out in London some 17 years ago as part of a three-and-a-half-year study which explored the adaption of French, German and Spanish nationals to the English educational system and how they worked as language teachers and lived their lives in Greater London (Block 2001, 2005, 2006). The speaker is Elena, a 29-year-old Spanish woman who at the time of the interview was working as a French and Spanish teacher in a secondary school south of London. As is the case with all excerpts from interviews, there is a lot going on, some of it immediate and of the here-and-now and some of it out of sight. Thus, one might read meaning off the transcribed words but there is also the need to consider how the meaning of Elena's words is out of sight, embedded in the rich sociohistorical context which underlies and shapes the very moment when Elena relates this particular part of her life. Thus while we may understand from her transcribed words that she is a feminist and that she is not someone who takes a slight lying down, there is so much more that does not leap off the page because it is part of the rich texture of her past and present experiences which both precede and surround her account of this part of her life. This paper is about what may be read off immediately from accounts provided during life story interviews, but it is also about the phenomenological layers of life story interviews which we need to consider in a thorough and rigorous way if we are to arrive at a fuller understanding of the meaning of interviewees' words.

The backdrop to my discussion here is the 'narrative turn' in the social sciences and educational research which has taken hold over the past three decades (Bruner 1986; Clandinin 2007). This turn has meant that researchers are showing more and more interest in how individuals self-present through productions of what count (in the context of research) as their life stories. These life stories are elicited from informants by a variety of means, from more traditional pen-and-paper written diaries to, in more recent times, electronic logs. However, it is by far the face-to-face interview which has been the elicitation mode of choice over the past three decades. In such research, life-story interviews are generally lengthy, lasting up to three hours, and they are by nature open-ended, resembling day-to-day conversations. They are often organized around particular stages in the interviewee's life, such as early childhood, early primary school and early adolescence, but they may also be more specifically focussed on short-term experiences such as a teacher training course. The researcher may conduct a single one-off interview with an informant, or he/she may conduct a set of two or three interrelated ones, fairly close together in time (Wengraf 2001). Alternatively, he/she may adopt a longitudinal approach, which involves multiple interviews, carried out at intervals over a long period of time (Block 2006). Whatever the number of interviews per informant, in the end, the goal is generally the same: 'the story a person chooses to tell about the life he or she has lived, told as completely and honestly as possible, what is remembered of it, and what the teller wants others to know of it …' (Atkinson 1998: 3). In previous publications (e.g. Block 2000, 2006, 2015), I have taken on the problematic nature of interviews as a means of 'getting at' the life stories of individuals, questioning the view that things said during interviews reflect the deepest inner thoughts of informants and/or constitute true representations of their experiences. Following Kvale (1996), I have instead suggested that they are often more symptomatic of deeper feelings and/or a product of the immediate interaction between interviewer and interviewee. In this chapter, I continue with this tack, but add a layer to my thinking about interviews as I consider the potential usefulness of *positioning theory* (Harré and van Langenhove 1999a) as a methodological framework for understanding the communicative processes unfolding during interviews. As I have done in my past work, I aim to shed some light on how we might understand interviews as socioculturally-situated co-productions.

2.2 Positioning Theory

According to Davies and Harré (1999: 37), '[p]ositioning is the discursive process whereby people are located in conversations as observably and subjectively coherent participants in jointly produced storylines'. By 'discursive process', the authors mean individuals' day-to-day participation in communicative events involving one or more other individuals, drawing not only on language but also other forms of semiotic activity such as direction of gaze, posture, gestures and other embodied behaviour. Being 'located … as observably and subjectively coherent participants' is about the kind of image management engaged in by participants in face-to-face conversations (Goffman 1981). It is about how, for example, individuals draw on a range of communicative resources to portray themselves as what Gee (2008: 3) calls 'types of people'. Or, in Judith Butler's (1990) terms, it is about performativity, or how constellations of communicative resources in use create the effect of particular possible, plausible and recognisable subjectivities. At the same time Harré (2004: 4) points out that positioning theory also entails 'the study of the way rights and duties are taken up and laid down, ascribed and appropriated, refused and defended in the fine grain of the encounters of daily lives'. In recent years, positioning theory has been employed in range of contexts, ranging from conflict resolution (Moghaddam et al. 2008) to public relations (James 2014).

van Langenhove and Harré (1999) suggest that any communicative event can be framed as a mutually determining triad with each point impacting on the other two (see Fig. 2.1). On the righthand side is the 'storyline' which emerges in the interaction between interlocutors, understood to be 'the conversational history and the sequence of things already being said' (Harré and van Langenhove 1999b: 6). In the middle of the triangle is 'position', which as we have just observed is about 'the moral positions of the participants and the rights and duties they have to stay certain things' (Harré and van Langenhove 1999b: 6). Positions may be manifested in binary alternatives such as 'powerful or powerless, confident or apologetic, dominant or submissive, definitive or tentative, authorized or unauthorized, and so on' (van Langenhove and Harré 1999: 17). Important here is how the characters in the storyline being developed are portrayed. As Wortham and Gadsden (2006: 319) put it, ‘narrators “voice” or position people represented in their narrative, including their own various narrated selves, as recognizable types of people’ (see the reference to Gee’s work below). In addition, as Wortham and Gadsden (2006: 319) explain, ‘while voicing themselves and other characters, narrators also evaluate these voices, such that the narrator him or herself often takes a position on the types of characters represented’. In these circumstances, there might be a simplistic form of heroes and villains or there might be an altogether more sophisticated and nuanced character development at work.

Finally, on the left hand side of the triangle, there are what Austin (1962) would have called ‘speech acts’, that is, words uttered with purpose and effect as the minimal units of human communication. In the development of speech-act theory, Austin famously distinguished between illocutionary and perlocutionary speech acts, where the former term refers to the functional meaning of utterances (e.g. relating one’s thoughts on a matter) and the latter is about the effect of utterances. However, positioning theorists have expanded on the notion of speech act from Austin’s original linguistics-based definition considerably, making room for the larger notion of communicative acts, which would include, for example, a handshake:

> Every socially significant action, intended movement, or speech must be interpreted as an act, a socially meaningful and significant performance. A handshake is an intended action. Does it express a greeting, a farewell, congratulations, seal a bet, or what? It is only significant as far as it is given a meaning in the unfolding episode of which it forms a part. Once interpreted it falls under rules of propriety and standards of correctness, not only in itself but also in what are its proper precursors and consequences. (Harré and Moghaddam 2003: 6)

Taking into account the discussion thus far, it is possible to construct a positioning triangle such as the one in Fig. 2.1.

In the interview excerpt which opens this paper, we see how Elena develops a storyline around her experiences in Germany, specifically how she found acceptance among students but generally felt rejected by university staff, and how the latter experience lead to her subsequent rejection of all things related to Germany. She adopts the position of a no-nonsense, independent Spanish woman who accepts neither facile stereotypes nor slights to her self-esteem, be these individual or institutional. The notion that ‘Spanish women are an inexhaustible well of bodily

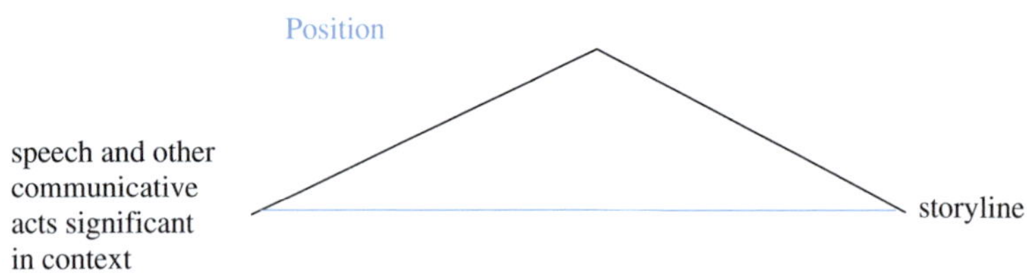

Fig. 2.1 The Positioning Triangle (based on van Langenhove and Harré 1999: 18; Harré and Moghaddam 2003: 5–6)

joy' (a nice turn of phrase, to be sure) is dispatched without reservation as 'completely false', and Elena very compellingly reveals her refusal to accept some of the positions identified by van Langenhove and Harré (1999): powerless, submissive, tentative or unauthorized. She strengthens her positioning vis-a-vis her interlocutor (me) by beginning with a description of harmony among students. This move grants her a warrant as a fair assessor of her own experiences, which in turn becomes important when we come to her withering criticism of the higher echelons of the German university, ultimately portrayed as sexist and even xenophobic.

In this way (and very briefly), I might apply the positioning triangle described and illustrated above to Elena's account of her German experiences. However, in doing so, I am engaging with what is on the surface, the words uttered by Elena, but I am not going too far beyond them (or *under* them).[1] To be fair to the originators of positioning theory (Harré and his associates), I am also applying a fairly basic model here. And to stay at this level of analysis would be to ignore work in recent years which has either challenged some of the foundations which undergird positioning theory or which has attempted to clarify aspects of positioning theory (e.g. work by Harré and his associates). In the next section, I examine some of this critical and clarifying work as I attempt to improve positioning theory for the purpose of making sense of life-story interviews.

2.3 Extending Positioning Theory

Butler (2004 [1997]) develops an incisive critique of Austin's original speech act theory and most significantly queries what it means to say that *things can be done with words*, or if we follow Harré and Moghaddam's (2003) expanded version, we might add: *things can be done with any semiotically mediated act*. She wonders how words, or indeed other modalities of communication, can both name or signify something while also being constitutive of, or enactments of, or performances of, actions. The issue is that in such a theory, a speech/communicative act is framed as an 'intended action', as Harré and Moghaddam put it, and therefore it is an individual act for which only the individual is responsible. In addition, a speech/communicative act is said to be 'only significant as far as it is given a meaning in the unfolding episode of which it forms a part', which makes it emergent in the ongoing flow of interaction while stripping it of any synchronic embeddedness in any social structure or diachronic embeddedness in any historical structure. For Butler this way of framing communication is problematic: in the former case, it is asocial; in the latter case, it is ahistorical. Butler explains her position as follows:

[1]Crucially, as one reviewer of an earlier version of this chapter noted, I am also limited somewhat by the fact that my transcription captures minimal information about how the exchange took place: while it indicates the rhythm of what was said and pauses where relevant, it does not represent a wide range of semiotic elements such as gaze and gestures.

> If a performative provisionally succeeds (and I will suggest that "success" is always and only provisional), then it is not because an intention successfully governs the action of speech, but only because that action echoes prior actions, and *accumulates the force of authority through the repetition or citation of a prior and authoritative set of practices*. It is not simply that the speech act takes place *within* a practice, but that the act is itself a ritualized practice. What this means, then, is that a performative "works" to the extent that it *draws on* and *covers over* the constitutive conventions by which it is mobilized. In this sense, no term or statement can function performatively without accumulating and dissimulating historicity of force. (Butler 2004 [1997]: 221; italics in the original)

Butler's views find resonance in Mikhail Bakhtin's notions of voice and intertextuality when she attributes the success of the performative to how it 'echoes prior actions' and 'accumulates the force of authority through the repetition or citation of a prior and authoritative set of practices'. While voice is about how words uttered by individuals in communicative acts are imbued with the meanings invested in them in the past by other speakers in communicative acts (Bakhtin 1981), intertextuality is about how texts, as more extended productions of words, are interlinked in terms of meaning and interpretability with previously produced texts (Bakhtin 1986). In short, we cannot understand communication as a strictly individual action, the product of individual intentions (between, say, an interviewer and interviewee); rather, all communication is sociohistorical situated such that the past weighs as heavily as the volatility of the immediate context in exchanges taking place on a moment-to-moment basis.

However, it can be argued that something akin to attention to the sociohistorical does arise in the second point on the triangle in Fig. 2.1, position, which is defined as follows:

> … a cluster of rights and duties to perform certain actions with a certain significance as acts, but which include prohibitions or denials of access to some local repertoire of meaningful acts. In a certain sense in each social milieu there is a kind of Platonic realm of positions, realized in current practices, which people can adopt, strive to locate themselves in, be pushed into, be displaced from or be refused access, recess themselves from and so on, in a highly mobile and dynamic way. (Harré and Moghaddam 2003: 6)

This ties in with notions of discourse, as developed by authors such as Weedon (1997, 2004), and in particular Foucault's (1979) notion of 'discursive fields' as the 'competing ways of giving meaning to the world and of organizing social institutions and processes' (Weedon 1997: 34). A discursive field is understood to be a social space in which not only language, but also a range of other semiotic resources ranging from dress to body movement, are deployed as individuals participate in activity either alone or in the company of others. In addition, similar to Terry Eagleton's concept of 'discursive formation', a discursive field 'can be seen as a set of rules which determine what can and must be said from a certain position in social life, and expressions have meaning only by virtue of the discursive formations within which they occur, changing meaning as they are transported from one to another' (Eagleton 2007: 195). In this sense, discourse comes to be conceived in very broad terms, as what Gee (2008) calls capital 'D' discourse, that is, '"ways of being in the world" … "forms of life" … [and] socially situated identities' (Gee 2008: 3), which are emergent in ongoing interaction but also relatively stable. This effect of stability emergent in interaction is explained by Harré and Moghaddam when they discuss the third component of the positioning triangle, the storyline:

> We have emphasized the enormous importance of the dynamics of social episodes, how they unfold as this or that person contributes to the pattern, episodes do not unfold in any random way. They tend to follow already established patterns of development, which for convenience have come to be called story lines. Each story line is expressible in a loose cluster of narrative conventions (Harré and Moghaddam 2003: 5–6)

It is also worth noting that as the different components of the positioning triangle come to life, there are reciprocal actions of positioning and being positioned, As I suggest elsewhere (Block 2007) participants in an interaction situate themselves through their discursive practices and at the same time, they are situated by others. During such activity, there is a sense of what constitutes a coherent socially-situated identity, one which makes sense for the context. In other words, all actors will position themselves and others according to their sense of what constitutes a coherent narrative for the particular activity, time and place in which they find themselves.

While being situated by others, individuals may find themselves the subjects of structuring and disciplining discourses. An early example of what structuring and disciplining discourses might mean is to be found in Marx's *Capital 1*. In the chapter entitled 'The working day', Marx (1990 [1867]) describes in great detail the ways in which factory owners are able to subject workers to their will via their control over time and space. However, a more recent (and more relevant) discussion of discipline can be found in Michel Foucault's work on the clinic. Foucault charts a shift from a medical profession which relied purely and strictly on an academic knowledge to cure patients, to a policing role, which included taking decisions regarding what was normal and what was abnormal, and what was legitimate and what was illegitimate. He explains:

> Medicine must no longer be confined to a body of techniques for curing ills and of the knowledge that they require; it will also embrace knowledge of *healthy man*, that is, a study of *non-sick man* and a definition of the *model man*. In the ordering of human existence it assumes a normative posture, which authorizes it not only to distribute advice as to healthy life, but also to dictate the standards for physical and moral relations of the individual and of the society in which he lives. (Foucault 1973: 34)

The key to making this normative behaviour effective in medical practice is the right of doctors to impose their 'gaze', a technical term used by Foucault in reference to how observation is not just about taking in and documenting what is happening before the observer's eyes; it is also about categorising and shaping others according to dominant discourses of normativity. This change in how gaze might work is summed up by Foucault as follows:

> …. the medical gaze was also organised in a new way. First, it was no longer the gaze of an observer, but that of a doctor supported and justified by an institution, that of doctor endowed with the power of decision and intervention. Moreover, it was a gaze that was not

> bound by the narrow grid of structure (form, arrangements, number, and size) but that could and should grasp colours, variations, tiny anomalies, always receptive to the deviant. Finally, it was a gaze that was not content to observe what was self-evident; it must make it possible to outline chances and risks; it was calculating. (Foucault 1973: 89)

Crucially, Foucault is not so much interested in how individual doctors enact or impose the medical gaze on patients, or how a prison official enforces the judicial gaze on a prisoner; rather, 'it is the anonymous medical fraternity that has a gaze, as does the anonymous legal fraternity' (Boxer 2003: 257). In this sense, gaze is about power residing in institutions as discursive fields. It is a discursive resource as opposed to an individually-held right or entitlement, even if individuals are invested with the right and entitlement to gaze by virtue of occupying social positions of which the gaze is one of many constituent features. Where there is gaze, there is often compliance, acquiescence and acceptance; however, there is also often resistance, or the 'intentional, and hence conscious, acts of defiance or opposition by a subordinate individual or group of individuals against a superior individual or set of individuals' (Seymour 2006: 305). Resistance always exists as a counter to hegemony and uneven power relations and it may or may not be successful as an attempt to challenge and overturn such relations. This means that in any analysis of interview data, it is interesting not only to consider instances in which the gaze is, in effect, accepted and owned by the gazed-upon, but also instances in which it is resisted, and beyond this, the effect of resistance.

To summarise the discussion thus far, positioning theory, in the expanded form presented here, offers a suggestive way of making sense of interview data and it is no doubt for this reason that it is often drawn on in narrative research. However, 'drawing on' positioning theory in many cases means merely mentioning it in passing. Or, it is explained briefly to make the point that individuals through their actions during interactions adopt different subject positions on a moment-to-moment basis. Of course, to make the latter point one does not need positioning theory as one might more fruitfully refer to Erving Goffman's work on footing and framing (e.g. Goffman 1981).[2] Here I have attempted to get behind some of the basic tenets of positioning theory and in doing so I have managed to include the work of scholars who have discussed discursive fields, gaze and resistance. In this sense, I have emphasized the sociohistorically-situated nature of positioning while injecting a power dimension into the framework. Revisiting the positioning triangle presented above, perhaps there is room for an expansion of it to take into account some of the extensions which I have discussed. I attempt to capture how such a triangle might look in Fig. 2.2.

In her detailed discussion of narrative methods, Riessman (2008) describes different ways of analysing narratives and it is perhaps interesting to see how the

---

[2]Footing is 'the alignment we take up to ourselves and the others present as expressed in the way we manage the production or reception of an utterance' (Goffman 1981: 128) and framing is the interlocutor's 'understanding of what it is that is going on' and how 'individuals fit their actions to this understanding and ordinarily find that the ongoing world supports this fitting' (Goffman 1974: 247).

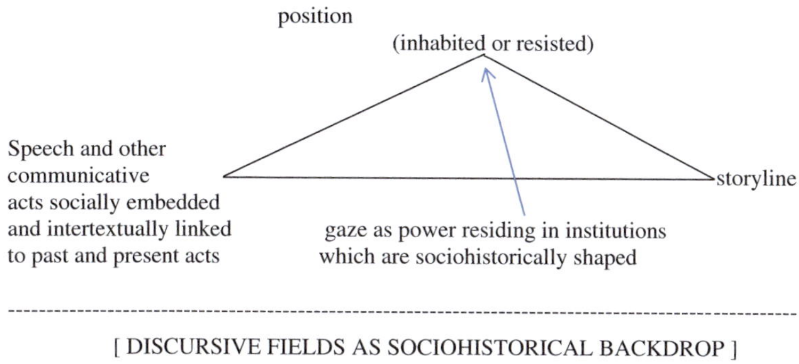

Fig. 2.2 The positioning triangle extended

model presented here articulates with her discussion. First, there is what she calls *thematic* analysis, which is primarily a focus on the content of what is said. Although this approach may be seen as overly intuitive and even simplistic (reading meaning off words), Riessman makes clear that it requires a great deal of rigour, as the researcher has to identify key themes and strands in the data and make sense of them, drawing on history, sociology, anthropology and other social sciences disciplines in the process. Second, there is *structural* analysis, which addresses how narratives are produced. On the one hand, this approach may focus on the micro-level linguistic phenomena, such as grammar, lexis and accent; on the other hand, it may examine how different clauses are assembled to produce a story line or the strategies adopted by the story teller as the story is told. The third approach, which Riessman calls *dialogic/performative*, draws on elements of the previous two approaches, but goes beyond being a mere combination of them. As Riessman explains, 'if thematic and structural approaches interrogate "what" is spoken and "how", the dialogic/performative approach asks "who" an utterance may be directed to, "when," and "why," that is, for what purposes?' (Riessman 2008: 105). Thus, the analyst works from the immediate context, in terms of the minutiae of interaction, discourse patterns, the background of interlocutors, the general socio-historical backdrop and so on, eventually working up to border social categories, related to institutions and cultures, and the identity inscriptions outlined earlier in this chapter (e.g. social class, gender, ethnicity, etc.).[3]

In the extended positioning theory triangle presented in Fig. 2.2, content analysis is certainly in evidence, as this is what is done when a storyline is interpreted. There is also a degree of structural analysis implied in the examination of speech acts, although we would need to be clear about exactly what kind of structural analysis is appropriate for the research being done here (multimodal, pronoun use, speech acts

[3]It should be noted that there is a fourth approach discussed by Riessman, what she calls *visual analysis*. This approach builds on the previous three approaches and is concerned with what images are produced, how they are produced and why they are produced. It is not of direct relevance to my discussion here.

as linguistic phenomena and so on). Finally, there is a move beyond the what and how of stories and an attempt to understand positioning as discursively constructed with relation to discursive fields and as connected to larger social structures. And here a concern with '"who" an utterance may be directed to, "when," and "why," that is, for what purposes?' (Riessman 2008: 105) may be addressed.

A more in-depth understanding of Elena's account of her experiences in Germany arises if we apply some of the ideas introduced in this section and reflected in Fig. 2.2. In the story that she tells about Germany, we have her portrayal of what we might call, for lack of a better term, the German university gaze.[4] In Foucault's (1973: 34) terms, this gaze is about 'the ordering of human existence' at a German university. The university 'assumes a normative posture, which authorizes it not only to distribute advice as to [university] life …, but also to dictate the standards for [academic] relations of the individual' in the university context. In Elena's account of her time in Germany, the university gaze positioned her as an 'airhead' and generally as an unworthy interlocutor.

For her part, in the midst of what Seymour (2006: 305) terms 'differential power relationships', Elena rejects and resists this gaze, in the end, by leaving Germany and finding somewhere else to study where she feels validated. Of course, as Seymour (2006: 305) notes, acts of resistance may be 'counter-hegemonic but may not succeed in effecting change' and one has to wonder about the effect of Elena's evasive action as regards its potential to undermine authority and ultimately the German university gaze which she felt herself to be the victim of.

Moving to another level of analysis, I might apply the triangle not to the story inside Elena's life story interview but to the interaction between her and me, that is, to the most immediate, on-the-surface, interactive level, and the different positionings that emerge as interviewer and interviewee interact. Georgakopoulou (2006, 2007; De Fina and Georgakopoulou 2012) offers us much food for thought in this regard in her work with Greek adolescent girls. She noted how her informants took on 'telling identities' in group interviews, that is, they adopted subject positions related to their role—active, less active, relatively silent and so on—in the ongoing development of a storyline and overall conversational management. These more immediate, situational identities are linked by Georgakopoulou to 'larger social identifies that are consequential for the construction and interpretation of stories … have[ing] to do with the participants' group-internal roles, relations and hierarchies on the one hand and their gender on the other' (Georgakopoulou 2006: 99)

In Gee's (2008: 3) words, in this excerpt Elena presents herself *discursively* as the embodiment of particular 'ways of behaving, interacting, valuing, thinking, believing, [and] speaking … that are accepted as instantiations of particular identities (or "types of people") by [the interviewer]'. Specifically, she inhabits the position of an empowered individual, in control of her story. And as was observed

[4]While Elena does make reference to Germany and Germans in general in the excerpt, she is clearly talking specifically about her experiences at a Germany university in this part of the interview.

previously, she is able to dispatch the entirety of German higher education (and indeed Germany and its language and culture) with a few well-chosen phrases. The core to all of this, and indeed, the essential backdrop to it, is a discursive field of gender theory and practice which has arisen worldwide in recent years, and which Elena is able to tap into. Among other things, she 'flips the script',[5] or challenges some established thinking, in her assessment of Germany with regard to gender relations. I say this because Germany is a country which is generally favourably compared with the countries of southern Europe when it comes to gender relations. Elena positions herself an independent-minded and intelligent woman, and also as a Spanish woman, who encountered a degree of sexism in Germany.

2.4 More Thoughts and Conclusion

This discussion of positioning theory could end with Fig. 2.2 and my discussion of Elena's German story, as we have made Harré's original postulation more socio-historically embedded as opposed to individual and intention driven. However, there are other issues to consider in narrative research that might be addressed through this expanded model of positioning theory. Here I will cite three.

The first issue is related to timescales and when a story is being told and how the story is placed in terms the past and the teller's personal ongoing life narrative. Linde (1993) reminds us that all accounts of life experiences are told in the present and therefore perhaps tell us more about how interviewees wish to position themselves now than what really happened in the past. Elsewhere, Mishler (2006) has very perceptively written about how story tellings may be more about their endings. He cites the work of Ricoeur (1980) who questioned the strict chronological, clock-based approach to narrative analysis, what he called the 'arrow of time' metaphor. Narratives, in Ricoeur's view, have two dimensions, one 'chronological' and the other 'non-chronological'. The former is about events tied together in sequence to constitute a coherent account of an episode in life with a beginning, middle and end (one supposes that these latter constituents can be juggled around, as in films with flashback scenes). This dimension is evident in approaches to narrative which include the notion of sequenced events, such as Labov and Waletzky's (1967) oft-cited model, according to which a narrative begins with a quick synopsis of the story to be told, followed by the provision of key background information, the development of a complicating action, an evaluation of what happened, a resolution and a coda in the form of a return to the ongoing conversation in the present. The second dimension in Ricoeur's thinking, the non-chronological, is about how plot is made out of what might well be

---

[5]'Flippin the script', or semantic inversion, 'refers to turning a meaning into its opposite or divesting a concept of its received meaning to inscribe one reflective of the speaker's experience' (Richardson 2006: 11).

scattered and unrelated events in the past. In this case, it is the necessity which comes with knowing the ending which drives the process. The point I wish to make here is that with Elena and any other interviewee, this temporal aspect needs to be born in mind. The Elena I spoke to in September 2001 relives her experiences from five years earlier not as the 24-year-old Elena of the time but as the 29-year-old Elena who was sitting in front of me. And this 29-year-old Elena has had the benefit of five more years of experience as she makes sense of what happened to her during her stay in Germany.

This discussion of position in time is related to the credibility of the interviewee and it brings to mind a second consideration worth mentioning, and that is how Elena's words might be treated as truth or as something else. Elsewhere (Block 2000, 2006), I have dealt with this issue in the following way. First, I would argue that the extent to which the notion of accuracy of storytelling or truth comes to be a central issue is proportional to the extent to which the interviewer is concerned with obtaining a veridical account of past events. Interviewees are engaged in the process of postioning themselves in the present via the accounts of events and experiences that they provide. And with this in mind, the researcher may adopt a position whereby he/she is not dependent on whether or not an interviewee is telling the truth about his/her life, or about what he/she has done or whether or not what he/she has said about any number of topics is *really* what he/she thinks. Indeed, there are very few cases in life (and the same applies to research contexts) in which we can verify with third parties accounts provided by interlocutors.[6]

Instead, there is a view of interview talk as the enactment of Weedon's (1997) *discursive fields*. As we observed above, discursive fields are defined as "competing ways of giving meaning to the world and of organizing social institutions and processes." (Weedon 1997: 34). For Weedon, any version of events provided by an interlocutor is the expression of a position (in Harré's model) which is linked to a particular *discursive field*. What is actually said and how it is said may be classified as plausible or reasonable within that particular *discursive field*. It is, therefore, a particular voice which a particular speaker has adopted perhaps momentarily, though it may also be more permanent, with a view to projecting a particular position in the ongoing storyline being produced. In Elena's case, the veracity of what she said happened to her is less important than how her storyline is used to construct her as a particular type of person in this case, as an intelligent, independent woman.

A third and final issue to consider in narrative research is what counts as narrative and what does not. This is a good question, especially because I have called

[6]One reviewer of an earlier version of this chapter pointed out that here I open a can of worms with regard to the notion of truth in narrative research (and indeed empirical research in general), noting how scholars such as Polanyi (1958) have for some time highlighted the difficulties in making sense of the personal knowledge manifested by informants in word and deed. Elsewhere (Block 2000, 2006), I have dealt with this issue in more detail (albeit with limitations), but here find that there is not ample space to do justice to this topic.

my interview with Elena a 'life-story' interview which could imply that everything she said was 'narrative' in that it was about events in her life. I had, after all, opened the interview by asking her to tell me her life story. At one point in the interview, Elena said the following:

> the more I go back to Spain / well the more you realise / that life there is a lot easier / but at the same time/ what I said / you live well / but you don't work well / and here it's the other way round / so I don't know / also at this point (.5) it's a joint venture / (Elena 27/09/01)
>
> cuanto más vuelvo a España / pues más te das cuenta / de que la vida allí es mucho más fácil / pero al mismo tiempo / lo que he dicho / se vive muy bien / pero no se trabaja muy bien / y aquí pasa lo contrario / entonces no sé / además a estas alturas (.5) es una situación conjunta / (Elena 27/09/01)

I should mention that Elena uttered these words in response to my question about how long she thought she would live in London. So it is first of all useful to consider that I had momentarily interrupted the flow of her story-telling to get her to comment on a more general point. Also, the mention of a 'joint venture' cannot be understood unless the reader knows that Elena had incorporated her boyfriend into her storyline immediately prior to this part of the interview. In any case, while this excerpt could be classified as the expression of an opinion arising from the bald comparison of the UK and Spain (one speech act in a larger flow of other speech acts), it contributes to a fairly coherent position that Elena constructs for herself during the course of the interview. So here we can add to 'feminist' and 'intelligent, independent woman', the notions of 'highly mobile', in that she does not seem reticent about changing countries again, and 'cosmopolitan', as she is not tied to her home country of Spain.

But perhaps the big issue here is how this comment by Elena in response to a question posed by me, constitutes an evaluative comment relevant to a key aspect of her life story, her move from Spain to the UK. As Labov and Waletzky (1967) note, evaluation in narrative is directly about a narrated event and it examines the consequences of this event in both cognitive and affective terms. It may be embedded in ongoing story-telling or it may occupy a kind of taking-stock position in the narrative as a whole. Here the latter applies as Elena offers a partial evaluation of her life in the UK via her comparative comments. She obviously could offer a broader more comprehensive evaluation of this part of her life were she prompted not do so, but as it stands, this excerpt is, as I explain above, the response to a specific question. In any case, my point is that as an evaluation, it may be seen to constitute a part of the ongoing story-line being constructed. And as for the issue I originally raised—where narrative begins and ends in an interview—I will have to be non-committal if we are referring to interviews in general. However, in the case of the transcription of my interview with Elena in September 2001, I would say that it is all narrative.

There are obviously more auxiliary issues which I could add to my list here. And they would all serve to complicate still further the implementation of my expanded positioning theory triangle, as laid out in earlier sections of this paper. In a paper of this type, where the goal is more to problematize than resolve, it is often hard to bring matters to a clean and clear conclusion. Suffice it to say that in this paper I have tried to offer a working model (which is very much a work in progress, I might add) for making sense of life-story interviews, and I have endeavoured to exemplify how it might work by examining an excerpt from an interview I carried out some years ago. But my conclusion is that reflecting on interviews as a means of collecting data in narrative research is a task that is never finished.

References

Atkinson, R. (1998). *The life-story interview*. London: Sage.

Austin, J. L. (1962). *How to do things with words*. Oxford: Oxford University Press.

Bakhtin, M. (1981). *The dialogic imagination: Four essays*. Auston: University of Texas.

Bakhtin, M. (1986). *Speech*. Austin: University of Texas.

Block, D. (2000). Problematizing interview data: Voices in the mind's machine? *TESOL Quarterly, 34*(4), 757–763.

Block, D. (2001). Foreign nationals on PGCE in modern languages course: Issues in national identity construction. *European Journal of Teacher Education, 24*(3), 291–312.

Block, D. (2005). Convergence and resistance in the construction of personal and professional identities: Four French modern language teachers in London. In S. A. Canagarajah (Ed.), *Reclaiming the local in language policy and practice* (pp. 167–196). Mahwah, NJ: Lawrence Erlbaum Associates.

Block, D. (2006). *Multilingual identities in a global city: London stories*. London: Palgrave.

Block, D. (2007). *Second language identities*. London: Continuum.

Block, D. (2015). Researching language and identity. In B. Paltridge & A. Phakiti (Eds.), *Research methods in applied linguistics* (pp. 337–349). London: Bloomsbury.

Boxer, L. (2003). Assessment of quality systems with positioning theory. In R. Harré & F. M. Moghaddam (Eds.), *The self and others: Positioning individuals and groups in personal, political, and cultural contexts* (pp. 251–277). Westport, CT: Praeger.

Bruner, J. (1986). *Actual minds, possible worlds*. Cambridge, MA: Harvard University Press.

Butler, J. (1990). *Gender trouble: Feminism and the subversion of identity*. New York: Routledge.

Butler, J. (2004 [1997]). Burning acts, injurious speech. In S. Salih (Ed.), *The Judith Butler Reader* (pp. 212–239). Oxford: Blackwell.

Clandinin, J. (Ed.). (2007). *Handbook of narrative inquiry: Mapping a methodology*. London: Sage.

Davies, B., & Harré, R. (1999). Positioning and personhood. In R. Harré & L. van Langenhove (Eds.), *Positioning theory* (pp. 32–52). London: Sage.

De Fina, A., & Georgakopoulou, A. (2012). *Analyzing narrative: Discourse and sociolinguistic perspectives*. Cambridge: Cambridge University Press.

Eagleton, T. (2007). *Ideology* (2nd ed.). London: Verson.

Foucault, M. (1973). *The Birth of the clinic. An archaeology of medical perception*. London: Routledge.

Foucault, M. (1979). *Discipline and punish*. Harmondsworth, UK: Penguin.

Gee, J. P. (2008). *Social linguistics and literacies: Ideology in discourses* (3rd ed.). London: Falmer.

Georgakopoulou, A. (2006). Small and large identities in narrative (inter)action. In A. De Fina, D. Schiffrin, & M. Bamberg (Eds.), *Discourse and identity* (pp. 83–102). Cambridge: Cambridge University Press.

Georgakopoulou, A. (2007). *Small stories, interaction and identities*. Amsterdam: John Benjamins.

Goffman, E. (1974). *Frame analysis*. Cambridge, MA: Harvard University Press.
Goffman, E. (1981). *Forms of talk*. Oxford: Blackwell.
Harré, R. (2004). Positioning theory. www.massey.ac.nz/~alock/virtual/positioning.doc/. Accessed September 10, 2013.
Harré, R., & Moghaddam, F. M. (2003). Introduction: The self and others in traditional psychology and in positioning theory. In R. Harré & F. M. Moghaddam (Eds.), *The self and others: Positioning individuals and groups in personal, political, and cultural contexts* (pp. 1–11). Westport, CT: Praeger.
Harré, R., & van Langenhove, L. (1999a). *Positioning theory*. London: Sage.
Harré, R., & van Langenhove, L. (1999b). The dynamics of social episodes. In R. Harré & L. van Langenhove (Eds.), *Positioning theory* (pp. 1–13). London: Sage.
James, M. (2014). *Positioning theory and strategic communication. A new approach to public relations research and practice*. London: Routledge.
Kvale, S. (1996). *Interviews*. London: Sage.
Labov, W., & Waletzky, J. (1967). Narrative analysis: Oral versions of personal experience. In W. Labov (Ed.), *Language in the inner city: Studies in the Black English vernacular* (pp. 354–396). Philadelphia, PA: University of Pennsylvania Press.
Linde, C. (1993). *Life stories: The creation of coherence*. New York: Oxford University Press.
Marx, K. (1990 [1867]). *Capital: A critique of political economy* (Vol. 1). Harmondsworth, UK: Penguin.
Mishler, E. (2006). Narrative and identity: The double arrow of time. In A. De Fina, D. Schiffrin, & M. Bamberg (Eds.), *Discourse and identity* (pp. 30–47). Cambridge: Cambridge University Press.
Moghaddam, F. M., Harré, R., & Lee, N. (Eds.). (2008). *Global conflict resolution through positioning analysis*. Berlin: Springer.
Polanyi, M. (1958). *Personal knowledge: Towards a post-critical philosophy*. Chicago: University of Chicago Press.
Richardson, E. (2006). *Hiphop literacies*. London: Routledge.
Ricoeur, P. (1980). Narrative time. *Critical Inquiry, 7*, 188.
Riessman, C. K. (2008). *Narrative methods for the human sciences*. London: Sage.
Seymour, S. (2006). Resistance. *Anthropological Theory, 6*(3), 303–321.
van Langenhove, L., & Harré, R. (1999). Introducing positioning theory. In R. Harré & L. van Langenhove (Eds.), *Positioning theory* (pp. 14–31). London: Sage.
Weedon, C. (1997). *Feminist practice and poststructuralist theory* (2nd ed.). Oxford: Blackwell.
Weedon, C. (2004). *Identity and culture: Narratives of difference and belonging*. Buckingham, UK: Open University Press.
Wengraf, T. (2001). *Qualitative research interviewing: Biographic narrative and semi-structured methods*. London: Sage.
Wortham, S., & Gadsden, V. (2006). Urban fathers positioning themselves through narrative: An approach to narrative self-construction. In A. de Fina, D. Schiffrin, & M. Bamberg (Eds.), *Discourse and identity* (pp. 314–341). Cambridge: Cambridge University Press.

Author Biography

David Block is ICREA Research Professor in Sociolinguistics at the University of Lleida. In his current research, he focusses on multimodal phenomena such as identity, social movements, multiculturalism and multilingualism, drawing on scholarship in political economy. He is author of *Social class in applied linguistics* (Routledge, 2014) and *Political economy and sociolinguistics: Neoliberalism, inequality and social class* (Bloomsbury, 2018), and edits the Routledge book series *Language, Society and Political Economy*.

Chapter 3
Refusing What We Are: Communicating Counter-Identities and Prefiguring Social Change in Social Movements

Paul McIlvenny

3.1 Revisiting Identity

In the mid-1990s, my own research investigated the relatively new question of the relationship of discourse and identity, focusing on the performativity of gender, race and national identities as well as online identities in a variety of settings (McIlvenny 1996, 1998, 1999, 2001). Since then I have increasingly felt that we need to revisit and challenge how we conceptualise *identity*.[1] Some scholars have sought to problematize identity (as well as identification, subjectivation and individualisation) in interesting ways, and I would like to quote and paraphrase those who I have found to be both challenging and inspiring, namely Michel Foucault, Michel Serres, Bruno Latour, Nikolas Rose and Ron Scollon.[2] Their understandings of the dispersed composition or assemblage of the individual have great relevance for rethinking studies of discourse and identity. Also, it is noteworthy to consider how much they have in common, despite their very different disciplinary backgrounds.

[1]Key works include Hall and Gay (1996), Antaki and Widdicombe (1998), Benwell and Stokoe (2006), Caldas-Coulthard and Iedema (2007). There have also been heated debates about the study of identity in research on language and sexuality (Bucholtz and Hall 2004; Kulick 2005).

[2]I could add many others, such as Deleuze and Guattari, who write that "you are a longitude and a latitude, a set of speeds and slownesses between uniformed particles, a set of nonsubjectified affects. You have the individuality of a day, a season, a year, a life (regardless of its duration)—a climate, a wind, a fog, a swarm, a pack (regardless of its singularity). Or at least you can have it, you can reach it" (1987: 162).

P. McIlvenny (✉)
Department of Culture and Global Studies, Aalborg University, Aalborg, Denmark
e-mail: paul@cgs.aau.dk

S. Bagga-Gupta et al. (eds.), *Identity Revisited and Reimagined*,
DOI 10.1007/978-3-319-58056-2_3

First, Foucault (1980: 98) writes that

> the individual is not to be conceived as a sort of elementary nucleus, a primitive atom, a multiple and inert material on which power comes to fasten or against which it happens to strike, and in so doing subdues or crushes individuals. In fact, it is already one of the prime effects of power that certain bodies, certain gestures, certain discourses, certain desires come to be *identified* and constituted as *individuals*. The individual, that is, is not the vis-á-vis of power; it is, I believe, one of its prime effects. The individual is an effect of power, and at the same time, or precisely to the extent to which it is that effect, it is the element of its articulation. [emphasis added]

As a consequence, Foucault notes that a critique of the political technology of the individual is necessary. In contrast to his more ambiguous work on the ethical technologies of the self, Foucault (1988) is critical of the ways in which the individual and individuality are harnessed by governmental projects. In one of his lectures, he highlights "the ways by which, through some political technology of individuals, we have been led to recognise ourselves as a society, as part of a social entity, as part of a nation or of a state" (404). Moreover, Foucault (1983: 215) argues that "the state can be seen as a modern matrix of individualization, or a new form of pastoral power." He notes that this new form of individualisation took on the form of a series of powers—e.g., those of the family, medicine, psychiatry, education, and employers—and the target "nowadays is not to discover what we are but to *refuse what we are*" and "to promote new forms of *subjectivity* through the refusal of this kind of individuality that has been imposed on us [by the state] for several centuries. [emphasis added]" (216). Thus, for Foucault writing in the early 1980s, "the political, ethical, social, philosophical problem of our days is not to try to liberate the individual from the state, and from the state's institutions, but to liberate us both from the state and the type of individualisation linked to the state" (216).

Writing about the eclectic work of Michel Serres, Brown (2002: 21–22) notes that

> we become subjects through the way in which we are caught up in the circulation of that which will make us 'it' – the 'moving back and forth of the "I"'. Sociality is neither an atomistic adding together of individuals, nor an abstract contractual arrangement. It is a collectivity assembled and held together by the circulation of an object.

In the same vein, Bruno Latour (2005: 208) contends that

> we should be able to observe empirically how an anonymous and generic body is made to be a person: the more intense the shower of offers of *subjectivities*, the more interiority you get. Subjects are no more autochthonous than face-to-face interactions. They, too, depend on the flood of entities allowing them to exist. To be an 'actor' is now at last a totally artificial and fully traceable gathering. [emphasis added]

Within studies of governmentality, Rose (1996: 6) proliferates the number of ways in which 'we' can be composed:

> These links between the molar and the molecular have taken a variety of forms, not merely or principally paternalistic attempts at the micro-management of conduct, but more complex and subtle procedures for establishing a delicate and complex web of affiliations

> between thousands of habits of which human beings are composed – movements, gestures, combinations, associations, passions, satisfactions, exhaustions, aspirations, contemplations – and the wealth, tranquillity, efficiency, economy, glory of the collective body.

In an online publication, Rose (no date) connects this idea to identity formation:

> nonetheless, if [one] construes power in terms of 'action upon action' [i.e. governmentality], one can see the ways in which through the kinds of mechanisms I have sketched out, therapeutic language, therapeutic techniques, therapeutic scenarios, the proliferation of the therapeutic through our culture, has a role in fabricating us as certain kinds of persons: certain human kinds who attend to ourselves in certain ways, value particular aspects of ourselves, take certain things as our truths, whether these be our desire or our *identity* or our skills, and act on those things in order to lead our own lives. [emphasis added]

Lastly, within the field of discourse studies, Scollon (2001: 158) stresses that we loosen up our understanding of identity when he writes that

> the production of communities of practice as bounded membership entities of inclusion and exclusion out of the nexus of practice must be studied to see how the transformation from practice, action and habitus to person, characteristics and *identity* is performed through discursive practices and other practices of technologisation and objectivisation. [emphasis added]

What these provocative quotations suggest is that we should not take identity (and the individual/subject) for granted. In fact, we should loosen up our understanding of the location of identity, and we ought to problematize the notion of the individual who claims an identity. In other words, we should think of identity as a contingent accomplishment and objectivisation. We should proliferate the means by which identity is constituted and distribute the constitution of identity over a diversity of actors, actants, artefacts, materialities, technologies and nexus of practice (see also Cooren 2010). If we do so, then it remains for us to show how, on every occasion, an 'identity' is constituted and maintained, or resisted and countered. The play of 'identity' and 'counter-identity' is what is explored in this chapter by analyzing a theatrical protest event using Ethnomethodological Conversation Analysis (EMCA).

3.2 Governmentality and Counter-Conduct

This chapter draws upon Foucault's later work, especially his studies of governmentality and the ethics of the care of the self. Foucault (2007: 193) carefully defines *conduct*. The translator notes that "when Foucault speaks of 'a conduct' (*une conduit*) the sense often embraces the activity by which some conduct others, the way in which some are conducted by others, and the way in which individuals conduct themselves within this form of 'conduct'" (193, footnote†). Davidson (2011: 26.27) notes that Foucault cleverly writes of "the double dimension of conduct, namely the activity of conducting an individual, conduction as a relation between individuals, and the way in which an individual conducts 'himself' or is conducted, 'his' conduct or behavior in the narrower sense of the term. Yet Foucault moves quickly from the quite specific form of power that takes as its object the conduct of individuals to the correlative countermovements that he initially designates as specific revolts of conduct." In one of his lectures, Foucault makes the case for using what he acknowledges as a badly constructed word 'counter-conduct' because it has the advantage of allowing reference to the *active* sense of the verb. Moreover, it points to the sense of struggle against the processes implemented for conducting others; he prefers it to "'misconduct' (*inconduite*), which only refers to the passive sense of the word, of behaviour: not conducting oneself properly" (Foucault 2007: 201).

In an interview, Foucault sketchily outlines what he means by the will not to be governed (*counter-conducts*) as "the will not to be governed thusly, like that, by these people, at this price" (1997: 72). Later he clarifies: "I was not referring to something that would be a fundamental anarchism, that would be like an originary freedom, absolutely and wholeheartedly resistant to any governmentalisation" (73). Indeed, Rose (1999) concludes his book on governmentality and 'powers of freedom' in advanced liberal societies by reiterating Foucault's warning about dichotomising power and resistance. He argues that we are required to abandon those binary divisions that have structured our political thinking and our theorizing about the political for so long, such as domination and emancipation, and power and resistance: "each such binary suggests a principle of division between those political, technical and ethical strategies that have made up our present and those that have opposed them. This way of dividing the matter is illusory. There is not a single discourse or strategy of power confronted by forces of resistance, but a set of conflicting points and issues of opposition, alliance and division of labour" (277).

In order to examine the discourse and interactional practices of *counter-conducts*, and also the *identities* that are co-constituted, particularly in relation to social movements, I combine Ethnomethodological Conversation Analysis with Death's (2010) analytics of protest derived from Dean's (2010) analytics of government. A first step in an analytics of protest is to uncover how fields of visibility, forms of knowledge, and subjectivities and identities are negotiated and collaboratively accomplished by the protestors and the people they encounter.

3.3 Prefiguration and Identity

There is one last notion I wish to introduce in relation to counter-identity and that is *prefiguration*. The saying "Be the Change You Want to See in the World", attributed to Gandhi, has been adopted as a slogan by many social movements. Maeckelbergh (2009, 2011) argues that prefiguration is a strategic practice of recent social movements, especially alterglobalisation movements in the 2000s and the

Occupy movement in the 2010s. With the concern for modes of horizontal organisation in social movements, one can look at how movement actors experiment with a range of communicative and social interactional practices that support more democratic forms of social organising, deliberation and decision-making. For instance, spokescouncils, 'process' and consensus can stop the formation of a vanguard or elite core group who organise vertically. We can ask how an event is made prefigurative, and how prefiguration is accomplished successfully and how are prefigurative identities accomplished discursively.[3] And we can explore the ways in which political prefiguration and the communicative practices of counter-conduct reimagine *identity* as a process of self-transformation. For instance, some members of new social movements such as Anonymous have donned the stylised Guy Fawkes mask of the graphic novel and film adaptation *V for Vendetta*.[4] What does this gesture tell us about how claims to individual identity can be disrupted in embodied communication? What are the conditions of possibility for individuals to recognize themselves as particular kinds of person and to reflect upon their own and others' conduct, i.e. to problematize it? What are the connections between discursive processes of identification, desire and subjectivation in contemporary political life? These are important questions that can be empirically addressed from a discourse studies perspective.

3.4 Discourse, Governmentality and Counter-Identities

There is only a small body of work that incorporates into discourse and social interaction studies some of the concepts and methods suggested by Foucault (Dent 2009; Harris 2005; Hodges 2003; Lindegaard 2012; McIlvenny 2009a, b; Rasmussen 2011, 2013; Salskov-Iversen et al. 2000; Summerville 2007; Summerville and Adkins 2007). For example, Hodges (2003) uses discursive psychology to explore the ways in which the ethical subject is regulated by therapeutic discourse in the media as a political strategy of governmentality. Summerville and Adkins (2007) use membership categorisation analysis to investigate the common-sense and methodical ways in which 'the citizen' is produced and enrolled as an active participant in 'sustainable' regional planning. Lindegaard (2012) also uses membership categorisation analysis to analyse the accomplishment of rationalities of government as they unfold within the continuously contested, discursive field of 'green driving' in an automobile society.

[3]Maeckelbergh (2011) argues that social change is a matter of practice and experience, but she does not do any detailed analyses of actual practices from a discourse studies perspective.

[4]https://en.wikipedia.org/wiki/Guy_Fawkes_mask.

As an ethnomethodologist, Lynch (1993: 131) cautiously notes that

> Foucault's descriptions nevertheless can be exemplary for ethnomethodological investigations, because they so clearly identify how material architectures, machineries, bodily techniques, and disciplinary routines make up coherent phenomenal fields. Whereas Foucault problematizes the diachronic continuity of historical discourses, ethnomethodology explodes the contemporaneous landscape of language games into distinctive orders of practice, which are neither hermetically sealed from one another nor expressive of a single historical narrative.

Using Foucault's recently discovered later work combined with Ethnomethodological Conversation Analysis (EMCA), I examine how 'counter-conducts' and 'counter-identities' are achieved and made accountable in the interactional practices of prefigurative demonstrations and protest events. EMCA helps us document the ways in which fields of visibility and modes of rationality are sequentially organised. However, we also need to examine critically in what ways it can help trace the practices that are endemic and endogenous to conducting the conduct of others, and thus which constitute or contest counter-identities:

- What are the relations between practice, conduct and identity?
- Is sequential and categorial analysis *enough* to investigate counter-conducts and counter-identities?
- What particular sequential, interactional, embodied and categorial practices are relevant to this investigation?

The data corpus I am working with includes in situ video recordings of the Occupy movement, radical clowning by the Clandestine Insurgent Radical Clown Army (CIRCA) and other creative protest events.[5] For example, McIlvenny (2017) documents some of the ways in which practices of 'horizontal' communication, organisation and participation in the Occupy movement—e.g. the participatory communicative practice known as the 'human microphone' (Costanza-Chock 2012; Mitchell et al. 2013)—are trialled and transformed by participants. In the photograph in Fig. 3.1, one can see the spatial configurations and participation frameworks of several Occupy events in which hand signals and the 'human microphone' are being used to communicate collectively without electronic amplification.

In addition, one can explore how the playful discursive crossings of characters and roles—e.g. clowns, mock officials—are communicated and practised as a form of tactical reversal, often in liminal encounters with the police, proxies and bystanders. In Figs. 3.2 and 3.3, one can see a variety of members of CIRCA (Bogad 2011; Klepto 2004) engage with the authorities who are policing the scene in question.

[5]Similar types of events can be described as "tactical carnival" (Bogad 2006), "electoral guerilla theatre" (Bogad 2005), "serious play" (Peacock 2009), and "Impro Everywhere" (Todd and Scordelis 2009).

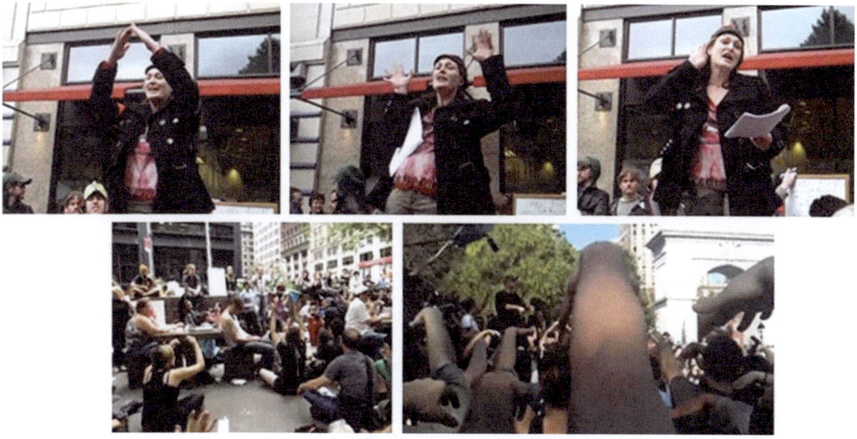

Fig. 3.1 Hand signals at various Occupy events (*source* YouTube)

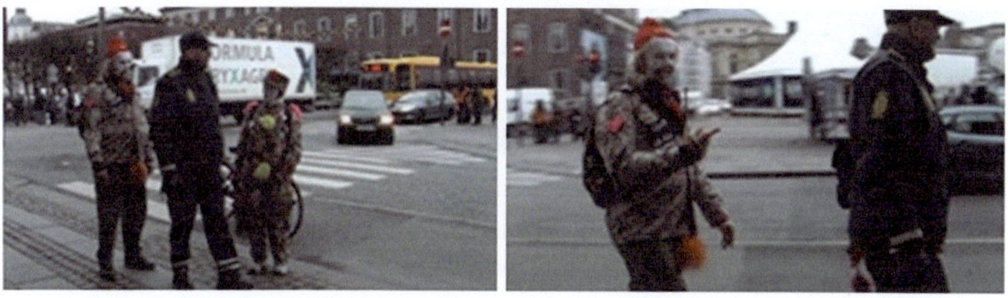

Fig. 3.2 CIRCA members engage with a police officer at COP15 in Denmark (*source* private)

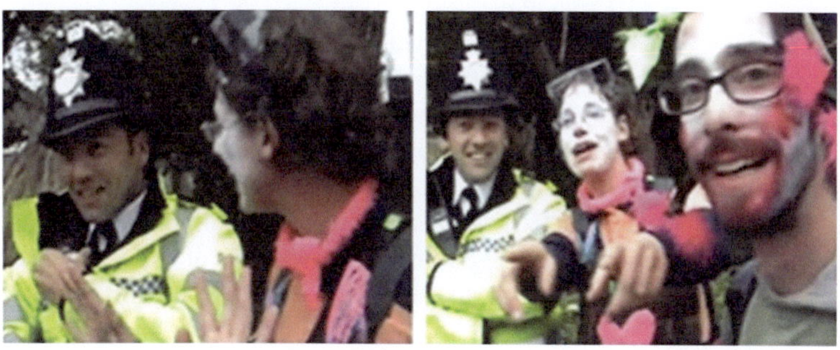

Fig. 3.3 CIRCA members engage with a friendly police officer in the UK (*source* YouTube)

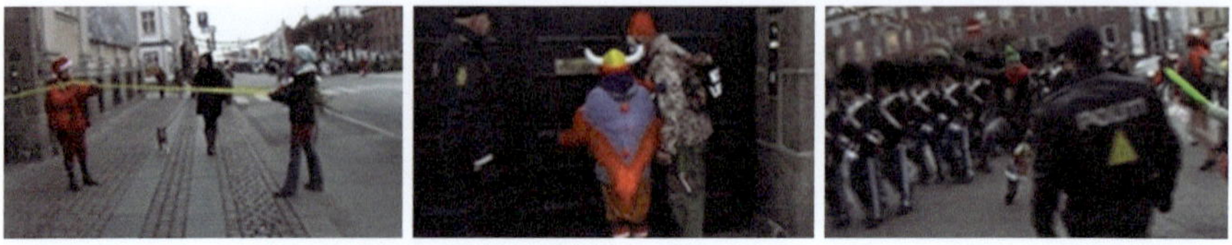

Fig. 3.4 CIRCA members engage with space, institutions and culture at COP15 (*source* private)

In Fig. 3.4, various stages in a CIRCA event at the United Nations' Conference of the Parties conference (COP 15) on climate change in Copenhagen in 2009 are documented as the clowns enroll other actors, agencies and materialities in the urban space of the street outside the French embassy.

Issues that are topicalised by these social movements include climate change, racism, war and international conflicts, the financial crisis and austerity. And they are all, like the "United Nathans weapons inspectors", a kind of theatrical social protest which has the power to reorganize identity relationships, due to the deployment and disruption of taken-for-granted arrangements.[6]

3.5 Case Study: "United Nathans Weapons Inspectors"

The main case study in this chapter is a theatrical protest event that took place on 13th February 2003. The data was collected in order to document the actions of a peace group in Denmark protesting against the imminent invasion of Iraq by the United States of America (USA) and its coalition forces, which in fact took place on 19th March without the authorisation of the United Nations (UN). On 5th February, U.S. Secretary of State Colin Powell addressed the UN General Assembly, producing what later turned out to be false evidence for Weapons of Mass Destruction (WMD) in an effort to gain UN authorization for an invasion. The protest event took place eight days later, two days before the global peace protests on 15th February, which were heralded as the largest peace demonstrations the world has ever seen before a war began.[7] The protest event was called "United Nathans weapons inspectors" [sic], and it was conducted to highlight the lack of transparency on the part of the USA regarding its own stock of WMD, and thus the hypocrisy of the USA and its allies to demand that another country, namely Iraq,

[6]One can compare such amateur political theatre by social movement activists to the professional political theatre associated with the Brazilian theatre director Augusto Boal (1974/2008, 1998) and others.

[7]https://en.wikipedia.org/wiki/February_15,_2003,_anti-war_protests.

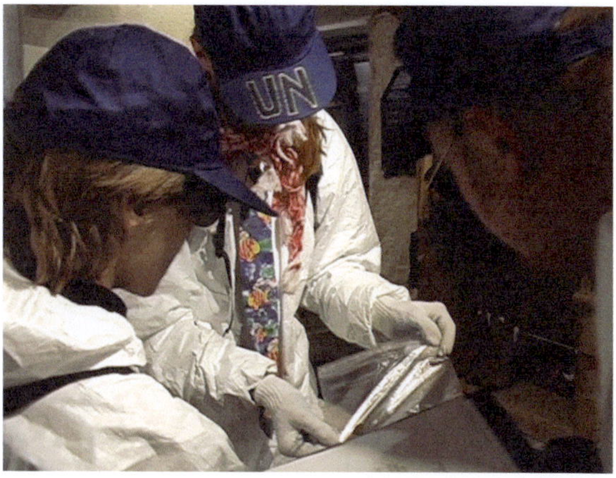

Fig. 3.5 Members of United Nathans inspecting an object in *Malboro Classics* (*source* private)

open up to inspections by UNMOVIC (United Nations Monitoring, Verification and Inspection Commission) and the IAEA (International Atomic Energy Agency) as a pretext for invasion.

A group of activists decided as a serious 'prank' to inspect US and corporate businesses unannounced for WMD in order to focus attention on the matter, and to promote the upcoming peaceful demonstration. They dressed uniformly and visibly as 'inspectors' (see Fig. 3.5), donning white overalls, blue caps, clipboards, gloves and logos that echoed the United Nations. However, each was called, and referred to each other as, "Nathan", from the "United Nathans". The group was shadowed by a reporter and video camera operator from the local division of a national TV station, as well as a student radio reporter. The group travelled by local bus (informing passengers of the rationale of the protest event and inspecting the bus) and visited and inspected, with no warning, several businesses in the city, including a *Shell* garage, a *Levi's* shop, a *Malboro Classics* shop, a *McDonald's* restaurant, a pharmacy, and *Blockbusters* video rental shop. The analysis will focus on the events in the *Malboro Classics* shop.[8] The group entered from the street and stayed for five minutes, with the permission of the shop assistant in charge, who was oblivious to the protest performance that was about to begin.[9]

The video recordings of the "United Nathans weapons inspectors" event are transcribed using the conventions used in Conversation Analysis (Jefferson 2004). Text in italics is spoken in Danish, with an English translation in the line below.

[8]A more detailed empirical analysis comparing the protest action by the Nathans in *Levi's* with the one in *Malboro Classics* can be found in McIlvenny (2016).

[9]A shorter, edited video made by the group can be found online: https://www.youtube.com/watch?v=DRFk1xLFZSw.

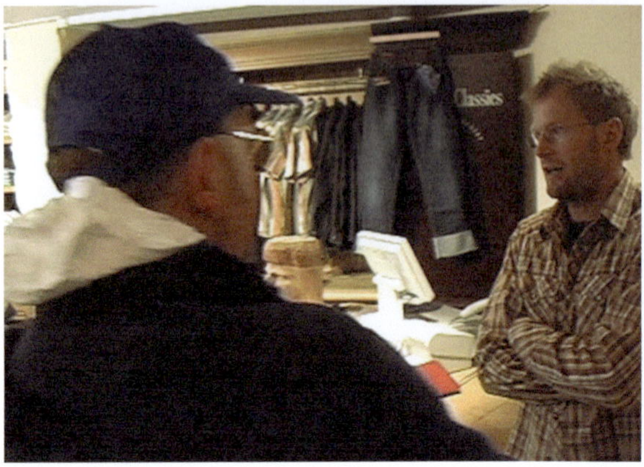

Fig. 3.6 A first encounter with the shop assistant in *Malboro Classics* (*source* private)

3.5.1 From Customers to Inspectors

Once in the shop, what could easily have been a routine service encounter is step-by-step transformed into a type of inspection—the prank in question. This is initiated by gaining permission to search for a particular item (hearable as associated with that shop) as a condition and pretext for conducting the stylised mock inspection.

In Transcript 3.1 below, K enters *Malboro Classics* and walks towards the shop assistant, who is presently talking with a customer in Danish. The opening sequence consists of paired greetings (in two languages) and identifications (see Fig. 3.6), followed by a question by K to determine the competence, and gain the consent, of the assistant to speak English. K does not introduce himself yet as an agent of a particular organisation, but he quickly establishes a dialogue with A1, and he treats A1 as the gatekeeper from whom it is necessary to secure consent. K asks A1 whether or not there are cigarettes present on the premises (line 16). After a jocular exchange, in which A1 seems remarkably calm and tolerant, K requests permission to search the shop, and then instructs the other Nathans (line 37) to see if any samples of "cigarettes" can be found. Thus, K unilaterally moves into the inspection phase by instructing the Nathans to begin their search for a specific object. Up until this point, the participants try to sustain the impression that K is a potential customer with rights to independently peruse the goods on offer in an appropriate manner without further assistance.

Transcript 3.1: Entrance and first encounter (Malboro Classics)

((K enters shop))
((A1 is talking in Danish to a customer))
((K walks up to A1))
A1: *god dag*
good day
K: good afternoon
how are you:.
A1: i a:m fi:ne? ((A1 looks over at who enters the shop))
K: good.
how is your engli:sh
A1: i: don't kno::w=you can tell me la:ter
A1: =[maybe]
K: =[ah it] sou:nds [quite goo:d
(): [hahahahahah •hh
((A1 scans those who have entered and looks to K))
K: have you got any cigare:ttes
A1: no.
K: =[malboro
A1: =[no. ((A1 twists to left))
A1 no. ((A1 twists further to left))
K: cigarettes
A1: sure ((A1 turns back to K))
K: it says ((K points to door))
=[malboro]
A1: =[no problem]
K: =[it says malboro] on the door
A1: =[>yeah yeah yeah<]
(): ( )
K: can we ((points to right)) look for some cigare:ttes?
A1: yeah [sure]
K: [can y-] can w- heheh thank youhuhuh
((K pats A1 on shoulder))
A1: look ou:t in the ba:ck *(selv tak)*
(you're welcome)
K: yeah
K: CAN YOU t'SEE IF YOU FI:ND ANY CIGARE:TTES?

In the shop, the protestors have to negotiate and sustain the consent of the assistant to 'inspect' the property. In *Malboro Classics*, K asks an apparently innocent question of the shop assistant, namely if he has any cigarettes (line 16). Given the service encounter frame and the inferences that can be drawn from the name of the shop, this is hearable as a reasonable question. But this time, K more actively pursues the accountability of the shop to reasonably have cigarettes on the premises. After A1 acknowledges the logic of the question based on the assumption that a shop with the name "Malboro" will also sell cigarettes, K makes a request in line 29 to inspect the shop—to "look for some cigarettes". A1 gives consent, and even suggests they look in the backstage space of the shop "in the back".

We can see from these early stages of the notional service encounter that the protestors are seeking to destabilise the normative identities in play in the consumerist setting, and thus to politicise what are ostensibly apolitical corporations/local franchises. This can be bewildering to the shop assistants in the corporation concerned, e.g. in the *Levi's* shop they also visited.

3.5.2 Doing Being 'Mock Inspectors'

Once they have moved into the 'mock inspection' frame, they need to maintain roles, rights and permission to inspect, to conduct the inspection in an open and transparent manner, to search and locate objects of suspicion. Yet they ultimately fail to find WMD at each site, much as the evidence for WMD in Iraq was speculative and such weapons were never found. Maintaining the illusion of a mock inspection is difficult when decisions have to be made collectively. Once in the frame of the inspection, one must either play in character or find an opportunity to shift frame. Once the inspections start, the group chose to refer to each other anonymously as Nathans—everyone is identified in the same way, except the chief inspector who the other Nathans address as "Sir". This preserves their anonymity, yet it instantiates a hierarchy typical for an inspection team. Both the protestors and the other participants not only have to maintain a background institutional 'role' and associated discursive identities—e.g. the inspector and the inspectee, the customer and the shop assistant—they also have to negotiate the voices of the 'global justice/peace movement' and the corporation.

In Transcript 3.2, after instructing the Nathans, they disperse and K moves to the back of the shop (line 42). He talks to customers noting the discrepancy between the name of the shop and the lack of cigarettes. After a brief search, K proposes that the shop is clean (line 75), a pre-closing that attempts to move the mock inspections to completion.

Transcript 3.2: The inspection proceeds

37 K: CAN YOU t'SEE IF YOU FI:ND ANY CIGARE:TTES?
38 where's nathan ((K turns to look at the back))
39 K: ↑NAthan
40 check the rubbish bins for cigarettes
41 ((Nathans spread out over shop))
42 ((K walks to back of shop where three customers are standing))
43 K: anybody got any cigarettes
44 K: *har i cigaretter*
45 do you have cigarettes
46 K: and ((K points up and back)) *det er ↑ma:lboro*
47 it is ↑ma:lboro
48 K: heheh
49 C1: heheheh
50 K: *det siger* malboro
51 it says malboro
52 C1: *(°det er rigtigt°)*
53 (°it is right°)
54 *K:* ↑uh
55 A1: *og vi kan ikke en gang vise en prince eller noget*
56 and we can't even show a single prince or something
57 ((K turns around and looks at A1))
58 C2: *jamen [jeg har da*
59 but i have
60 K: [hahahahah
61 ((L hands A1 a flyer))
62 L: *( ) demonstration på lørdag*
63 ( ) demonstration on saturday
64 L: *tak ska'du ha'*
65 thanks
66 (2.5)
67 K: can you see any fi:nnish cigarettes
68 P: *ei en näe yhtään suomalais(ia) ((in Finnish))*
69 no i can't see any finnish ( )
70 L: finnish cigarettes no si:r
71 K: no: finnish cigarettes
72 L: no finnish cigare:ttes
73 ((they search the shop))
74 ((J finds a small piece of brown material))
75 ((the search continues))
76 K: o::kay the place looks clea:n to me
77 ((K walks towards the front))
78 K: IS THIS PLACE CLEA:N,
79 i think this place is clean=no cigarettes

Soon after, in Transcript 3.3 another Nathan (J) finds a suspicious object (line 90) and it is bagged as a sample. It is suggested it might be a fragment of chewing tobacco. A1 humorously denies this when presented with the evidence (line 111).

Transcript 3.3: A suspicious object is discovered

90 ((J is holding a transparent bag containing a fragment))
91 L: si:r this could be chewing tobacco
92 K: ↑che:wing tobacco
93 ((J, L and K bend forward to examine the fragment))
94 S: it's wo:rse
95 K: oh it's worse
96 L: it's very hard
97 L: it came out of a pot
98 (): shall we give it t'them
99 K: let's::
100 K: (   )
101 K: can you ask him if that's che:wing tobacco
102 J: yeah
103 K: that's a:lmo:st a cigarette isn't it tha:nk you
104 K: could you er: Cha- Chris could you (.) just
105 ((K points towards A1))
106 ((J walks up to A1 talking to C2 and C3))
107 K: oka:y na:thans
108 ((J shows the bag to A1))
109 J: sorry (   )
110 ((A1 shakes his head))
111 A1: t- try to (.) try to ta:ste it
112 J: ah yeh
113 (): ((laugh))

Over the course of the event, the protestors have to sustain the right to inspect gained in the initial sequence which K negotiated with the shop assistant. Moreover, for an inspection regime to work, the inspectors must be seen as neutral. This was always a problem in Iraq, especially when it was revealed that some of the inspectors were spying for Western governments. The group take care to complete the inspection successfully with the cooperation of the local caretaker of the business. It is important for the success of the protest actions that the police are not called to the site. If an owner or shop assistant becomes agitated and refuses permission, then the group planned to leave immediately. This happened at one site when the group left quickly, giving the reason that the site was not complying with inspections. By the end of the mock inspection, the protestors may or may not have found evidence of suspicious objects that need further attention. In *Malboro Classics* it may be the shred of "chewing tobacco" that is bagged and held up as evidence. Nevertheless, the group close the inspections amicably and they leave the premises.

In Transcript 3.4, even though some evidence is being removed from the site, supposedly for further examination, K this time explicitly commends the shop for a clean inspection (lines 143–51). This has a double function: it makes explicit the ulterior motive for their presence, and it reinforces the play-frame of the whole encounter. After mutual thanks and appreciation, the mock inspection frame is cooperatively and playfully extended into the future when K invokes the threat of satellite surveillance and continuous monitoring (lines 168–74). After a brief round of termination pairs, they exit.

Transcript 3.4: the inspection is concluded

143 K: (your sa:d) but i'd like to sa:y
144 i'd like to sa:y ((K turns to A1)) that this site (.)
145 in ma:lboro (.) classic is rega- absolutely
146 ((K shakes hand of A1)) clea:n
147 not a si:ngle cigarette
148 A1: nice
149 K: not a si:ngle cigarette of mass destruction
150 on the whole si:te.
151 ve:ry good. thank you. ((shake hands))
152 H: *det var meget samarbejdsvillig*
153 it was very cooperative
154 L: *mange tak*
155 many thanks
156 A1: *selv tak*
157 thank you too
158 H: *tak*
159 thanks
160 A1: *og tak for besøg*
161 and thanks for visiting
162 (): *( )*
163 (): *( )*
164 (): *( )*
165 K: but we'll be er::: ((finger raised))
166 L: *vi håber [at se dig på lørdag*
167 we hope to see on saturday
168 A1: [you'll be ba:ck or: what
169 K: we'll be watching you
170 ((A1 nods to L))
171 K: we'll be watching with satelli:tes
172 A1: ok ( )
173 K: if there's a cigarette in this sho:p
174 ↑BOO BOO:P
175 A1: you're welcome
176 P: mind our ( )
177 A1: never
178 ((the Nathans exit))

In this case the mock inspection is completed, and the head inspector explicitly states that the site is "clean". Rather than finding evidence and accusing the shop assistant or the corporation of hiding something like WMD, the protestors move on to the next site.

3.5.3 Analytics of Protest

An analytics of protest uncovers how fields of visibility, forms of knowledge, technologies and apparatuses, and subjectivities and identities are negotiated and accomplished collaboratively by the activists and the people they encounter. A number of subjectivities and identities are produced and contested in this case. In such protest events, the participants are compelled to negotiate and temporarily sustain the particular relational identities that enable the analogy to work. Participants accomplish the 'citizen-inspector' who inspects on behalf of everyone, the 'inspector-hero' who perseveres to reveal a hidden 'truth', and the shop assistant, the representative of the compliant business governed by international law.[10] Moreover, in terms of scale, the protest group members are peaceful protestors, global citizens *and* neutral inspectors. The local shop assistants are also employees of a large multinational corporation that is presumed to be identified as American. Thus, the protest attempts to stabilise particular counter-identities—e.g. the citizen-inspectors—in order to resonate analogically with a particular interpretation of the international political conflict at hand. This is quite an achievement of scale. These citizens can inspect this local instance of a retail chain store on behalf of a global public. This business and therefore all American businesses are accountable as political entities. This local inspection parallels the inspection practices of international bodies. Thus, the protestors (and other participants) need to connect the local actions taking place in situ with the actions of distant others. As Latour (2005: 252) argues, "action is possible only in a territory that has been opened up, flattened down, and cut down to size in a place where formats, structures, globalisation, and totalities circulate inside tiny conduits and where for each of their applications they need to rely on masses of hidden potentialities." Further, Latour (2005: 202) contends that in studies of 'interaction' "the number and type of 'actions' and the span of their 'inter' relations has been vastly underestimated. Stretch any given inter-action and, sure enough, it becomes an actor-network." One could also, by extension, stretch any 'identity' and, sure enough, it becomes a more dynamic relationality, making visible 'counter-identities'. In this case, participants stitch together disparate local practices in order to scale up the routine practices of

[10]Membership Categorisation Analysis (MCA) offers a way to understand how categories are worked up by participants as part and parcel of particular moral orders. For example, the membership device of [inspector, inspectee] and the activities that get bound to the incumbents of these categories are crucial elements for amplifying the moral force of the inspection regime.

'citizens' inspecting a site on behalf of a global public to the scene of international politics and the official United Nations inspection regime.[11]

3.5.4 Governing Inspection: Counter-Identities

There are two ways in which this event can be analysed in relation to the conduct of conduct and counter-identities. First, there are the ways in which the group govern their own conduct and in so doing enrol and perform particular counter-identities.[12] In this case, because they are simulating a UN inspection team, they are also appropriating some of the styles, genres and discourses as well as interactional routines that most easily accomplish 'inspection'. This is a form of discursive 'crossing', in which participants draw upon a range of resources to do discursive work of which they are not fully competent.[13] When they slip out of the inspection frame to coordinate their next actions, then there are the alternative forms of conducting their own conduct as 'protestors'.

Second, there is the practical logic of the demonstration and how it interfaces with a particular regime of international governmentality that uses the inspection as one of many means to conduct the conduct of other countries. In the event, a diversity of 'local' actions and practices are redistributed and stitched together according to a rationality of global justice in which hypocrisy and transparency are produced. The inspection is localised, appropriated and turned on the governors who have used it asymmetrically. The protest attempts in a playful fashion to construct a temporary alternative space of governmentality—a counter-conduct with counter-identities—in which new objects and spaces of governance are produced and new governors (e.g. citizens—the anonymous Nathans of the United Nathans) do the governing. One could say that the protestors offer up a regime of governmentality fit for and constitutive of a global assembly of peoples, and not an inter-national club of countries (e.g. the UN security council), and this results in a rather rarefied 'atmosphere of democracy' in which certain 'truths' are made public (Latour and Weibel 2005).

Blühdorn (2006: 36) argues that "the significance of social movement politics lies not so much in the demonstration of protest and opposition for the purpose of

[11]See the work of Barad (2003: 819), which ties in nicely with Foucault, Latour and Scollon: "Discourse is not what is said; it is that which constrains and enables what can be said. Discursive practices define what counts as meaningful statements. Statements are not the mere utterances of the originating consciousness of a unified subject; rather, statements and subjects emerge from a field of possibilities. This field of possibilities is not static or singular but rather is a dynamic and contingent multiplicity."

[12]In his anthropological study of the clowning of members of the Western Apache in relation to 'the white man' and symbolic domination, Basso (1979) shows how impersonation can create a safe space for different interpretations.

[13]See Rampton (1995) for a discussion of the similar concept of 'language crossing'.

political change, but in the demonstration, performance and experience of something that is desperately needed in the late modern condition but that has no place in the established socio-economic system: autonomy, identity, and agency." One could also argue that prefiguration intrinsically involves a demonstration of alternative autonomies, agencies and *identities* that do not yet exist or are not stabilised. The protestors show autonomy in that they carry out the inspections independently of any governmental body. Their legitimacy and authority are accomplished in their local encounters with onsite officials (e.g. shop assistants). And the protestors inspect the sites acting as concerned citizens with rights and obligations that are prefigurative. They can do this partly because the group avoids personal names, preferring Nathan as their uniform address term.

3.6 Conclusion

Using Ethnomethodological Conversation Analysis (EMCA), the chapter has examined some of the ways in which 'counter-identities' are achieved and made accountable in the interactional practices of a specific prefigurative protest event. Combining conversation analysis and studies of governmentality—the conduct of conduct—means we have some analytical tools to open up the 'black box' of identity and challenge the orthodoxy of mainstream 'identitarian' approaches. For example, such an approach can document the ways in which fields of visibility and modes of rationality are sequentially and categorially organised in the contingent and precarious accomplishment of counter-identities (that is, t*o be identified in other ways, by other means and by other actors*) as part and parcel of a counter-conduct. Moreover, it was documented that the United Nathans protest is prefigurative in that it imagines counter-identities as it performs an equitable inspection regime. Ultimately, the protest event was designed to prefigure an alternative world in which concerned citizens could act autonomously to expose publicly the hypocrisy of nation-states acting in their own interests. In a creative and playful fashion, the protestors take on stylised institutional identities (*discursive crossing*) in order to attempt to make plain the hypocrisy of the USA to demand inspections of another sovereign country yet refuse inspections of its own installations/territory. Through a variety of communicative practices and interactional routines, the United Nathans manage to 'pull off' a mock inspection in American businesses without causing a disturbance and with what seems, and ironically requires, the full consent of the transnational corporation's local employees. The mock inspections by the United Nathans are, in fact, a disguise for real citizens' inspections, i.e. for citizens themselves, in the name of transparency and global justice, to inspect what governments and the UN are unwilling or unsure of undertaking. We can think of the prefigurative protest as both a form of counter-conduct, with accompanying counter-identities, as well as an attempt by analogy to repair the tainted international inspection regime as an instrument of governmentality.

Rose (1999: 279) suggests that "something might be learnt from those insurgent, minority or subaltern forces that have often refused to codify themselves, that have resisted the temptations of party and programme, that have taken shape in the shadows, interstices and oversights of conventional politics and that have so often acted as *laboratories for alternative futures* [emphasis added]." Instead of looking for heroic agents or acts of bravery against power, "one would examine the ways in which creativity arises out of the situation of human beings engaged in particular relations of force and meaning, and what is made out of the possibilities of that location" (1999: 279). He notes that they frequently arise in 'cramped spaces'—"within a set of relations that are intolerable, where movement is impossible, where change is blocked and voice is strangulated. And, in relation to these little territories of the everyday, they seek to engender a small reworking of their own spaces of action" (280). For him, it is in feminist politics that was conducted under the slogan of 'the personal is political' that we find the most obvious example from our recent past of "the ways in which such a molecular and minor engagement with cramped space can connect up with a whole series of other circuits and cause them to fluctuate, waver and reconfigure in wholly unexpected ways" (280).

These cramped spaces and everyday spaces of actions, such as also seen in the "United Nathans weapons inspectors" protest, are important to study because they are interactional micro-laboratories for experimenting with contemporary modes of identity formation and disruption. They are also prefigure future radical transformations in the practices of everyday life and institutional settings (see Bayat 2010). We can compare them with, for example, the often forgotten Gandhian inspired 'sit-ins' of the 1940s at sites of consumption by members of CORE, the Congress of Racial Equality, which foreshadowed the more famous civil rights movement of the 1960s and the resulting challenges to pervasive racial inequality in everyday life and institutions that still play out today in the USA (Scalmer 2011).

References

Antaki, C., & Widdicombe, S. (Eds.). (1998). *Identities in talk*. London: Sage.

Barad, K. (2003). Posthumanist performativity: Toward an understanding of how matter comes to matter. *Signs: Journal of Women in Culture and Society, 28*(3), 802–831.

Basso, K. (1979). *Portraits of 'the Whiteman': Linguistic play and cultural symbols among the western Apache*. Cambridge: Cambridge University Press.

Bayat, A. (2010). *Life as politics: How ordinary people change the Middle East*. Stanford, CA: Stanford University Press.

Benwell, B., & Stokoe, E. (2006). *Discourse and identity*. Edinburgh: Edinburgh University Press.

Blühdorn, I. (2006). Self-experience in the theme park of radical action?: Social movements and political articulation in the late-modern condition. *European Journal of Social Theory, 9*(1), 23–42.

Boal, A. (1974/2008). *Theatre of the oppressed*. London: Pluto Press.

Boal, A. (1998). *Legislative theatre: Using performance to make politics*. London: Routledge.

Bogad, L. M. (2005). *Electoral guerrilla theatre: Radical ridicule and social movements*. London: Routledge.

Bogad, L. M. (2006). Tactical carnival: Social movements, public space and dialogical performance. In J. Cohen-Cruz & M. Schutzman (Eds.), *A Boal companion: Dialogues on theatre and cultural politics* (pp. 46–58). London: Routledge.

Bogad, L. M. (2011). Clowndestine maneuvers: A study of clownfrontational tactics. *Thamyris/Intersecting: Place, Sex and Race, 21*(1), 179–198.

Brown, S. D. (2002). Michel Serres: Science, translation and the logic of the parasite. *Theory, Culture and Society, 19*(3), 1–27.

Bucholtz, M., & Hall, K. (2004). Theorizing identity in language and sexuality research. *Language in Society, 33*(4), 469–515.

Caldas-Coulthard, C. R., & Iedema, R. (Eds.). (2007). *Identity trouble: Critical discourse and contested identities*. Basingstoke: Palgrave Macmillan.

Cooren, F. (2010). *Action and agency in dialogue: Passion, incarnation and ventriloquism*. Amsterdam: John Benjamins.

Costanza-Chock, S. (2012). Mic check! Media cultures and the Occupy movement. *Social Movement Studies, 11*(3–4), 375–385. doi:10.1080/14742837.2012.710746

Davidson, A. I. (2011). In praise of counter-conduct. *History of the Human Sciences, 24*(4), 25–41.

Dean, M. (2010). *Governmentality: Power and rule in modern society* (2nd ed.). London: Sage.

Death, C. (2010). Counter-conducts: A Foucauldian analytics of protest. *Social Movement Studies: Journal of Social, Cultural and Political Protest, 9*(3), 235–251.

Deleuze, G., & Guattari, F. (1987). *A thousand plateaus: Capitalism and schizophrenia*. London: Continuum.

Dent, C. (2009). Not all practices are equal: An exploration of discourses, governmentality and scale-free networks. *Social Semiotics, 19*(3), 345–361.

Foucault, M. (1980). Two lectures. In M. Foucault & C. Gordon (Eds.), *Power/knowledge: Selected interviews and other writings, 1972–1977* (pp. 78–108). Brighton: Harvester.

Foucault, M. (1983). The subject and power. In H. Dreyfus & P. Rabinow (Eds.), *Michel Foucault: Beyond structuralism and hermeneutics* (pp. 208–226). Chicago: The University of Chicago Press.

Foucault, M. (1988). The political technology of individuals. In L. H. Martin, H. Gutman, & P. H. Hutton (Eds.), *Technologies of the self: A seminar with Michel Foucault* (pp. 403–417). Amherst: The University of Massachusetts Press.

Foucault, M. (1997). *The politics of truth* (L. Hochroth & C. Porter, Trans.). Los Angeles: Semiotext(e).

Foucault, M. (2007). *Security, territory, population (Lectures at the Collège De France 1977–1978)*. Basingstoke: Palgrave Macmillan.

Hall, S., & Gay, P. D. (Eds.). (1996). *Questions of cultural identity*. London: Sage.

Harris, A. (2005). Discourses of desire as governmentality: Young women, sexuality and the significance of safe spaces. *Feminism & Psychology, 15*(1), 39–43.

Hodges, I. (2003). Assembling the soul: Self and media consumption in alternative spirituality. *International Journal of Critical Psychology, 8*, 34–54.

Jefferson, G. (2004). Glossary of transcript symbols with an introduction. In G. Lerner (Ed.), *Conversation analysis. Studies from the first generation* (pp. 13–31). Amsterdam: John Benjamins.

Klepto, K. (2004). Making war with love: The clandestine insurgent rebel clown army. *City, 8*(3), 403–411.

Kulick, D. (2005). The importance of what gets left out. *Discourse Studies, 7*(4–5), 615–624.

Latour, B. (2005). *Reassembling the social: An introduction to actor-network-theory*. Oxford: Oxford University Press.

Latour, B., & Weibel, P. (Eds.). (2005). *Making things public: Atmospheres of democracy*. Cambridge, MA: The MIT Press.

Lindegaard, L. B. (2012). *Automobility at the Intersection of Discourse and Governmentality: A study of the accomplishment of rationalities that co-constitute car-dependent mobility in the face of climate change*. Doctoral Dissertation, Aalborg University, Aalborg.

Lynch, M. (1993). *Scientific practice and ordinary action: Ethnomethodology and social studies of science*. Cambridge: Cambridge University Press.

Maeckelbergh, M. (2009). *The will of the many: How the alterglobalisation movement is changing the face of democracy*. London: Pluto Press.

Maeckelbergh, M. (2011). Doing is believing: Prefiguration as strategic practice in the alterglobalization movement. *Social Movement Studies, 10*(1), 1–20.

McIlvenny, P. (1996). Popular public discourse at Speakers' Corner: Negotiating cultural identities in interaction. *Discourse & Society, 7*(1), 7–37.

McIlvenny, P. (1998). Talk is sexy! normalising gender/sex/sexuality in new media (Plenary lecture). In I. L. Pedersen & J. Scheuer (Eds.), *Sprog, køn og kommunikation [Language, gender & communication]: Proceedings of the 3rd Nordic conference on language and gender, Copenhagen, 11–13 October 1997* (pp. 19–33). Copenhagen: C.A. Rietzels Forlag.

McIlvenny, P. (1999). Avatars R Us? Discourses of community and embodiment in intercultural cyberspace. *Intercultural Communication (electronic journal), 1*.

McIlvenny, P. (2001). Do 'opposites always attract'?: Doing gender/sexuality in intercultural encounters. In K. G. Andersen (Ed.), *Communicating culture: Proceedings of the 3rd Nordic symposium on intercultural communication, October 1996 [Language & cultural contact 28]* (pp. 81–99). Aalborg: Centre for Languages and Intercultural Studies, Aalborg University.

McIlvenny, P. (2009a). Communicating a 'time-out' in parent-child conflict: Embodied interaction, domestic space and discipline in a reality TV parenting programme. *Journal of Pragmatics, 41*(10), 2017–2032.

McIlvenny, P. (2009b). "Your light switch is your vote": Mediating discourse and participation in the 'Vote Earth' campaign to foster awareness of anthropogenic climate change. *Journal of Applied Linguistics, 6*(3), 303–332.

McIlvenny, P. (2016). Governmentality, counter-conduct and prefigurative demonstrations: Interactional and categorial practices in the strange case of the United Nathans weapons inspections. In P. McIlvenny, J. Z. Klausen, & L. B. Lindegaard (Eds.), *New perspectives on discourse and governmentality* (pp. 265–294). Amsterdam: John Benjamins.

McIlvenny, P. (2017). Mobilising the micro-political voice: Doing the 'Human Microphone' and the 'mic-check'. *Journal of Language and Politics, 16*(1), 110-136.

Mitchell, W. J. T., Harcourt, B. E., & Taussig, M. (2013). *Occupy: Three inquiries in disobedience*. Chicago: The University of Chicago Press.

Peacock, L. (2009). *Serious play: Modern clown performance*. Bristol: Intellect.

Rampton, B. (1995). *Crossing: Language and ethnicity among adolescents*. London: Longman.

Rasmussen, J. (2011). Enabling selves to conduct themselves safely: Safety committee discourse as governmentality in practice. *Human Relations, 64*(3), 459–478.

Rasmussen, J. (2013). Governing the workplace or the worker? Evolving dilemmas in chemical professionals' discourse on occupational health and safety. *Discourse & Communication, 7*(1), 75–94.

Rose, N. (1996). The death of the social? Refiguring the territory of government. *Economy and Society, 25*(3), 327–356.

Rose, N. (1999). *Powers of freedom: Reframing political thought*. Cambridge: Cambridge University Press.

Rose, N. (n.d.). Power in therapy: Techne and ethos [online article]. http://www.academyanalyticarts.org/rose-power-in-therapy. Accessed March 26, 2014.

Salskov-Iversen, D., Hansen, H. K., & Bislev, S. (2000). Governmentality, globalization and local practice: Transformations of a hegemonic discourse. *Alternatives: Global, Local, Political, 25* (2), 183–222.

Scalmer, S. (2011). *Gandhi in the West: The Mahatma and the rise of radical protest*. Cambridge: Cambridge University Press.

Scollon, R. (2001). *Mediated discourse: The nexus of practice*. London: Routledge.

Summerville, J. (2007). *Governmentality, pedagogy and membership categorization: A case of enrolling the citizen in sustainable regional planning*. Doctoral Dissertation, Queensland University of Technology, Brisbane.

Summerville, J., & Adkins, B. (2007). Enrolling the citizen in sustainability: Membership categorization, morality and civic participation. *Human Studies, 30*(4), 429–446.
Todd, C., & Scordelis, A. (2009). *Causing a scene: Extraordinary pranks in ordinary places with Improv Everywhere*. New York: William Morrow & Company.

Author Biography

Paul McIlvenny is a full Professor in the Department of Culture and Global Studies, as well as Director of the Centre for Discourses in Transition (C-DiT) and Director of the Interdisciplinary Discourse Studies doctoral programme, at Aalborg University, Denmark. His current research interests include the everyday practices of vélomobility, skimobility and assisted e-mobility, the mediated discourses and micro-politics of prefigurative protest movements, and Big Video methodologies.

Chapter 4
Center-Staging Language and Identity Research from *Earthrise* Positions. Contextualizing *Performances* in Open Spaces

Sangeeta Bagga-Gupta

4.1 Introduction

4.1.1 Two Dominant Views

The moon journeys across the emptiness of open space, circulating the earth, while the latter rotates on its axis and journeys around the sun. Various forces of nature keep these three celestial bodies relationally *situated* in the vastness of space and relationally *mobile* in different trajectories. It is the moons trajectory around the earth, and the fact that it does not spin on its axis, that gives rise to the illusion of different moon-phases (for an observer on the earth). Lasting approximately 28 days, a full phase cycle consists of the transition from one full-moon to new-moon to full-moon. The phenomena called "Moonrise", may involve the moon rising in the sky in the middle of the day (when it is, at best, only faintly visible) or it may not be visible at all if its lighted side (facing the sun) is away from the earth, thus remaining relatively unmarked for human beings.

In contrast, it is the rotation of the earth on its axis that gives rise to the phenomena we recognize as "Sunrise". The sun (appears to) rise in the east, making its daily appearance known first in geopolitical land spaces on the west of the international dateline, rising subsequently across our planet, even though it is the rotation of the earth itself that creates sunrises. While a moonrise is less explicitly experienced as compared to a sunrise, and it is the latter that is significant for humankind,[1] both are experienced *from the* earth.

[1]The moon, however also significantly shapes life on earth (Resource, TestTube Video "But we've had a moon for 4.5 billion years", 4 November 2015).

S. Bagga-Gupta (✉)
School of Education and Communication, Jönköping University, Jönköping, Sweden
e-mail: Sangeeta.bagga-gupta@ju.se

S. Bagga-Gupta et al. (eds.), *Identity Revisited and Reimagined*,
DOI 10.1007/978-3-319-58056-2_4

In this chapter, I will use the moonrise-sunrise phenomena metaphorically to explicate two perspectives that highlight the ways in which we *commonly* approach and/or understand communication and identity (including culture). Represented by moonrises, the first position highlights a relatively less "visible" norm that nevertheless potently shapes our understandings of communication and identity. This *dominant* default norm is marked by a monolingual—monocultural or monoethnic perspective. It is "naturalized" (Säljö 2002) in Eurocentric global North discourses and is often *not made* visible in either mundane discourses or the academic literature (Bagga-Gupta 2007a). In other words, this position 1 is taken as the given. In contrast, the more visible second position, represented by sunrises, highlights the common human condition vis-à-vis communication and identity. This condition however, paradoxically gets marked as the deviant, *margin*alized, not-*norm*al in global North discourses. Position 2 gets framed in academic discourses and commonsensical thinking through concepts like bi/multi/pluri/translingualism, bi/multiculturalism and multiethnicities. Recent terminology that has emerged within European literature on globalization, framed by migration flows into European geopolitical spaces (and digitalization) include concepts like super/hyperdiversity (Vertovec 2006). In other words, the more common human condition of diversity gets *deviantly* framed, marking and making visible (albeit as the not-normal) multiple language varieties and membership in multiple cultures and ethnicities. These two positions, I argue, represent normative global North discourses where communication, identity, including culture, are approached through, as well as reduced to, technicalities and essentialistically framed epistemologies. Such understandings are critically relevant for the organizing of institutionalized learning for children and adults across geopolitical spaces generally, and in global North contexts like those of Sweden especially.

4.1.2 Going Beyond Binary Hegemonic Positions

Going beyond these two hegemonic positions and informed by decolonial alternative epistemologies (Hasnain et al. 2013), I center-stage a third perspective wherein language-use or languag*ing* (Garcia 2009; Linell 2009) and identity-position*ings* (Butler 1999) or identit*ing* (Bagga-Gupta 2016a), including cultur*ing,* represent dynamically different ways of approaching and/or understanding human behavior and the human condition. Drawing upon the iconic images seen and captured on film by Frank Borman, James Lovell and William Anders, astronauts on Apollo 8 on 24 December 1968 (http://www.nasa.gov/multimedia/imagegallery/image_feature_1249.html, 14 July 2014), I use the phenomenon of "Earthrise" (see Fig. 4.1) to substantiate such an alternative position. Earthrise is a phenomenon that, for my purposes here, contrasts in significant ways with moonrise and sunrise.

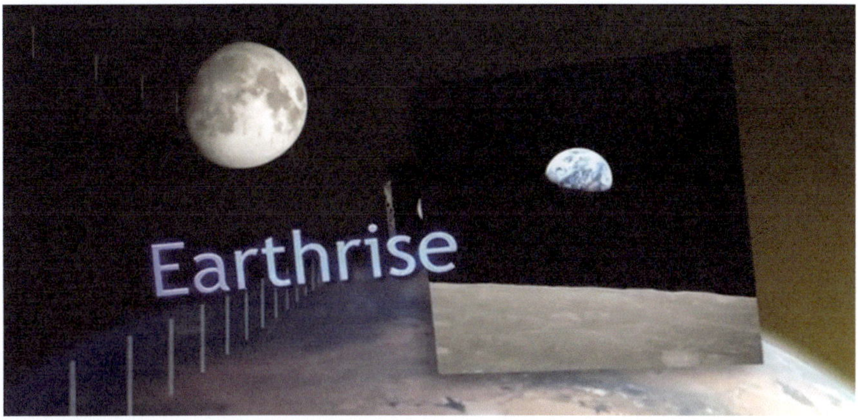

Fig. 4.1 Earthrise—a new paradigm in human history (http://www.nasa.gov/multimedia/imagegallery/image_feature_1249.html, 15 July 2014)

To begin with, earthrise was made possible through space explorations and the collaborated *inter*actions of three astronauts[2] as well as specific human-technological interfaces.[3] It was experienced by humans *from* the vastness of open spaces, and subsequently, by humankind mediated through the iconic pictures of the earth taken by those in space. Here it was the situatedness in space as well as the relational rotating mobile trajectory of a spacecraft relative to the celestial bodies of the moon, sun and earth, which allowed the astronauts to "see" and "document", from their spacecraft, a view of their home planet. These viewings subsequently became labeled "Earthrise". Using earthrise to represent a third position, my aim is to highlight the need to radically *re-think* issues of communication and identity through a focus upon recorded and archival "naturalistic" empirical data (Guba and Lincoln 1994). I argue that such data, in comparison with reported or experimental data, opens a window to understand the complexities of contexts where more than one language variety, modality are in play and where different kinds of tools are deployed across *timespace* (Edwards 2012; Oostendorp 2017).

[2]This collaboration included a large number of human beings who made the technologically savvy missions to the moon possible in the first place.

[3]NASA, on the occasion of its 45th anniversary in 2013, released a 6.53 min re-created simulation of the viewings of earthrise by the three astronauts (see http://www.nasa.gov/content/goddard/nasa-releases-new-earthrise-simulation-video); my discussion builds upon this simulation as well as other NASA resources (http://www.nasa.gov/content/goddard/nasa-releases-new-earthrise-simulation-video; http://www-tc.pbs.org/wgbh/amex/moon/media/sf_audio_pop_01b.mp3).

4.1.3 Aims and Chapter Structure

This theoretically framed chapter aims to make visible the discourses regarding conceptualizations of language and identity in the moonrise-sunrise positions 1 and 2 on the one hand (in Sect. 4.3), and in the earthrise position 3 on the other hand (see Sects. 4.2 and 4.4). I argue that the fundamental assumptions that frame and substantiate position 3 earthrise viewings (see Sect. 4.2) are not new but rather are in need of revitalization. These viewings are eclipsed in large parts of the current research that focuses and discusses language varieties, modalities, identity, including culture in global North spaces. Here I note some of the shifts in the webs-of-understandings (Bagga-Gupta 2012, 2014a) related to the areas of language and identity across timespace.

Building upon Lakoff and Johnson's (1984) seminal work on metaphors and concepts "we live by", I highlight the similar and different ways in which the webs-of-understandings and assumptions related to the moonrise-sunrise positions 1 and 2 are framed in global North hegemonies (see Sect. 4.3). I also present ideas related to the theoretical and methodological emphasis *in* and framings *of* the research that can be characterized as falling into these positions (see Sects. 4.3 and 4.4). Earthrise perspectives are illustrated by drawing upon (i) some classical projects from the late 1970s in the area of communication studies, and (ii) by pointing towards research that I have been (or am currently) involved in, since the end of the 1980s, in the geopolitical spaces of Sweden and India, including digital spaces. This body of research is also relevant in the area of identity. Framed in terms of a critical humanistic social orientation that includes (i) a sociocultural perspective on communication and learning and (ii) a decolonial framing of communication and identity, the next section highlights some salient assumptions that build upon specific theoretical-methodological perspectives, salient for equity work and the organization of learning in institutional settings.

4.2 Critical Humanistic Socially Oriented Conceptual Framings

This section first discusses the parameters of research, highlighting Eurocentric biases in conceptual framings of communication and identity. Central assumptions that encompass specific theoretical-methodological framings, salient for equity work and the organization of learning in institutional settings, are discussed thereafter.

4.2.1 A Note on Alternative Epistemologies and Research Agendas

Research as well as institutionally organized learning in spaces, such as K-12 schools or adult education, are shaped by strong collective traditions across timespaces. It was the establishment of a compulsory one-school-for-all institution in the post-World War II period that itself made visible issues of human diversity and difference (Bagga-Gupta 2007; 2014b; Winzer 1993; Winzer and Mazurek 2000). This spearheaded societal concerns with regards to equity, difference and marginalization, which in turn has shaped research endeavours. Such research is not uncommonly understood in terms of a tool for identifying better methods to integrate immigrants, include the functionally disabled or create gender equality in different societal institutions, not least those shaped by metaphors of a one-school-for-all and life-long-learning. In addition to research, institutions such as that of the Ombudsman have been established in Scandinavian spaces to monitor the integration, inclusion and equity work in society at large. For present purposes, the following two issues are salient with regards to such institutions.

Firstly, there is need to highlight the relationship between centres and margins with regards to for whom, by whom and in what spaces such relationships get operationalized. The emergence of the knowledge society, increased global-local migration flows, the explosion of social media and disparate regional power and resource shifts, including current societal conflicts have shaped not only the sociocultural fabric of human existence on our planet, but also the parameters of the research enterprise itself (Appadurai 1996). Taking decolonial points of departure, Bagga-Gupta and Surian (2014) call attention to the following questions: what (newer) global North hegemonies can be identified that are involved in the research enterprise in itself in present day glocalization spaces? What framings allow for understanding new-old concepts such as superdiversity and bi/multi/pluri/translingualism? Are the largely Eurocentric conceptions regarding super/hyperdiversities, bi/multi/pluri/translingualism and inclusion/exclusion, that have re-emerged or are re-emphasized, an entrenchment of the colonial order under a new guise?

In similar fashion, raising concerns regarding the colonization of recent ways of conceptualizing globalization, Omoniyi (2015) emphasizes that there is "debate waiting to be heard along the lines of Northern versus Southern conceptualisations of 'globalization'". Calling for a new range of questions, he suggests that scholarship needs to investigate,

> ideas about how we conceptualise/perceive The Centre and how The Centre perceives and constructs itself. Perhaps what we ought to be calling for in the Global Academy is a reconfiguration of The Centre such that it is not simply a synonym for a collection of Northern Intellectual elites.
>
> What alternative articulations of The Centre can we postulate? How does that postulate define and delimit diversity? What have the Northern scholars missed out on by not sufficiently engaging with Southern multilingual realities? How does 'superdiversity' apply

> to [complex language southern spaces…]? What is there on 'rural multilingualism' - transient farm labour, farm product retailers across sub-Saharan Africa? What Southern authored literature can we call on to challenge the dominant Northern articulation? […] To what extent has the sociolinguistics of globalization scholarship been ethical in its methodologies and theorizations? (Omoniyi 2015; see also Pavlenko 2017).

These types of recent articulations call for the recognition of alternative epistemologies that shake and dislodge the stability of global North moonrise and sunrise knowledge framings. "What is at stake is the larger task of the very decolonization of knowledge, and being, including institutions such as the university" (Maldonado-Torres 2011: 1). Drawing upon various "turns", especially the Decolonial Turn (Maldonado-Torres 2011; Mignolo 2009, 2012), the Mobility Turn (Landri and Neuman 2014; Sheller and Urry 2006) and the Boundary-Turn (Bagga-Gupta 2013a), Bagga-Gupta and Surian (2014) "center-stage the growing disparity in newer-colonial power relationships in research, including access to and the acknowledgement of different epistemologies in the learning sciences, not least when cultural and linguistic diversity are in focus" (see also Apple and Buras 2006). This then lays the point of departure for calling attention to the need for transgressing global North hegemonies and turning towards "alternative voices" (Hasnain et al. 2013) where global South scholarship comes into dialogue in its own terms with dominant conceptualizations vis-à-vis communication and identity, including culture.

The second issue that is significant here relates to a need for making visible an important distinction between a research enterprise on the one hand and equity work carried out by institutions like schools and the Ombudsman on the other. While being an institutional activity system in itself, research—or as I have previously highlighted, the "re"-searching or "re"-viewings of different phenomena—constitutes an activity that differs (or should do so) in fundamental ways from other institutional activity systems. By deploying (i) analytically pushed questions, (ii) methodologies that have been refined over time and (iii) theoretical framings, research is entrusted with systematically illuminating phenomena under scrutiny against the backdrop of previously accumulated knowledge in and across a domain (see also below). However, epistemologies are themselves historically framed into different disciplines and these become stratified across time. Recent calls for multi-, cross-, inter- and transdisciplinary research aim to break loose from such boundedness, drawing attention to the centrality of analytical viewings in *re*search or the knowledge *re*building enterprise. This not-withstanding, the issue at hand is that research into communication and identity, including culture, differs significantly from the work done in institutions like the one-school-for-all, life-long-education or the Ombudsman. Thus, what is glossed in terms of a bilingual pupil or adult, or gender or functional disability or immigrant pupil/adult in institutional activity fields such as bilingual education, special education, equality work, equity monitoring work, etc. has significantly *different agendas* when compared to research work where bilingual education, special education or equality and equity work constitute phenomena under scrutiny. In the latter, the analytical enterprise calls for critically re-viewing and re-searching not only specific institutional activity fields, but also the very assumptions that underlie the analytical enterprise of research in itself. It is this line of thought that frames the ideas that I explore in this chapter.

Language education or special education or the work in institutions for equity are thus, both *research fields* as well as *activity and institutional fields* constituted by social practices (see also below). The *research enterprise* where the searching and viewing of the activity that is glossed as bilingualism or bilingual education, or gender or functional disability is in focus, critical analysis and reflections on the institutional activity field of bilingual education or identity-positionings (glossed as gender or functional disability) is the fundamental agenda. Key assumptions vis-à-vis communication, identity, learning and development shape research agendas and work that constitutes the lenses with which different methodological and conceptual tool-kits are deployed by researchers. It is these assumptions vis-à-vis moonrise, sunrise and earthrise positions that are tweezed out here.

While my arguments so far analytically differentiate between (i) reflecting critically upon the work carried out in the institutional fields of education and equity (i.e. doing research) from the (ii) activity of being engaged as a professional within the same institutional fields, there is acute need to also highlight a significant limitation of the research enterprise itself. While research builds upon a web of interlinked fundamental assumptions (that may or may not be articulated explicitly), on a specific or more general phenomena, it is far from a neutral tool from which we can distil methods for achieving equity and equality. The nature of the research task implies that research in itself cannot (at least not in the short-term) be deployed to fix or cure issues related to marginalization and inequality. Having said that, it is equally significant to emphasize the potency of research to illuminate issues in focus in newer ways, not least by drawing inspiration from "eureka moments", cross-disciplinary projects and cross-sector endeavours.

4.2.2 Boundary-Turn, Hybridity and Intersectionality

The perspectives on decoloniality discussed so far represent a call for a new reflexivity. Here a Boundary-Turn is significant (Bagga-Gupta 2013a, 2015; Surian 2015). Decoloniality recognizes that the colonial project is alive and thriving in *both* the global South as well as the global North. In other words, it highlights the colonial underpinnings in and across timespaces and calls for understanding power relations that frame human lives in terms of *open spaces* and not merely geopolitical *places*. Thus, there is a South in global North geopolitical places and global North spaces exist in large parts of global South places. What is relevant for present purposes is that decoloniality offers an important vantage viewing point for discussing key interrelated ideas that emerge through concepts such as boundaries, hybridity and intersectionality. These concepts, I argue, are salient in the areas of communication and identity and relevant in the domains of learning and equity work. For instance, the location and constitution of language and identity (focused below) is related to the threshold and in-between spaces that Bhabha (1994) calls "liminality". In-between spaces or border-spaces, instead of boundaries, become the interesting sites of beginnings (and endings) including what lies beyond,

> there is a sense of disorientation, a disturbance of direction, in the 'beyond': an exploratory, restless movement [...] here and there, on all sides [...] hither and thither, back and forth (Bhabha 1994: 2, see also Bagga-Gupta 2013a).

It is such liminal alternative spaces where complexity and hybridity are the norm that non-linear processes of languaging and identiting can be observed and studied. The move from "fixity" to complexity and hybridity points to "openings between spaces of uncertainity [...and indexing] a break with essential colonial categories" of identity and culture (Jones 2011: 30). Such verb-related performative understandings of language and identity (see Fig. 4.2) are related to discourses in academic domains within emancipatory postcolonial discourses (like feministic postcolonialism; see also Jones 2011; Mohanty 2004), ethnicity and cultural studies. Other areas where static, fixed notions of identity and language are challenged include performance pushed analytical positions within feminism (Butler 1999; Coates 1996; Tannen 1993), sociocultural theory (Bagga-Gupta 2014a, b; Linell 2009; Simao and Valsiner 2007; Säljö 2005) and branches within anthropology.

Marked by a Boundary-Turn, decolonially framed research is related to other turns that have emerged in the literature on education, language, culture and identity (see also Clifford 1997; Hasnain et al. 2013; Khubchandani 1997, 1998; Scollan and Scollan 2004): the Decolonial Turn and the Mobility Turn (Landri and Neuman 2014; Sheller and Urry 2006), the Multilingual Turn (May 2013) and the Complexity Turn (Hult 2010). A Boundary-Turn highlights the paradoxical invisibility accorded to boundaries in global North epistemologies where bounded*ness* explicitly and implicitly dominates conceptualizations of language, identity (individual, group and nation-state) and culture (at least in the geopolitical spaces of

Moonrise and Sunrise Positions	**Earthrise Position**
• Knowledge • Language • Learning = stuff • Music • Culture • Identity	• Knowledging + plural • Languaging • Learning = meaning making • Musicing/musiking • Culturing • Identity-positionings, identiting
AS	*AS*
• Transfer, storage • Individual capacity • Localized, place (head, school) • Bounded, static with boundaries	• Activities, practices, everyday • Reconstruction of experiences • Interaction everywhere • Linked, continuum
Focus on the unmarked norm and Others	*Focus on interaction (with others and tools)*

Fig. 4.2 Noun- and verb-focused understandings related to moonrise, sunrise and earthrise positions

Sweden since the 1990s; see Bagga-Gupta 2004a, 2010, 2012). The need to revisit concepts like hybridity and intersectionality arises from paying attention to this paradox.

Hybridity and intersectionality have become central in anti-essentialistically framed discourses in the human sciences generally and identity research particularly. However, while hybridity encompasses individual, collective identity, culture and race, it itself retains a large dose of essentialist framings; it builds upon the key assumption that a hybrid state arises by mixing two previously distinct, demarcated states of being. Furthermore, academic discourses that draw upon hybridity seep into everyday parlance where it further gets consolidated with the sense of "mixing". Intersectionality on the other hand, arises in and continues to be individual-centered. It too focuses border-spaces where power-structures and individual identity categories are salient. While intersectionality center-staged gender with race and color, other identity categories have become salient in its context more recently. Like hybridity, it too builds upon distinct states of being that intersect (Gunnarsson 2015). Despite efforts to elaborate on the entwined and performative nature of identity (see Butler 1999; McCall 2005), an essentialist individual-centered point of departure frames discussions vis-à-vis intersectionality as well.

Furthermore concepts like hybridity and intersectionality continue to exist in, what in other academic contexts has been called, an "empirical ghetto" (Clark et al. 1998). Thus, while both concepts are used in theoretical discussions to counter essentialist framings, they are marginally, if at all, deployed in empirical research in the language and educational sciences. In addition, current emancipatory discussions related to "gender mainstreaming" within feminism (Rees 1998; Walby 2003), do not engage with intersectional framings. A recent shift in how the concept hybridity is shaping domains in the human sciences as well as in the public imagination relates to discourses of globalization. Hybridity here gets related to the "cultural logic" of the effect of globalization in that current population mobility and digitalization precludes essentialist conceptualizations of identity and culture (Kraidy 2005). This concept nevertheless remains contested and exists at the periphery of many mainstream theoretical discourses in the human sciences. Bringing a Boundary-Turn perspective into dialogue with hybridity and intersectionality and engaging them in empirical investigations (of for instance, communication and identity) has, I argue, the potential to contribute to both theoretical-methodological framings and to alternative epistemologies.

4.2.3 The Centrality of Communication—Hybridity-Continuum and Expanded-Intersectionality

Moving beyond a focus on characteristics or divisions that mark individuals and communication, but also activities, places or specific scales, a Boundary-Turn perspective recognizes the need for a *hybridity-continuum* and an *expanded-intersectional* point of departure where the irreducibility of social action across timespace is recognized (Bagga-Gupta 2013a; Khubchandani 1997, 1998). This resonates with the socioculturally framed conceptual discussions on the irreducible nature of "individual(s)-acting/operating-with-mediational-means" (Wertsch 1998), including the human-tool continuum. Such a stance calls for the need to have mundane languaging data inform discussions related to institutional equity issues and work. It also calls attention to pre- or weakly-theorized noun based ideas (see Fig. 4.2) that inform popular thinking, policy vis-à-vis communication and identity as well as the organization of learning and equity work in global North settings such as Sweden (see below).

Scholars across timespaces have highlighted the relevance of understanding communication or the *usage* of linguistic resources—i.e. different language varieties, different modalities (including written, oral, signed) and embodiment, including the deployment of tools—as central to identity formation and learning. Such conceptualizations tend to flourish in the realm of so called theoretical or philosophical scholarship (Hasnain et al. 2013; Khubchandani 1997, 1998; Linell 2009; Wittgenstein 1999) as well as in disciplines where anthropological tenants are salient. Furthermore, as outlined above, scholarship in literature, postcolonial theory, feminism, etc. also implicitly or explicitly draw upon such *performative* conceptualizations that build upon fluidity and processes rather than fixed essentialist framings.

Salient here is that the *location* of language and identity (see Finnegan 2015) continues to engage scholarship in these traditions. Thus boundaries between different language's' and different identit'ies' are discussed at length and their very existence is challenged (Bhaktin 1981; Khubchandani 1997, 1998; Landri and Neuman 2014; Wittgenstein 1999). Finnegan eloquently highlights the issues that lie at the heart of these new-old discussions in the first chapter "Where is language?" of her recent book:

> It is common to assume we know what language is and what is needed to capture and describe it; hence, by implication, what 'language' in essence is. But there are many contending theories, too easily forgotten in the understandable rush to document and describe. These need to be considered at the outset, above all the performance approach to linguistic action entailed in pragmatic perspectives, and the issue of how and for whom linguistic accounts are constructed in the first place.
>
> I too was once confident of what 'language' was, where its boundaries lay, and hence what might count as data for documenting it. But I am no longer sure. Nor am I clear where information about a given language should be found, or how, by, and for whom a language should be documented (2015: 1, emphasis added).

4.2.4 Language and Identity "as" Action

The constitutive and mediational functions of language mark a larger shift underway in the human and social sciences. Contributions to (what I call) an earthrise position can currently be seen within multidisciplinary domains such as Communication

Studies, Literacy Studies, Deaf Studies, Gender Studies, etc.[4] Conceptual framings that draw upon the Linguistic Turn (and other related turns highlighted above), and *dialogical-action* theories and perspectives that pay allegiance to the social (social-psychology, social-cognition, socio-historical, etc.) frame this larger shift. Significant here is the call to replace boundary-marked *noun-dominated* dimensions connected to language and identity, including culture with *verb-focused* framings (see Fig. 4.2; Bagga-Gupta 2013b, 2016a, b, 2017). The latter are marked by the relatively recent emergence of and focus upon concepts such as languaging, language-use, social practices, performativity, identity-positions/ings, identiting or language and identity *as* action (Bagga-Gupta 2016a, 2017).

A performative stance on communication where language and identity are understood *as* social action, differs significantly from essentialist, static, bounded understandings. This constitutes a central point of departure in both a theoretical sociocultural perspective and a decolonial framework. Terminology shifts in the literature—knowledging, instead of knowledge (as stuff), musicing and musiking, instead of music, culturing, instead of culture, together with languaging (instead of language) and identity-positioning and identiting (instead of identity categories)—mark key ways of framing the very nature of knowledge, learning and communication (see Fig. 4.2). Thus, and marking a paradigmatic shift in conceptual framings, knowledge and learning are recognized as participation in communities of *practices* and communities of *practitioners* where reframings of experiences occurs in and through social interactions. Here communication is recognized as being seamless, constituted by a continuum across varieties and modalities that humans deploy *to language*.

Language thus, "comes to life in the real world and changes from words and sentences into discourse" (Agar 1994: 6; see also Blommaert 2015). Furthermore, it is through languaging that identity-positionings receive meanings in social practices (at least temporarily). Framed in a sociocultural decolonial perspective, such a shift implies that an understanding of human behaviour needs to build upon the nitty-grittyness of mundane life processes and actions, including langauging and identiting in textual data (for instance, archives, policy) across timespaces. In other words, such a shift calls attention to the need for empirically framed re-viewings and re-searchings where recognition needs to be accorded to the constitutive boundary-marking role of language when it comes to communication and identity.

4.2.5 *Language as a Constitutive and Boundary-Marking Tool in Social Practices*

While human beings "language for many reasons" (Garcia 2009: 31) and "are a *languaging* species" (Jørgensen et al. 2011, emphasis in original), language—"the

[4]This does not mean that all scholarship from these domains contribute to an earthrise position.

tool of tools" (Wertsch 1998) itself creates boundaries, including a we-them dichotomy in different ways (Bagga-Gupta 2013a). This constitutive and boundary-marking function of languaging creates categories where the inclusion of some people constitutes a process that in itself excludes others. One could potentially dissolve a specific boundary or a specific criteria for a specific boundary, if one makes relevant another criteria which in turn would create other new boundaries (Bagga-Gupta 2010, 2012, 2013a). To label a secondary school pupil as a computer-nerd, sport-interested, internet-junkie creates identity-positionings of a youngster that differ from images that emerge if s/he were identified with labels such as talkative, disruptive, weak in Swedish or English. Alternative labels could create completely different identity-associations: mathematics genius, interested in physics, immigrant, ADHD, deaf. An individual or a community of practitioners could thus be understood in a number of different ways. A critical ethnographic "seeing" (Wolcott 1999) thus highlights that viewings are shaped through linguistic labels. Languaging potently, explicitly and implicitly, demarcates *things*, *feelings*, *actions* and *attributes* in a very similar manner.

Thus, etiquettes, labels, words, etc. demarcate something from something else and constitute a key ingredient in how meaning and understanding are created. A *stone*—or *stein*, *pietra*, *pierre*, *piedra*, *ἀγήρατος2*, *לררך*, *sten*, पत्थर, http://teckensprakslexikon.su.se/ord/02090,[5] https://www.signingsavvy.com/sign/STONE/2369/1[6]—are a bunch of written signs as well as manual signs deployed in different communities of practitioners that enable members of those specific communities to collectively mark a thing through linguistic behavior.[7] The semantic sign stone (or the other labels for the same object in other specific communities of practitioners) has little affinity to the object that it labels. The significant issue here is that it is in actions that a stone gets shaped into something specific and it is through its embeddedness in social practices that specific qualities become subscribed to it: a catapult where an object can be used to hunt prey, a curling event where a large round object is gracefully released on icy sports arena surfaces, a personal memory of objects collected during a walk on the beach, status or symbols of love mediated by expensive objects, etc. Weapons, sports events, beach souvenirs, and precious stones: specific criteria and aspects related to a physical object are targeted in specific social practices framed by linguistic behavior. It is in this manner that physical things—but also emotions, actions and attributes—become infused with meanings. Languaging in this sense does not mirror the world; it constitutes and mediates the world (Säljö 2005). Communication, the deployment of the oral/written/signed/medialized word, in symbiosis with artefacts and embodied actions, are thus people's most central tools (Bagga-Gupta 2017). Etiquettes and tags are used and identities are both inscribed and subscribed to human beings in and via such processes.

---

[5]Manual three-dimensional sign for stone/sten in Swedish Sign Language.

[6]Manual three-dimensional sign for stone in American Sign Language.

[7]Such markings occur in a similar manner in oral linguistic behavior as well.

4.2.6 Languaging "as" the Nexus of Identity-Positionings. on Human Diversity

The shift from a noun- to a verb-focus (see Fig. 4.2) pays allegiance to a larger consensus regarding the key role that language-use itself plays in shaping human identity: "the discursive approach sees identification as a construction, a process never completed—always 'in process'" (Hall 1996: 16). This means that an individual is not a *woman* or *deaf* or *long*, but that s/he *becomes* a woman, deaf or long within specific social practices. As discussed above, this is highlighted in scholarship where the *doing of* or the *performance of* identity is made salient. 'Diversity' is central here and needs some commentary in that it both encompasses everyone/all and marks difference. While human diversity is celebrated, at least rhetorically within policies and laws in geopolitical spaces like Sweden, and includes minority, marginalized identity positions, I will raise a couple of issues for present purposes.

Firstly, there is a clear regression to *Otherness* (not least in terms of ethnicity and race) today as compared to more open meanings that the concept was infused with previously (at least in the Swedish context). *Furthermore*, discussions regarding intersectionality and hybridity not-with-standing, diversity continues to be conceptualized in essentialized ways when it comes to domains such as support services, special education and equality work. In other words, intersectionality and hybridity discussions, as noted above, appear to flourish primarily in philosophical and theoretical arenas, and intersectionality has, so far, primarily focused individual human identity. *Finally*, diversity discourses have become prominent in European geopolitical spaces in the 21st century in novel ways. Difference-hood, not least spurred by re-viewings of old and new migrations from previous colonies and more recent conflict related population mobility are increasingly marked through concepts such as "super- and hyper-diversity" (Vertovec 2006; see also Blommaert 2010). The editors of the "International Journal of Education for Diversity" raise concern with some aspects of these new diversity discourses in a recent editorial (see also Pavlenko 2017): There exists a,

> 'hijacking' of the concept of diversity which is often misused to merely highlight 'racial'/'ethnic'/'cultural' differences, instead of integrating individuals' many complex facets such as gender, language(s), religion, social class, etc. […] the way people identify, appropriate and live a same social identity (e.g. religion) varies among individuals (Machart et al. 2014: i).

Taking cognizance of a performatory nature of identity-positionings, brings center-stage the fluidity and continuum to which attention is being (re)drawn in Machart et al's words. Recognizing the essentialism of etiquettes and labels on the one hand and recognizing the intersectional, hybrid and multifaceted nature of diversity—both at the individual *and* community levels, are thus key to leaving aside noun based boundary marked essentialist epistemologies.

4.2.7 Final Note on Conceptual Framings

In summary, while ideas about equity, diversity, pluralism etc. build upon fundamental democratic notions of everyone's equal rights in today's globalized world, there exists a need to relate as well as down-scale these lofty ideals to the boundary-marking and representational functions of languaging in mundane everyday social practices. Language represents, creates categories and identity-positionings in and through linguistically framed embodied actions. It is in this sense that identity can be understood as action. Significant here are the scientific and methodological perspectives that have contributed to the shift from noun- to verb-focused concepts were scholarship has seen the emergence of concepts like *languaging*, *situated* and *distributed learning* (Lave and Wenger 1991; Rogoff 1990; Säljö 2005) and *identity-positionings* and *identiting*. Herein lies the importance of recognizing the "imagined" (Anderson 1991) existence of all communities of practices, including the arbitrariness of specific individual and community traits that shape essentialist identity-positions and imagined communities.

Another specific point of departure that guides an earthrise position 3 discussion, is that humans communicate with one another, and the meaning-making they thus engage in occurs irrespective of whether they deploy one or more language varieties, dialects, modalities, etc. Humans language, irrespective of which and how many varieties, modalities, etc they engage with. This means, among other things, that naturalizing a moonrise position 1—monolingual, mono-modal, mono-identity norm is problematic. It also means that emphasizing the use of two or more varieties, modalities wherein boundaries are taken as a 'natural' point of departure in a sunrise position 2 is equally problematic. Thus the multidimensional nature of languaging, here represents a hybrid complexity and a hybridity-continuum that goes beyond both mono (moonrise) and bi/multi (sunrise) positions. Such complexities, I argue, need to be illuminated through a closer analysis of language-in-use and identity-as-action in mundane social practices across timespaces; research that represents such analysis is discussed further below. But before doing that, lets return to the binary hegemonic moonrise and earthrise positions with the intent of un-packaging current dominant webs-of-understandings in the human sciences.

4.3 Moonrise and Sunrise: Dominant Viewings in the Global North

The dichotomized viewing of communication and identity, including culture in terms of the hegemonic default moonrise norm position (of monolingualism, monoculturalism, etc.) and a paradoxically framed deviant sunrise position (of bi/multilingualism, biculturalism, etc.) are focused here. This section first discusses two principles that frame how society organizes institutions for the given, non-marked default moonrise *normal* citizen and the deviant *marginal*ised sunrise human being. After that the moonrise-sunrise positions are illustrated by research in the fields of language and identity. Finally, webs-of-understandings related to the key notion of bilingualism are focused in relation to how these understandings shape equity work in the educational sector.

4.3.1 Two Principles that Enable and Maintain Moonrise and Sunrise Positions

The principles of "sameness" and "difference" (Rees 1998; Walby 2003, 2011) illuminate discourses that frame how equity work in institutions such as the one-school-for-all, life-long-learning and the Ombudsman are conceptualized. Thus for instance, institutional and societal work for including the functionally disabled and integrating immigrants builds upon the idea of a metaphoric as well as a real expectation that the not-normal Other moves from the margins to the center of an "imagined community" (Anderson 1991). This idea rests upon a sameness principle where slogans regarding everyone's equal worth and a rights and justice discourse are taken as points of departure. Gender equality work rests on the notion that men and women are equal (Rees 1998; Walby 2003, 2011); deaf individuals are required to be able to hear and talk as a significant dimension of normalization (Bagga-Gupta 2004a, b; Bagga-Gupta and Holmström 2016; Holmström 2013); immigrants are required to master a national language so that they can become integrated in schools, workplaces and become normal, mainstream citizens (Rosén 2013, 2017).

Segregation (and special treatment) as an organizational strategy builds, on the other hand, upon differences that are regarded as important for a range of reasons. For instance, in the context of gender, differences between men and women are recognized and demands are made to value their different spheres of work in equal terms (Rees 1998; Walby 2003, 2011); the deaf are marked in terms of a separate community that has its own-language, different from the language of hearing people and this raises the need for segregating deaf children in separate schools (Bagga-Gupta 2004a); immigrants are stratified into different communities based upon religion, what is glossed as ethnicity and race or the tag of a nation-state they have come from; this then is seen as requiring special language and culture related education that cannot be made available in mainstream settings (Rosén 2013); new neuropsychiatric categories like ADHD create segregation since pupils with these diagnoses are seen as requiring training in order to be able to function subsequently in a mainstream context (Hjörne 2004). In other words, a principle of difference becomes a point of departure for special treatment of different groups and is seen as a necessary step for (later) integration or inclusion or mainstreaming in schools and society at large.

4.3.2 Webs-of-Understandings that Frame Moonrise and Sunrise Positions

The webs-of-understandings and assumptions that frame the two dominating positions vis-à-vis language and identity research in the global North are presented in Fig. 4.3. The default *norm*, for instance, in the ways in which monolingualism and (mono)identity are understood, has played a dominant role in how othering of the common human condition has taken place. A moonrise position highlights an invisible norm that potently shapes understandings of communication and identity. Building upon an explicit boundary-marked one-nation-one-language myth, this *dominant* default position is "naturalized" (Säljö 2002) in Eurocentric global North discourses and is rarely *made* visible in mundane discourses or in scholarship. In other words, it is taken as the given. While the use of only one language or dialect or sociolect is an uncommon human condition, it is this position that sets the standard. An essentialist, prescriptive-ideological framing of language, identity, including culture marks this position and shapes how equity work has developed across timespaces in global North spaces like Sweden and elsewhere. It builds upon the principle of sameness and thus integration and mainstreaming are seen as ways of achieving equity. The placement of native children in white families in the global North spaces of North America and Australia in the past and the education of deaf children in mainstream monolingual hearing schools currently, constitute examples of how the sameness principle gets operationalized. Mainstream support is provided

Moonrise Position	Sunrise Position
• Use of only one language: uncommon human condition in the world	• Use of more than one language: common human condition in the world
• Default norm, not marked	• Deviant, generally marked as the Other, marginalized
• Focuses mono: monolingualism, monoculturalism, single identity	• Focuses bi/multi: bi/multilingualism, bi/multiculturalism, single identity
• Dominant view in the global North	• Dominant view in the global North
• Essentialist view of language, identity, culture	• Essentialist view of language, identity, culture
• Prescriptive and ideological view of language, identity, culture	• Prescriptive and ideological view of language, identity, culture
	• Recent concepts: Superdiversity, hyperdiversity, translingualism
• Focuses the unmarked Norm, and thereby creates the Other	• Focuses the marginalized Other, and thereby creates the Norm
• Central concept bilingualism	• Central concept bilingualism

Fig. 4.3 Webs-of-understandings: assumptions and underlying features of moonrise and sunrise positions

to research that takes a moonrise position as a point of departure. In scholarship, the position is represented in traditional linguistics, language studies and separate fields of identity research such as disability research, gender research and research that focuses upon any individual who can be labelled immigrant.

The deviant point of departure in the ways in which bilingualism and biculturalism are conceptualized have also played a significant role in how othering of the common human condition continues to take place, not least in global North spaces. A sunrise position makes visible the normal human condition in a paradoxical manner, since the condition gets marked as belonging to the marginalized Other. It constitutes the dominant view in the global North and represents an essentialist view of language, identity and culture. This paradox is made visible in both mundane discourses and flourishes in the scholarship. It builds upon, as discussed above, the principle of difference and implicit or explicit segregation and special treatment are seen as ways of creating equity. The placement of immigrant children in special language streams, the education of deaf children in segregated bilingual or oral schools constitute examples that represent the operationalization of a difference principle. Mainstream support is provided to research that takes a sunrise position as a point of departure. In scholarship, the position is represented in traditional linguistics, language studies and separate fields of identity research such as disability research and research that focuses upon immigrants.

4.3.3 On Bilingualism and a Monolingual Bias. Horizontal, Vertical and Other Reinforced Boundaries

Bilingualism is a key concept that either implicitly or explicitly frames the moonrise and sunrise positions (see Fig. 4.3). It has, during the last quarter of a century, become an important area of study in global North settings and is perhaps one of the most central concepts in the language sciences today. It lies at the center of a web-of-understandings, where boundary-marking shapes a flora of concepts in language education. The latter include both areas of research inquiry and subjects that are currently taught in schools and focused upon in higher education. In Sweden, these include, ‘home language’, ‘mother tongue’, ‘foreign language’, ‘Swedish’, ‘first language’, ‘second language’, ‘Swedish as a second language’, ‘Swedish for the deaf/hard of hearing’, etc.

The conceptual framings discussed in Sect. 4.2 above imply that the use of two or more language varieties—glossed in the term bilingualism, can scarcely be understood in terms of competencies in two language ‘codes’. Researchers situated within an earthrise position today acknowledge that a competencies view of two or more language varieties, modalities, registers, etc. is problematic and misleading and that such a view builds upon a *monolingual bias*. As has already been noted, monolingualism, especially in the global North, continues to be (incorrectly) taken as a point of departure as the human norm (see Fig. 4.3; see also Gramling 2016).

A monolingual (largely) Eurocentric position makes invisible the global norm, wherein people live lives using more than one language variety, modality, register etc. Linguist scholars (especially in global North spaces) however tend to mark such complex but normal languaging as novel. What is relevant for present purposes is that both (i) mono- and bi-lingualism—as extensions of moonrise and sunrise positions—are related and reductionist, and (ii) these are consequential for how identity positions get framed.

The webs-of-understandings related to the boundary-marked and the boundary-marking concept bilingualism become elaborated though organizational divisions in educational institutions. Thus, in addition to the strict boundaries that are made relevant between *different language varieties* (such as Swedish, Finnish, Hindi, Italian, Swedish Sign Language, British Sign Language, American Sign Language, etc.), webs-of-understandings related to bilingualism have enabled the naturalisation of explicit and implicit ideas regarding *different codes for different learner categories* (Bagga-Gupta 2004a, 2012; see Fig. 4.4). These two organizationally framed stratifications—the *horizontal division* (i.e. different language codes) and the *vertical division* (i.e. different codes for different human beings)—are exemplified in Fig. 4.4 by the different language subjects and the explicit or implied learner category for each in the Swedish national syllabi (see also Bagga-Gupta 2004a, 2012).

Such horizontal and vertical boundaries illustrate a reductionist tendency that creates, mediates and functions as structuring resources for specific ways of understanding identity and learning within institutions on the one hand, and the organization of research on the other. In other words, such institutional conceptualisations have a bearing on the organisation of (i) language research within academia, (ii) language areas in higher and professional education and (iii) language teaching in schools (including policy).

The creation and subsequent linking of bounded language varieties to specific student groups is contentious for a range of reasons (see particularly Bagga-Gupta 2004a, 2012; Myndigheten för skolutveckling 2004). A couple of issues are relevant for present purposes. *Firstly*, a weak link to learning theories can be noted in the emergence and development of such institutional stratifications. *Secondly*, the distinctions spelled out earlier vis-à-vis research agendas and institutional agendas often collapse into one here. *Finally*, the horizontal and vertical boundary-marked and boundary-marking categorizations present a mismatch when compared to pupils and adults languaging and identiting (see further below). This continuing instrumental conceptualisation—the vertical division in the language sciences generally and the organisation of teaching and learning of language varieties, i.e. the horizontal division in educational settings more specifically—in this manner constitutes a more explicit selective reductionist position (in at least the geopolitical spaces of Sweden).

Webs-of-understandings linked to bilingualism also create other simplistic and reductionist boundaries. Figure 4.5 presents four *metaphor clusters* that emerge from revisiting previous, and conducting, linguistic-landscape based content analysis of the policy data in the language curricula across timespaces in the Swedish

Horizontal boundaries: language classification	***Vertical boundaries: explicit or implied learner category***
Swedish (first compulsory language) Swedish as a second language Swedish for immigrants	Ethnic Swedish pupils Ethnic minority or immigrant pupils Adult immigrants
Swedish for the deaf/hard of hearing	Deaf & heard of hearing pupils in segregated special schools
Mother tongue, home language Nationally recognised minority languages (Finnish, Meänkieli. Romani, Sami, Yiddish)	Ethnic minority or immigrant pupils Pupils who can make a claim to a nationally recognized minority language
English (second compulsory language)	All pupils
Swedish Sign Language	Deaf & hard of hearing pupils in segregated special schools
Swedish Sign Language for hearing	Hearing pupils in mainstream schools
Danish, Norwegian, Icelandic (neighbouring language)	All pupils
French, German, Spanish (foreign language)	All pupils

Fig. 4.4 Language varieties and learner-categories in the Swedish education landscape (adapted from Bagga-Gupta 2012)

Numerical or mathematical metaphors: first/second/third etc. language, bilingualism
Ownership metaphors: our/my language, their/his/her language, language background, native language
Geographical or place-bound metaphors: home language, native language, nation*al* language, roots, background
Gendered metaphors: mother tongue, home language

Fig. 4.5 Boundaries and metaphor clusters in the Swedish educational landscape that reinforce selective understandings related to identity

context (see also Bagga-Gupta 2004a). A *numerical*, mathematically framed connotation (e.g. first, second, third, bilingual, etc.) arises in the national curricula in the mid-1990s and continues to frame identity currently. A *relational* signification ín terms of ownership metaphors (e.g. my language, your language, their language, mother tongue, native language, language background, etc.) also marks understandings of both identity and of what and where language is. Place bound *geographical* emphasis (e.g. national language, native language, home language, foreign language, roots and background) constitute a third cluster that frames and reinforces language and identity related boundaries. A fourth metaphor that gets reinforced relates to gendering of language and the gendered spaces of language (e.g. mother tongue, home language). These four metaphor clusters overlap and are reinforced through boundaries that mediate understandings pushed by a selective individual-centred tradition vis-à-vis learning and development.

These types of demarcation processes get reinforced across the activity systems of research, higher education and schools and include sub-divisions within a specific language, e.g. Swedish, Swedish as a second language, Swedish for deaf/hand of hearing, Swedish for immigrants. In other words, the horizontal and vertical divisions in the language sciences flourish both as administrative categories in school sites and within higher education and research within the nation-state of Sweden. An issue that is salient here is that all these bounded concepts exist in relation to an imaginary static, correct and desired point of departure, i.e. "Swedish language", and/or in relation to a norm-identity, including how language learning takes place. Taking the identity-position of a monolingual native ethnic Swede as a natural point of departure, and particular understandings of language learning, thus gives legitimacy to other areas of language and identity in the curriculum.

The monolingual bias in the field of Bilingual Studies (especially in the global North) becomes compounded by the scarcity of researchers who themselves live lives wherein the deployment of multiple varieties, modalities, registers is common and mundane. These scholars potentially bring to their analysis an earthrise position. Creating spaces where such academic voices become mainstreamed in the field of Bi(multi)lingual Studies is thus an important way to address the monolingual bias in the scholarship. Thus, in addition to recognizing that patterned ways of meaning making or languaging in mundane activities are rich sites for research, there exists a significant need to research the use of different language varieties 'multilingually', or in other words, there exists a need to view such languaging *from* points of departure that go beyond moonrise and sunrise positions.

Bringing together the issues raised so far, one can say that the recurring use of the concept bilingualism across timespace—in daily life, social media, policy and in scholarship—needs to be critically re-viewed. Raising similar issues, but with a focus upon language registers and sociolects, Heath and her colleagues' in their studies from the 1970s in southern parts of the United States problematized the categorization of children and their families on the basis of class and race. Heath contended that linking such "categories to discrete language differences was to ignore the realities of the communicative patterns of the region" (1983: 3).

The issues raised here call for critical explorations of the dominant moonrise and sunrise positions in the language and identity domains from empirically framed earthrise positions. This draws attention to the need for studies of social practices, rather than studies that build upon people's reporting and accountings of social practices. Central assumptions here allow for viewings where mundane languaging (including languaging in academic discourses) is recognized as the location where our ever evolving realities are created and mediated. However, the kinds of studies that have emerged in such new positions (continue to) lie at the margins of the language and educational sciences landscapes. The next section revisits some classical studies from the 1970s and 1980s that illustrate an earthrise position. I discuss how such studies (have, but also need to) reshape academic thematic areas like bilingualism and identity research. Recent insights from research that I am engaged in, in the Deaf Studies and the Multimodality Studies fields, areas where a clear cut focus upon social practices, languaging and identiting is emerging, are also highlighted.

4.4 Earthrise Viewings in Open Spaces

Going beyond the notions of mixing demarcated entities, concepts such as hybridity-continuum and expanded-intersectionality, in their liminal and in-between sense, have the potential to acknowledge the open spaces of communication and identity on the one hand as well as open up novel "Third Spaces" (Bhabha 1994) of understandings in the fields of communication and identity. Focusing concepts like *chaining*, *expanded-intersectionality* and a *hybridity-continuum* together with empirically pushed research that forefronts mundane social practices, this section discusses peoples engagement with more than one language variety, modality, register, etc; here attention is paid to the performatory dimension of languaging and identiting. These, in important ways, counter the technification of language and identity, including culture in and through the proliferation of new-old boundary-marking concepts such as "bilingualism", "plurilingualism", "metrolingualism", "superdiversity", "hyperdiversity", "multiculturalism", "interculturalism", etc. in the (primarily) Eurocentrically framed globalization literature.

4.4.1 Descriptive-Analytical Research. Revisiting Some Studies of Social Practices

A number of specific models or ideologies of learning and communication are understood as having shaped the organisation of education for functionally disabled pupils and for pupils identified as bi/multilingual in school settings in the global North. Thus for instance, the label and the communicative rationale accounted for in a given bilingual education model tends to be equated with and is seen as representing the everyday communication or the social practices in that model. To underscore a key issue noted in the previous sections, there is a fundamental difference between the logic of the institutional field of bilingual education (including policies) or the ideologies of communication and identity that underlie a given model on the one hand and the activity of research which critically reflects upon this institutional field on the other. The studies that are used as illustrations in this section have, in terms of this distinction, focused the study of languaging in

Descriptive-analytical research agenda	***Prescriptive-ideological research agenda***
• Focuses *languaging* and communication in everyday life inside and/or outside institutional settings • Focuses communication-practices in educational settings and *language use* in a mono or bilingual educational model • Focuses when, how, together with whom and why language varieties and modalities are used inside and outside institutional settings • Focuses central assumptions regarding language, identity, culture, learning and development in a given educational model	• Aims to identify the most superior model or method of communication which is deemed to be applicable in all subjects and classroom situations • Focuses what should be done and what is considered as the correct method of instruction in a mono or bilingual school • An underlying assumption equates the communicative model with the communication-practices in that model
Some central empirically pushed concepts related to language and identity include chaining, expanded-intersectionality, hybridity-continuum, languaging, identity-positioning, identiting	Some central bounded new-old concepts related to language and identity include bilingual, intersectionality, hybridity, superdiversity, hyperdiversity, translingualism

Fig. 4.6 Descriptive and prescriptive research agendas in bilingual education (adapted from Bagga-Gupta 2012)

different communities both inside and outside institutional education. One can say that a *descriptive-analytical* agenda—and not a *prescriptive-ideological* agenda—is the point of departure in such studies (see Fig. 4.6).

A descriptive-analytical perspective focuses upon what is taken for granted in mundane social practices, including identity, and patterns in languaging where more than one variety, modality, sociolect, etc are deployed. Here, the primary focus goes beyond specific issues at the institutional field level: the significance of "best methods" for teaching different groups, and reinforced boundaries between different language varieties and modalities in the organization of teaching different groups. Furthermore, segregated or integrated organization of institutional services for marginalized groups of pupils or adults is here subordinate to issues of the content and patterns of languaging, who is involved in the teaching, what is being focused, etc. Such research concomitantly attempts to (i) illuminate patterned ways-of-being-with-words inside and outside institutional settings and (ii) understand central assumptions vis-à-vis communication, identity and learning that guide the social practices in a given bilingual educational model.

Such a theoretically significant distinction calls for the need to focus interaction and participation inside, outside and across educational settings, rather than the ideologies or models at institutional levels. Such a premise resonates with a sociocultural decolonial perspective. It is thus significant to go beyond understandings marked by bounded essentialized identities, including imaginary communities and attend to the languaging or ways-of-being-with-words in communities of practices where more than one language variety, modality, register, etc. are deployed.

Research focused since the 1970s on the everyday uses of oral, written and signed language varieties in a wide range of settings has put the spotlight on the situated, distributed, collective, chained ecology of communication and meaning making processes in settings where people use more than one language variety, modality, etc. These include early anthropological studies by Scribner and Cole (1981) of the Vai peoples in Liberia, by Heath (1983) and her colleagues in southern United States and Street (1984) of rural parts of Iran. Continuing in this tradition, research has focused on migrant groups in northern California (Vasquez et al. 1994), services for migrant groups (i) in urban India (Bagga-Gupta 1995, 2012, 2014c), (ii) in urban Sweden (Carlsson and Bagga-Gupta 2006; Rosén 2013) and in urban school settings in different geopolitical spaces where immigrant pupils are enrolled (Cromdal 2000; Gynne 2016; Knobel 1999; St John 2014). Taking sociocultural-decolonial and descriptive-analytical points of departure has seen research focus on languaging (and identiting) in (i) the Deaf Studies scholarship since the 1990s, in the United States (Erting 1999; Erting et al 2000) and in Scandinavia (Bagga-Gupta 1999/2000, 2002, 2004c, 2010; Hansen 2005; Holmström 2013; Holmström and Bagga-Gupta 2013; Holmström et al 2015; Tapio 2013) and in (ii) the multimodality area (see for instance, Gynne and Bagga-Gupta 2013, 2015; Holmström 2013; Holmström et al. 2015; Jewitt 2009; Messina Dahlberg 2015; Messina Dahlberg and Bagga-Gupta 2014, 2015). The focus on languaging in such scholarship has saliency for illuminating identiting.

While some of the early classical studies from the 1970s and 1980s focused children's and adult's usage of different language varieties in a range of geopolitical settings, their contributions have primarily been acknowledged within and have given rise to the area of (New) Literacy Studies in the language sciences. This body of research illustrates how formal schooling in global North settings makes extensive use of and reinforces practices in which written language becomes functional inside school settings, but that these experiences may not be functional in settings outside of it. In other words, reading and writing may play no, or a completely different role in another language variety or register outside schools. What is significant for present purposes is that while the early research by Scribner, Cole, Heath and Street was conducted in different communities of practices where more than one language variety, modality, including different scripts, sociolects, etc. were deployed by children and adults, this important body of work has not (as yet) shaped either the scholarship in bilingualism or identity research. In other words, while these kinds of early studies were conducted in contexts that in current Eurocentric vocabulary could be labeled as bi-, multi- or plurilingual and super-diverse, their contributions have mainly been acknowledged in (re)conceptualizations in the area of (New) Literacy Studies.

Work by Heath (1983), Scribner and Cole (1981), Street (1984) and others who have followed in their footsteps are acknowledged as showing that humans develop the language varieties, modalities, sociolects, etc. they use to the extent required in various life domains and arenas. In other words, these types of early studies in settings where people deployed more than one language variety, modality, etc. have shown that the capacity to deploy resources in oral, written or signed *languaging* cannot be seen as something neutral which humans use in social situations across language varieties, modalities and timespaces. Thus, such results have been taken to mean that developing oral, written or signed skills in a particular language variety, modality or register, requires contact with mundane tasks that mediate, support and make such skills functional and necessary. This, as I have argued above, has salience for identity-positionings.

Insights derived from other research fields where language and identity research gets center-staged from earthrise positions include the multidisciplinary fields of Deaf Studies and Multimodality Studies. Attending to issues related to the communities of practices and users in "visually-oriented" (Bagga-Gupta 2004c) settings since the 1990s has contributed to a new orientation in the literature pertaining to deaf education (see particularly Chap. 7 in Bagga-Gupta 2004b, 2016a, b). This contrasts clearly with the prescriptive tendencies of the two dominating perspectives and methodologies related to language and identity—oralism and manualism that have framed research for over a century in deaf education. This field has been highly polarized with two prescriptive tendencies: a medical-psychological perspective that views deafness and deaf human beings as handicapped (a moonrise position) and a cultural perspective that views deaf human beings in terms of a linguistic minority (a sunrise position). The prescriptive nature of the discussions in the deaf education literature, thus for instance, legitimizes one of these two traditions as the norm; this in turn gives rise to different, but superior or correct methods of communication in both the perspectives (especially in how education is organized).

The non-prescriptively oriented third research tradition that has surfaced since the 1990s is significant here. Leaving aside the previous focus upon oralism and manualism, researchers, often themselves users of one of the world's many different signed language varieties, engage in the analysis of visually-oriented everyday communication in different settings (Bagga-Gupta 1999/2000, 2004c, 2010, 2016b, 2017; Fjord 2003; Holmström 2013; Monaghan et al 2003; Tapio 2013). By focusing upon social practices where signed language varieties are routinely used together with one or more spoken and/or written language varieties has turned attention away from the binary hegemonic, normalizing discourses of an "oral tradition" and a "manual/sign language tradition". Academic disciplinary areas such as anthropology, sociolinguistics, history, social-psychology, as well as communication studies, currently contribute to an earthrise position in the literature on deaf education (Bagga-Gupta 2016b). Since this perspective takes its points of departure in multidisciplinary academic domains including a descriptive-analytical point of departure, it is not pushed by any specific instructional models. However, "inverted-inclusive" school models that build upon a language profile principle (for instance American Sign Language-English or Swedish Sign Language-Swedish, Italian Sign Language-Italian, etc. language profile schools)[8] can be considered examples that represent principles of an earthrise position.

The patterned ways of using manual signs from a specific signed language, manually representing written words through finger-spelling, visually linking manual signs of a signed language to the written signs of a written language system by pointing, underlining or otherwise highlighting, mouthing a word and linking it to other visual representations has, in this new scholarship, been recognized as a routine feature of languaging in visually-oriented settings. Concepts such as *chaining*, *linking*, *sandwiching*, etc. have emerged pointing to the complex, patterned ways in which different language varieties and modalities are routinely deployed in mundane communication. This parallel, patterned use of at least two language varieties—American Sign Language-English or Swedish Sign Language-Swedish or Norwegian Sign Language-Norwegian—in visually-oriented settings in many ways resembles the links between oral-written languaging that characterizes mundane communication discussed in the (New) Literacy Studies literature through concepts such as "literacy events" and "literacy practices". Making visible the deployment of different modalities in both *literacy events* (oral-written) as well as in *visually-oriented* (signed-written-oral) languaging thus enables viewings of chaining and a hybridity-continuum in languaging. Here it is the intertwined use of oral and written modalities or oral, signed and written modalities in one or more language varieties that constitutes the recurring patterns described in the (New) Literacy Studies field since the 1970s and Deaf Studies literature since the 1990s. These analytical developments and emically derived concepts have significance for illuminating identity-positionings.

Research that focuses language and identity and emerges in the multidisciplinary field of Multimodal Studies is more recent. Taking descriptive-analytical points of departure, a central dimension of multimodality also pertains to analysis embedded in a performatory languaging position: "A key aspect of multimodality is the analysis of language […] as it is nestled and embedded within a wider semiotic frame. This offers new ways to explore and understand language, and its place in a multimodal communicational landscape" (Jewitt 2009: 2). While an interest vis-à-vis

[8]Such institutional settings actively promote the participation of majority (or mainstream) pupils in schools where minority (or marginalized) pupils are members. In a visually-oriented language profile school, inverted-inclusion would imply the participation of hearing pupils and deaf pupils in educational settings where a given signed language and a majority language constitute the language varieties of learning and instruction.

multimodality emerged and focused the linkages between text and pictures on printed texts in the 1990s (Kress 2003; Kress and van Leeuven 1996), an explosion of interest in multimodality has taken place in the new millennium (Jewitt 2009). Scholarship that has engaged itself with children and adults' use of oral talk, body orientations such as gaze and gestures and the semiotic affordances of tools in different settings too has been framed in terms of multimodality research (Finnegan 2015; Goodwin 1994; Jewitt 2009; Machin 2013). Some of this focus is more recently being directed to learning institutional sites (Kress 2003; Messina Dahlberg 2015; Paulasto et al 2014; St John 2014; Tapio 2013; Säljö 2010). This type of literature in concert with analysis of interactions in digital spaces has deepened our understandings of embodiment and the materiality of human communication inside, outside and across institutional learning arenas. Here it is interesting to note that multimodal research that focuses signed-written-oral communication in visually-oriented social practices continues to be conducted in separate academic domains and remains, for the most, eclipsed from the mainstream academic scholarship on the complex multimodal nature of human communication across settings (Bagga-Gupta 2016b, 2017). The take-home message from the multidisciplinary field of multimodal scholarship, nevertheless, emphasizes the linked and chained hybridity-continuum of communication (Gynne and Bagga-Gupta 2013, 2015; Messina Dahlberg 2015) and an empirically explored expanded-intersectional identity-positioning.

Taking cognizance of a Multimodal Turn (Jewitt 2009), a multi-dimensional (as well as a multidisciplinary) approach to language and identity in the research enterprise thus highlights the need to focus social practices where humans deploy more than one language variety, modality, etc. through "an examination of different dimensions of modalities and language varieties in languaging practices" (Gynne and Bagga-Gupta 2015: 1). In other words, the field of multimodality has also recently seen calls to center-stage the complexities of languaging that are glossed in the concepts bi/multilingualism and multimodality itself (ibid, Messina Dahlberg 2015). While attention has been drawn to the complexities of learning trajectories of children and adults, including its performative dimensions across digital and in-real-life (henceforth IRL) spaces, this field has so far seen limited attention to (i) the ways in which humans deploy more than one language variety and modality across timespaces and (ii) the identity-positionings that such deployment entails (Messina Dahlberg and Bagga-Gupta 2014). The point that is relevant here is that analysis of mundane languaging across digital-IRL spaces has the potential to contribute to understandings of expanded-intersectionality as well as chaining and a hybridity-continuum (Bagga-Gupta 2017).

The brushstroke discussions of recent scholarship across disciplines presented above highlights a hybridity-continuum wherein different language varieties and modalities that characterize meaning making processes in languaging are chained. Furthermore, researchers who contribute to these new positions are themselves users of the language varieties and modalities as well as the tools and spaces that they focus upon. They bring with them ways of viewings and searchings that are salient to the analytical descriptive enterprise. Identity (potentially) gets explicated in terms of expanded-intersectionality positionings, rather than on the hearing levels or other a priori categorization of human beings. Thus for instance, displaying the heterogeneity and the "many ways of being deaf" (Monaghan et al. 2003) acknowledges the fact that hearing human beings (family members, professionals, etc.) are members of communities of practices where signed language is central, including the fact that some deaf people can deploy some oral language resources. Such a viewing, furthermore, illustrates an expanded-intersectionality understanding of identity at both the individual and the community level. This means that signed languages are not instrumentally connected to the deaf, but are understood as language varieties used by human beings—deaf and hearing—who are members of "Deaf-Hearing Worlds" (compare Lane et al. 1996; see Bagga-Gupta 2016b).

Taken together, the types of classical studies from the 1970s onwards and the more recent scholarship discussed here *exemplify* research that emerges from analysis of mundane social practices across timespace. Such earthrise framed research challenges the dominant moonrise and sunrise positions where emphasis lies upon bounded, formal, naturalized points of departure and research approaches that build upon global North hegemonic viewings and/or prescriptive-ideological framings of language and identity. The co-construction and situatedness of meaning, the social as pivotal, the need to focus social practices, attending to membership issues, taking into account the representative and interpretive nature of language, etc., make up some of the complex—though nevertheless important—issues that are attended to in the scholarship discussed in this section.

4.5 Some Concluding Reflections on Open Spaces. Communicating = Learning

Center-staging complexities and deploying a performative stance from sociocultural, decolonial framings where experiences of using more than one language variety, modality, etc. are privileged, allow for new viewings. Going beyond new-old terminology where language and identity are framed in naturalized, problematic concepts and focusing the doing of language and identity in social practices inside, outside and across institutional settings, including digital spaces, allows for alternative ways of framing empirically pushed concepts. Concepts such as *chaining*, *hybridity*-continuum, an *expanded-intersectionality*, *languaging* and *identiting* open up spaces for going beyond some of the static and stratifying terminology in the areas of language and identity discussed in this chapter.

Relevant research for language and identity from an earthrise position has been center-staged by going beyond the dominant and deviant points of departure in the webs-of-understandings related to mono- and bilingualism in moonrise and sunrise positions. This type of research lies at the margins of mainstream research in the language and education sciences. An earthrise position center-stages mundane human behavior and metaphorically recognizes the perils of boundaries and focuses upon the open spaces of languaging, spaces where identity-positionings are performed. It is in this sense that a focus upon open spaces (across institutions and disciplines) constitutes both a theoretical and a methodological enterprise. Such research (potentially) makes visible the complexity of languaging and identity-positionings without marking the use of more than one language variety, modality, register, sociolect or human identity in reductionist and exotic Othering concepts.

Such a perspective is currently recognized in global North academic discourses where recent concepts like plurilingualism, translingualism and superdiversity make attempts to deal with the complexities that frame communication and identification processes. However, my argument in this chapter underscores the boundary-marking as well as the prescriptive colonially marked flavor of some of these recent concepts. Such concepts risk missing the importance of seeings and (re)viewings from scholarship that arise in and from global South spaces. Furthermore, such concepts exotify new population mobilities in the global North and risk ignoring the complex nature of communication and identity everywhere.[9] Such concepts can become reductionist and continue to reproduce an Othering discourse. Echoing Omoniyi (2015; see above), it is pertinent to ask whether such scholarship recognizes the many-ways-of-being as well as the many-ways-with-words in the lives of humans in global South spaces: "What have the Northern scholars missed out on by not sufficiently engaging with Southern multilingual realities?".

The arguments presented in this chapter point towards a significant gap between the analytical assumptions that are prescribed to when language and identity are conceptualized "as" action, and the ways in which many branches of the language sciences are conceptualized, the resulting organization of language instruction in educational settings and in research itself. Linked to this gap is, as I have outlined in this chapter, a particular view of learning generally and language learning specifically. The specific, dominant traditions that allow us to categorize language varieties in numerical, relational, geographical, gendered etc. terms build upon the "brain as container" model where the underlying assumption is that an individuals' (singular) "mother tongue" or "home language" or "native language" should automatically form the basis for learning any other language/s. Human beings across global South spaces engage with plural "mother tongues" and multiple "home language varieties". However their rich languaging experiences continue to be made invisible through the deployment of a selective conceptual framework, not least when they migrate to global North places. An earthrise perspective argues that childrens' (and even adults') primary language varieties need to be understood in terms of parallel-chained deployment of language varieties, rather than "additive or subtractive (or other) bilingualism". The latter Eurocentric, linguacentric ideas disregard, as has been argued in this chapter, global human realities and the largely ethnographically oriented research that points to the patterned use of more than one language variety, modality, register, etc. across timespaces. Such scholarship builds upon recorded and archival data (rather than reported or elicited data) and privileges

[9]See also Pavlenko (2017) for an important discussion on the processes of "academic branding" in the area of identity and diversity.

mundane social practices; it illustrates an earthrise position that highlights the progression of language experiences and skills throughout the life span; and, recognizes that such skills tend to be domain specific in the lives of children and adults.

One can say that the analytical assumptions in an earthrise position are at odds with, for instance, linear trajectories that dominate framings of intellectual development in general and language learning in particular. The cluster metaphors and a "brain as container" metaphor reinforce how language development and learning are dominantly conceptualized. Such conceptualizations are reductionist and not in sync with a performative stance wherein complexities are centre-staged. Research that focuses everyday social practices where more than two or more language varieties and modalities are deployed illustrates how adults and children develop the language resources they use to the level of skills required in different domains and arenas in life. While these types of research findings suggest broader ways of understanding communication, identity and learning, they have perhaps only in limited ways shaped the very institution that is seen as being responsible for language teaching and learning.

Such research can potentially raise important issues vis-à-vis the organization of language instruction in school sites. Results from such research conducted in a diverse range of settings, both inside and outside educational institutions across global North and global South spaces and geopolitical places, including virtual sites, indicate that a demarcation is not uncommonly maintained between the formal teaching of language skills in language focused lessons/activities and the deployment of language resources in other subject lessons/activities (where language is itself often not in focus). Differences between focusing upon the form and function of languaging is reported[10] to be striking and it has been suggested that children and adults unwittingly are afforded more meaningful, dialogical and enriching ways of participation in the latter settings. Such earthrise framed research has important implications for learning different oral, written and signed language varieties across timespace (Bagga-Gupta 2017). The results from such studies and projects inside and outside different educational settings across global North and global South spaces seems to suggest that there is a tendency for language practices to become traditional and monological if and when pupils (children and adults), for any number of reasons, are viewed as deviating from normative understandings of a monolingual, functionally able, ethnic native human being. Thus for instance, immigrant pupils, deaf pupils in bilingual special institutional settings, ethnic minority Swedish pupils learning Swedish, all appear to receive more traditional language instruction if and when they are experienced as being weaker in the target language i.e. Swedish. It is such findings from descriptive-analytical framed research that demonstrate the dominance of a selective, traditional, narrow view of language instruction and identity in educational institutional settings.

[10]In research projects that I have been involved in and that has emerged at the CCD research group (www.ju.se/ccd) in Sweden. Some of this research has been discussed in Sect. 4.4 above.

The critique raised vis-à-vis mainstream understandings of language, identity and learning raised in this chapter bring to the forefront aspects of the common monolingual and monoethnic bias that has existed in language education, especially in the post-World War II period. Classifying language varieties in terms of a horizontal division, i.e. different language codes, in the educational curricula is, it can be argued, important from an institutional and administrative point of view. In other words, curricula, syllabi and the organisation of timespace in educational settings necessitates the differentiation between different language codes. However, there is need to recognize the selective nature of stratification of language varieties in relation to learners identity-positions, not least when it comes to marginalized children and adults in the educational system. Furthermore, based on essentialist identity categories that build upon pupil groups' (compare "imaginary communities") different learning abilities (i.e. the vertical division), is contentious. These latter conceptualizations draw upon particular assumptions related to views about "how language learning occurs" and "what language and culture are". An earthrise position challenges such categorizations (not least within academics and research itself) and conceptualizations since it is argued that (i) human attributes become meaningful within the context of everyday interactions in situated social practices, and (ii) language categories need to be freed from the constraints of identity categories themselves.

While institutional education in global North places and spaces like Sweden are traditionally understood as sites that socialize children and adults into (mono) lingual and (mono)cultural citizenship, I have in this chapter highlighted the fact that research into the social practices of human beings with a diverse range of linguistic and cultural experiences seems to have been dominated by the following tendencies. *Firstly*, research has focused communication in terms of different language categories rather than socialization processes more broadly. *Secondly*, issues related to culture, difference and identity are elaborated in terms of static essentialized understandings of marginalized groups and issues (and here it is not uncommon that language issues come center-stage). *Thirdly*, research inquiry has in large measure primarily focused school arenas and not peoples' everyday lives more broadly. In other words, critically understanding human beings' social practices (including new literacies, technologies and popular culture) in the changing contexts that characterize human life everywhere on the planet currently is important. *Fourthly*, research that focuses social practices, rather than accountings of these social practices lies at the margins of mainstream science. And *finally*, a critical earthrise perspective, including voices of scholars who routinely deploy multiple language varieties, sociolects, etc. are wanting in the bilingual research landscape. Making visible such epistemological hegemonies in the research enterprise itself has important implications for the work done by institutions like the one-school-for-all, life-long-learning, the Ombudsman, etc.

My line of argumentation illustrates the significance of a hybridity-continuum for understanding present day framings of language, functional abilities, gender and ethnicity positionings and other identity-positionings in educational institutional settings and institutions engaged in equity work. Noting the incongruence between institutional *accountings*, including accountings in the language sciences in the global North and research since the late 1970s that focuses upon languaging in the context of migrations, marginalization in and across the global South, as well as the *performance* of languaging and identity in and across the global North, challenges dominating understandings of language and identity generally and the organization of special support for marginalized individuals (immigrants, functionally disabled) more specifically. Here it is pertinent and interesting to note that while a "compensatory perspective" guides the activity and institutional field of bilingual education, *critical languaging, identiting* and *participatory perspectives* themselves make up marginal positions in the Bilingual Studies and identity research landscape. In other words, there exists both a dominance of monolingual and monoidentity points of departure and a parallel paucity of research that focuses upon social practices in the bulk of the research that informs the thematic areas of bilingual and/or identity research.

This raises concerns regarding the *technification* of both linguistic diversity and human diversity. One way of transcending such technification is by questioning the simplistic positions and problematic webs-of-understandings that frame mono-bi-multi/translingualism and super/hyperdiversity in global North spaces, and highlighting the need for (i) emic understandings of how accountings constitute a core dimension of "collective remembering" (Wertsch 2002) of "imagined communities" (Anderson 1991), and (ii) the need of "alternative voices" (Hasnain el al. 2013) where hybridity and intersectionality need to be approached empirically in the learning sciences. Framed against the backdrop of a critical humanistic socially oriented framework, an earthrise position challenges current dominant understandings of linguistic diversity and human diversity and highlights the largely Eurocentric hegemonies that currently frame discourses of globalization.

References

Agar, M. (1994). *Language shock. Understanding the culture of language*. New York: William Morrow.

Anderson, B. (1991). *Imagined communities. Reflections on the origin and spread of nationalism*. London: Verso.

Appadurai, A. (1996). *Modernity at large: Cultural dimensions of globalization*. Minneapolis: MN, University of Minnesota Press.

Apple, M. W., & Buras, K. L. (Eds.). (2006). *The subaltern speak curriculum, power, and educational struggles*. Routledge: New York.

Bagga-Gupta. S. (1995). *Human development and institutional practices: Women, child care and the mobile creches. Linköping studies in arts and sciences 130*. Doctoral dissertation. Linköping University, Sweden.

Bagga-Gupta, S. (1999/2000). Visual language environments. Exploring everyday life and literacies in Swedish deaf bilingual schools. *Visual Anthropology Review, 15*(2), 95–120.

Bagga Gupta, S. (2002). Explorations in bilingual instructional interaction: A sociocultural perspective on literacy. *Learning and Instruction, 5*(2), 557–587.

Bagga-Gupta, S. (2004a). Challenging understandings in pluralistic societies: Language and culture loose in school sites and losing sight of democratic agendas in education? *Utbildning och Demokrati, 13*(3), 11–36.

Bagga-Gupta, S. (2004b). *Literacies and deaf education. A theoretical analysis of the international and Swedish literature.* Forskning i Fokus. nr 23. Stockholm: Myndigheten för skolutveckling. (http://www.skolverket.se/publikationer?id=1843)

Bagga-Gupta, S. (2004c). Visually oriented bilingualism. Discursive and technological resources in Swedish deaf pedagogical arenas. In M. van Herreweghe and M. Vermeerbergen (eds) *To the Lexicon and beyond. Sociolinguistics in European deaf communities*, Volume 10—The sociolinguistics in deaf communities series. Editor Ceil Lucas (pp. 171–207). Washington DC: Gallaudet University Press.

Bagga-Gupta, S. (2007). Aspects of diversity, inclusion and democracy in education and research. *Scandinavian Journal of Educational Research, 51*(1), 1–22.

Bagga-Gupta, S. (2010). Creating and (re)negotiating boundaries. Representations as mediation in visually oriented multilingual Swedish school settings. *Language, Culture and Curriculum, 23* (3), 251–276.

Bagga-Gupta, S. (2012). Challenging understandings of bilingualism in the language sciences from the lens of research that focuses social practices. In E. Hjörne, G. van der Aalsvoort, & G. de Abreu (Eds.), *Learning, social interaction and diversity—exploring school practices* (pp. 85–102). Rotterdam: Sense.

Bagga-Gupta, S. (2013a). The boundary-turn. relocating language, identity and culture through the epistemological lenses of time, space and social interactions. In I. Hasnain, S. Bagga-Gupta, & S. Mohan (Eds.), *Alternative voices: (Re)searching language, culture and identity...* (pp. 28–49). Newcastle-upon-Tyne: Cambridge Scholars Publishing.

Bagga-Gupta, S. (2013b). Literacies som handling: den språkande människan och praktikgemenskaper [Literacy as action: The languaging human being and communities of practices]. In S. Bagga-Gupta, C. Liberg, A-C. Evaldsson, & R. Säljö (Eds.), *Literacy-praktiker i och utanför skolan* [Literacy practices inside and outside schools] (pp. 19–40). Malmö: Gleerups Utbildning AB.

Bagga-Gupta, S. (2014a). Languaging: Ways-of-being-with-words across disciplinary boundaries and empirical sites. In H. Paulasto, H. Riionheimo, L. Meriläinen, & M. Kok (Eds.), *Language contacts at the crossroads of disciplines* (pp. 89–130). Newcastle-upon-Tyne: Cambridge Scholars Publishing.

Bagga-Gupta, S. (2014b). A common education-for-all and life-long learning? Reflections on inclusion, equity and integration. In B. Hensen (Ed.), *Theory and methodology in international comparative classroom studies* (Vol. 2, pp. 225–243). Oslo: Cappelen Damm Akkademisk.

Bagga-Gupta, S. (2014c). Performing and accounting language and identity: Agency as actors-in-(inter)action-with-tools. In P. Deters, Xuesong Gao, E. Miller, & G. Vitanova-Haralampiev (Eds.), *Interdisciplinary approaches to theorizing and analyzing agency and second language learning* (pp. 113–132). Bristol: Multilingual Matters.

Bagga-Gupta, S. (2015, August 2015). *Language learners and learning language. Webs-of-understandings in the era of reinforced boundaries*. Paper presented in the invited symposium "The boundary turn: challenges in researching and theorizing learning and diversity from decolonial perspectives". 16th Biennial conference EARLI 2015. Limassol, Cyprus.

Bagga-Gupta, S. (2016a). Languaging, learning, identiting—The significance of everyday life. Inaugural lecture. Jönköping University Inauguration and Confernment Ceremony 20–21 May 2016.

Bagga-Gupta, S. (2016b). Signed languages in bilingual education. In: Stephan May (General Ed.), *Encyclopedia of education and bilingualism.* Ofelia García & Angel M.Y. Lin (Eds.), Volume 5: *Bilingual and multilingual education* (pp. 1–15). Rotterdam: Springer.

Bagga-Gupta, S., & Holmström, I. (2016). Language, identity and technologies in classrooms for the differently-abled. *Communication Disorders, Deaf Studies & Hearing Aids., 3*(4), 1–19. doi:10.4172/2375-4427.1000145.

Bagga-Gupta, S. & Surian, A. (2014). *Center-staging global north-south research in the glocal-virtual age: Challenges in researching and theorizing learning, communication and diversity.* Paper presented at EARLI, European Association of Research on Learning and Instruction conference: Open spaces for interaction and learning diversities.27–30 August 2014. Padova, Italy.

Bagga-Gupta, S. (2017). Going beyond oral-written-signed-virtual divides: theorizing languaging from social practice perspectives. *Writing & Pedagogy*, 9(1).
Bakhtin, M. (1981). *The dialogic imagination*. In C. Holmquist (Ed.) Austin: University of Texas Press.
Bhabha, H. (1994). *The location of culture*. London: Routledge.
Blommaert, J. (2010). *The sociolinguistics of globalization*. Cambridge: Cambridge University Press.
Blommaert, J. (2015). Commentary: Superdiversity old and new. *Language & Communication*. doi:10.1016/j.langcom.2015.01.003
Butler, J. (1999). *Gender trouble. Feminism and the subversion of identity*. London: Routledge.
Carlsson, R., & Bagga-Gupta, S. (2006). "Verktyg & lådor". En studie om språkfokuserade aktiviteter för minoriteter på förskolearenor ["Tools and boxes". A study of language focused activities for minorities in pre-school settings]. *Nordic Educational Researcher, 26*(3), 193–211.
Clark, C., Dyson, A., & Millward, A. (1998). Theorising special education. Time to move on! In C. Clark, A. Dyson, & A. Millward (Eds.), *Theorising special education* (pp. 156–173). London: Routledge.
Clifford, J. (1997). *Routes: Travel and translation in the late twentieth century*. Cambridge, MA: Harvard University Press.
Coates, J. (1996). *Women talk*. Oxford: Blackwell.
Cromdal, J. (2000). *Code-switching for all practical purposes. Bilingual organisation of children's play. Linköping Studies in Arts and Science 223*. Doctoral Dissertation. Linköping University, Linköping, Sweden.
Edwards, R. (2012). (Im)mobilities and (dis)locating practices in cyber-education. In R. Brooks, A. Fuller & J. Waters (Eds.), *Changing spaces of education. New perspectives on the nature of learning*. London: Routledge.
Erting, C. (1999). *Two languages at home and at school: Early literacy in ASL/english contexts.* Invited paper at the European Days of Deaf Education Conference: Bilingual Education with a Focus on Reading and Writing. Örebro, Sweden.
Erting, C. J., Thumann-Prezioso, C. & Benedict, B. S. (2000). Bilingualism in a Deaf Family. Fingerspelling in Early Childhood. In P. E. Spencer, C. J. Erting & M. Marschark (Eds.). *The deaf child in the family and at school. Essays in honor of Kathryn P. Meadow-Orlans* (pp. 41–54). Mahwah, NJ: Lawrence Erlbaum Associates.
Finnegan, R. (2015). *Where is language? An anthropologist's questions on language, literature and performance*. England: Bloomsbury.
Fjord, L. (2003). *Contested signs: Discursive disputes in the geography of the pediatric cochlear implant, language, kinship and expertise*. Doctoral dissertation. University of Virginia, USA.
Garcia, O. (2009). *Bilingual education in the 21st century: A global perspective*. Malden, MA: Blackwell.
Garcia, O., & Lin, A. (Eds.), (2016). *Bilingual and multilingual education. Volume 5.* Encyclopedia of language and education, General Editor Stephen May. Rotterdam: Springer.
Gramling, D. (2016). *The Invention of Monolingualism. Bloomsbury.*
Goodwin, C. (1994). Professional vision. *American Anthropologist, 96,* 606–633.
Guba, E. G., & Lincoln, Y. S. (1994). Competing paradigms in qualitative research. In N. K. Denzin & Y. S. Lincoln (Eds.), *Handbook of qualitative research* (pp. 105–117). Thousand Oaks, CA: Sage.
Gunnarsson, L. (2015). Why we keep separating the 'inseparable': Dialecticizing intersectionality. *The European journal of women's studies*. 1–14. doi:10.1177/1350506815577114
Gynne, A. (2016). *Languaging, learning and identities in glocal (educational) settings—The case of finnish background young people in Sweden*. Doctoral dissertation. Mälardalen University, Sweden.
Gynne, A., & Bagga-Gupta, S. (2013). Young people's language usage and identity positioning. Chaining in 'bilingual' educational settings in Sweden. *Linguistics and Education, 24,* 479–496.
Gynne, A., & Bagga-Gupta, S. (2015). Languaging in the twenty-first century. Exploring varieties and modalities in literacies inside and outside learning spaces. *Language and Education, 29*(6), 509–526. doi:10.1080/09500782.2015.1053812

Hjörne, E. (2004). Excluding for inclusion? Negotiating school careers and identities in pupil wefare settings in the Swedish school. Diss. Götenburg Studies in Educational Sciences 213.

Hall, S. (1996). Introduction: Who needs 'identity'?. In S. Hall & P. du Gay (Eds.) *Questions of cultural identity* (pp. 1–17). Thousand Oaks, CA and London: Sage.

Hansen, A. L. (2005). *Communicative practices in visually oriented classrooms: A study of a model education for deaf teacher candidates 1005:132*. Doctoral dissertation. NTNU University, Norway.

Hasnain, I., Bagga-Gupta, S., & Mohan, S. (Eds.). (2013). *Alternative voices: (Re)searching language, culture and identity*. Newcastle-upon-Tyne: Cambridge Scholars Publishing.

Heath, S. B. (1983). *Ways with words. Language, life and work in communities and classrooms*. Cambridge: Cambridge University Press.

Holmström, I. (2013). *"'Learning by hearing'. Technological framings for participation." Örebro Studies in Education 42*. Doctoral dissertation. Örebro University, Sweden.

Holmström, I., & Bagga-Gupta, S. (2013). Technologies at work. A sociohistorical analysis of human identities and communication. *Deafness and Education International, 15*(1), 2–28.

Holmström, I., Bagga-Gupta, S., & Jonsson, R. (2015). Communicating and hand(ling) technologies. Everyday life in educational settings where pupils with cochlear implants are mainstreamed. *Journal of Linguistic Anthropology, 25*, 256–284. doi:10.1111/jola.12097

Hult, F. (2010). The complexity turn in educational linguistics. *Language, Culture and Curriculum, 23*(3), 173–177.

Jewitt, C. (Ed.). (2009). *The Routledge handbook of multimodal analysis*. Abingdon; UK: Routledge.

Jones, R. B. (2011). *Postcolonial representations of women. Critical issues for education*. Rochester NY: Springer.

Jørgensen, N., Karrebaek, M. S., Madsen, L. M., & Moller, J. S. (2011). Polylanguaging in superdiversity. *Diversities, 13*(2), 25–38. www.unesco.org/shs/diversities/vol13/issue2/art2. June 2014.

Khubchandani, L. M. (1997). *Revisualizing boundaries. A plurilingual ethos. Language and Development—Volume 3*. New Delhi: Sage Publications.

Khubchandani, L. M. (1998). A plurilingual ethos: A Peep into the Sociology of Language. *Indian Journal of Applied Linguistics*, 24(1),5–37.

Knobel, M. (1999). *Everyday literacies. students, discourse and social practice*. New York: Peter Lang.

Kraidy, M. (2005). *Hybridity: Or the cultural logic of globalization*. Philadelphia: Temple.

Kress, G. (2003). *Literacy in the new media age*. London: Routledge.

Kress, G., & van Leeuven, T. (1996). *Reading Images: The grammar visual design*. London: Routledge.

Lakoff, G., & Johnson, M. (1984). *Metaphors we live by*. Chicago: University of Chicago Press.

Landri, P., & Neuman, E. (2014). Introduction. Mobile sociologies of education. *European Educational Research Journal, 13*(1), 1–8.

Lane, H., Hoffmeister, R., & Bahan, B. (1996). *A journey into the DEAF-WORLD*. San Diego: Dawn Press Sign.

Lave, J., & Wenger, E. (1991). *Situated learning. Legitimate peripheral participation*. Cambridge, MA: Cambridge University Press.

Linell, P. (2009). *Rethinking language, mind, and world dialogically. Interactional and contextual theories of human sense-making*. Charlotte, NC: Information Age Publishing.

Machart, R., Clark, J. B. & Dervin, F. (2014). Editorial. Perceived Differences, exhibited 'diversities' and overlooked individualities. *Internatinal Journal of Education for Diversity, 3*, I–vi.

Machin, D. (2013). What is multimodal critical discourse studies? *Critical Discourse Studies., 10* (4), 347–355.

Maldonado-Torres, N. (2011, Fall). Thinking through the decolonial turn: Post-continental Interventions in theory, philosophy, and critique—An introduction. *Transmodernity*, 1–15.

May, S. (Ed.). (2013). *The multilingual turn. Implications for SLA, TESOL and bilingual education*. New York: Routledge.

McCall, L. (2005). The complexity of intersectionality. *Signs: Journal of Women in Culture and Society., 3*(3), 1771–1800.

Messina Dahlberg, G. (2015). *Languaging in virtual learning sites: Studies of online encounters in the language-focused classroom.* Doctoral dissertation. Örebro Studies in Education 49. Örebro University, Sweden.

Messina Dahlberg, G. & Bagga-Gupta, S. (2014). Trajectories of learning and participation in online glocal communities. Languaging and identity positions at borderlands. *Learning, Media and Technology,* Special theme issue "Media and migration: learning in a globalized world", *39*(4), 468–487.

Messina Dahlberg, G., & Bagga-Gupta, S. (2015). Learning on-the-go in institutional telecollaboration: Anthropological perspectives on the boundaries of digital spaces. In E. Dixon, & M. Thomas (Eds.), *Researching language learner interaction online: From social media to MOOCs* (pp. 259–281). CALICO. Volume 13.

Mignolo, W. D. (2009). Epistemic disobedience, independent thought and decolonial freedom. *Theory, Culture and Society, 26*(7–8), 159–181.

Mignolo, W.D. (2012). *Local histories/global designs. Coloniallity, subaltern knowledges and border thinking*. New Jersey: Princeton University Press.

Mohanty, C. (2004). *Feminism without borders: Decolonizing theory, practising solidarity.* Durham, NC: Duke University Press.

Monaghan, L., Schmaling, C., Nakamura, K., & Turner, G. H. (Eds.). (2003). *Many ways to be deaf. International variation in deaf communities.* Washington DC: Gallaudet University Press.

Myndigheten för skolutveckling. (2004). *Kartläggning av svenska som andraspråk* [Overview of Swedish as a second language]. Dnr 2003:757. Stockholm: The Swedish National Agency for School Improvement.

Omoniyi, T. (2015). Illusions and delusions of the centre within the framework of globalization. Invited symposium at conference The Sociolinguistics of Globalisation: (De)centering and (de)standerdization. The University of Hong Kong. 3–6 June 2015.

Oostendorp, M. (2017). Extending resemiotisation: time, space and body in discursive representation. *Social Semiotics*. DOI: 10.1080/10350330.2017.1295849

Pavlenko, A. (2017). in press. Superdiversity and why it isn't. In S. Breidbach, L. Kuster & B. Schmenk (Eds.), *Sloganizations in Language Education Discourse. Bristol* UK: Multilingual Matters.

Paulasto, H., Riionheimo, H., Meriläinen, L., & Kok, M. (Eds.). (2014). *Language contacts at the crossroads of disciplines* (pp. 89–130). Newcastle-upon-Tyne: Cambridge Scholars Publishing.

Rees, T. (1998). *Mainstreaming equality in the European Union: Education, training and labor market policies*. New York: Routledge.

Rogoff, B. (1990). *Apprenticeship in thinking: Cognitive development in social context.* Oxford: Oxford University Press.

Rosén, J. (2013). *Svenska för invandrarskap?: Språk, kategorisering och identitet inom utbildningsformen Svenska för invandrare. [Swedish for immigrantness?: Language, categorization and identity within the education Swedish for immigrants]. Örebro Studies in Educational Sciences with an Emphasis on Didactics, 7.* Doctoral dissertation. Örebro University, Sweden.

Rosén, J. (2017). fortcoming. Becoming an immigrant in the language learning classroom. Intersections of gender and national identity. In S. Bagga-Gupta (Ed.), Marginalization Processes: *Studies of membership and participation across disciplines and sites.* Newcastle-upon-Tyne: Cambridge Scholars Publishing.

Scollan, R., & Scollan, S. W. (2004). *Nexus analysis. Discourse and the emerging internet.* London: Routledge.

Scribner, S., & Cole, M. (1981). *The psychology of literacy.* Cambridge, MA.: Harvard University Press.

Simao, L. M., & Valsiner, J. (Eds.). (2007). *Otherness in question. Labyrinths of the self.* Charlotte, North Carolina: Information Age Publishing.

Sheller, M., & Urry, J. (2006). The new mobilities paradigm. *Environment and Planning A, 38*(2), 207–226. doi:10.1068/a37268

St John, O. (2014). *Approaching classroom interaction dialogically: Studies of everyday encounters in a 'bilingual' secondary school.* Doctoral dissertation. Örebro Studies in Education 46. Örebro University, Sweden.

Street, B. (1984). *Literacy in theory and practice. Cambridge studies in oral and literate culture.* Cambridge: Cambridge University Press.

Surian, A. (2015, August). *Adressing the decolonial and boundary turn in transformative learning.* Paper presented at the invited symposium "The boundary turn: Challenges in researching and theorizing learning and diversity from decolonial perspectives". 16th Biennial Conference EARLI 2015. Limassol, Cyprus.

Säljö, R. (2002). My brain's running slow today—The preference for 'things ontologies' in research and everyday discourse on human thinking. *Studies in Philosophy and Education, 21* (4–5), 389–405.

Säljö, R. (2005). *Lärande och kulturella redskap: Om lärprocessser och det kollektiva minnet.* [Learning and cultural artefacts: On learning processes and collective memory]. Stockholm: Prisma.

Säljö, R. (2010). Digital Tools and challenges to institutional traditions of learning: Technologies, social memory and the performative nature of learning. *Journal of Computer Assisted learning, 26*(1), 53–64.

Tannen, D. (Ed.). (1993). *Gender and conversational interaction.* Oxford: Oxford University Press.

Tapio, E. (2013). *A nexus analysis of English in the everyday life of FinSL signers: A multimodal view on interaction.* Doctoral dissertation. Oulu University. Finland.

Vasquez, O. A., Pease-Alvarez, L., & Shannon, S. M. (1994). *Pushing boundaries: Language and culture in a mexicano community.* Cabridge: Cambridge University Press.

Vertovec, S. (2006). *The emergence of super-diversity in Britain.* Centre of migration, Policy and society. University of Oxford. UK.

Walby, S. (2003). Gender Mainstreaming. Productive tensions in theory and practice. Contribution to ESRC Gender Mainstreaming Seminars, 2003–4. http://www.unesco.org/new/fileadmin/MULTIMEDIA/HQ/SHS/pdf/Gender-Mainstreaming.pdf, 30 Apr 2015.

Walby, S. (2011). *The future of feminism.* Cambridge: Polity Press.

Wertsch, J. (1998). *Mind as action.* Oxford: Oxford University Press.

Wertsch, J. (2002). *Voices of collective remembering.* Cambridge: Cambridge University Press.

Winzer, M. A. (1993). *The history of special education. From isolation to integration.* Washington DC: Gallaudet University Press.

Winzer, M. A., & Mazurek, K. (Eds.). (2000). *Special education in the 21st century. Issues of inclusion and reform.* Washington DC: Gallaudet University Press.

Wittgenstein, L. (1999). *Philosophical Investigations* (G. E. M. Anscombe, Trans.). Prentice Hall.

Wolcott, H. (1999). *Ethnography. A way of seeing.* Walnut Creek, Calif: AltaMira.

Author Biography

Sangeeta Bagga-Gupta is Full Professor of Education since 2016 at Jönköping University, Sweden. She has been full professor at Örebro University, Sweden since 2007. She is also adjunct professor 2016–2017 at Aligarh University, India. Her multidisciplinary, multi-scalar ethnographically framed research focuses communication, learning and identity from sociocultural and decolonial framings. She publishes extensively and in a number of different research domains. She is the Principle Investigator of the new Swedish Research Council project *Participation for all? School and post-school pathways of young people* (2016–2020) and has been the leader of the research group CCD, *Communication, Culture and Diversity* since the end of the 1990s.

Part II
Making, Undoing and Remaking: Performing Identities

Part II of the volume "*Identity Revisited and Reimagined. Empirical and Theoretical Contributions Across Time and Space*" brings together three chapters that *empirically* focus upon the vulnerable, open, and fluid nature of identity (discussed in Part I) in different contexts. Here, the (re)making and (un)doing of identity performances are center-staged. The chapters in this part illustrate the ways in which human identity gets fossilized and constructed but also challenged by offering data-pushed examples.

In the first chapter in this part, Chap. 5, "Co-constructing the Adolescent's Identity: Agency and Autonomy as Interactional Accomplishments", Marina Everri and Laura Sterponi draw attention to the complexity and situatedness of processes where identity development gets played out. By focusing on the communicative exchanges between parents and adolescent children, they demonstrate how multiple identities are contingently performed, invoked, contested, and negotiated. Drawing on recent linguistic anthropological reflections on identity and discursive psychologists' theorizing on social positioning, Everri and Sterponi examine the dynamic and multifaceted enactment and transformation of identity in social interaction. They suggest that agency and autonomy, key dimensions of adolescent identity development, do not emerge solely from the individual but are co-constructed and transformed in interpersonal exchanges. They support these theoretical propositions through the discourse analysis of two family cases. Here, they illustrate the discursive co-construction of adolescent agency and autonomy as being continuously negotiated rather than being nonlinear. The examples presented in the chapter highlight that families oscillate between different interactional configurations, with individual family members claiming, declining, reclaiming certain roles and competencies vis-à-vis other members of the family. In addition to illustrating the value of bridging the gap between different disciplinary perspectives, Everri and Sterponi demonstrate the analytic purchase that a micro-examination of social interaction offers to adolescence and developmental psychology research.

In Chap. 6, the second chapter in Part II, “Rethinking Identity in Adult Language Learning Classrooms”, Jenny Rosén focuses on the performatory dimension of adult language learners’ identity-positions in institutional spaces. Learning a new language, Rosén argues, involves transformation and investment of identities, since people negotiate not only who they are, but also who they have been and who they are becoming. In this chapter, she investigates how participants in a Swedish language learning program, Swedish for immigrants (SFI), use multiple linguistic resources in the negotiation of identity in situ. The chapter aims to explore how participants in this specific setting use (multi)linguistic resources in the negotiation of identity generally and gender and national belonging more specifically. Rosén traces the development of the SFI program since the 1960s and its organization in Sweden. The chapter combines a sociocultural framework that emphasizes the relationship between learning, participation, and identity with a post-structural, intersectional understanding of identity. Grounded in an ethnographic framework, Rosén uses the work of Sangeeta Bagga-Gupta, Francis Hult and Ron Scollon and Suzanne Wong Scollon on a multi-scaled approach, which includes national policy of the SFI program and, interactional data from a SFI classroom. Rosén highlights how language learning is embedded in the socialization of students into certain values and norms which are perceived as specifically Swedish, tied to the geopolitical spaces of Sweden. She also shows how the participants constitute and negotiate meaning about the world and who they are through language-use. How linguistic and institutional identities in the classroom intersect and enforce the unequal distribution of power is another important contribution of this chapter.

Chapter 5
Co-constructing the Adolescent's Identity: Agency and Autonomy as Interactional Accomplishments

Marina Everri and Laura Sterponi

5.1 Introduction

In this chapter we leverage the insights of scholarship in linguistic anthropology and discursive psychology to re-examine dimensions typically associated with identity development in adolescence, i.e. agency and autonomy. While the traditional psychological perspective links agency to the developing individual and contrasts it with external structures, most frequently conceived of as constraining individual autonomy, we propose an interactional reappraisal of identity development during adolescence which brings to light the *situated* and *relational nature* of identity processes across the lifespan. Consistently, this paper aligns with post-modern perspectives which debunked the notion of identity as a stable and coherent structure located within the individual psyche and foregrounds the *dynamic* and *multifaceted* manifestation and transformation of identity in social interaction (e.g., Bucholtz and Hall 2010; Butler 1990).[1]

[1]The debate on subjectivity and identity issues is not new: it has characterized the fields of philosophy and critical theory for the past half century. In particular, psychoanalysis, feminism, late Marxism and post-structuralism have widely challenged the notion of free and autonomous individual. In this paper, we decided to focus on psychology and anthropology as they are the field in which we have been trained and currently working. Moreover, the empirical material we present in this paper was collected having in mind specific research questions guided by psychological and anthropological theoretical approaches.

M. Everri (✉)
Department of Psychological and Behavioural Science,
London School of Economics, London, UK
e-mail: M.everri@lse.ac.uk

L. Sterponi
Language Literacy and Culture at the Graduate School of Education,
University of California, Berkeley, USA
e-mail: Sterponi@berkeley.edu

S. Bagga-Gupta et al. (eds.), *Identity Revisited and Reimagined*,
DOI 10.1007/978-3-319-58056-2_5

Before outlining the contribution of linguistic anthropology and discursive psychology to our theoretical understanding of identity processes, we consider current psychological perspectives. Undoubtedly, developmental psychology has for long been the chief disciplinary reference for theoretical and empirical work on identity. We then provide empirical illustration and further support to situated and interactional understandings of identity processes by presenting some analyses of data extracts from an interview study of families with adolescent children. In the final section of the paper we discuss the potential of interdisciplinary approaches to identity processes, both from a theoretical and methodological standpoint.

5.2 Psychological Perspectives on Adolescents' Identity Development

One of the core research topics in psychology is identity. In particular, developmental and social psychology have provided various theories to shed light on both the multifaceted components of self and identity and the phases entailed in the formation processes since early stages of childhood.

Despite the ample theorizing, it is not easy to find a commonly agreed upon definition of identity in psychology; two assumptions can however be considered as traditionally underpinning general notions of identity:

(a) identity emerges from the progressive *self-other differentiation* in the interplay between individual characteristics and multiple relational contexts (e.g., Bronfenbrenner 1979; Ford and Lerner 1992; Vygotsky 1978);
(b) *adolescence* is a crucial developmental phase for identity formation and consolidation (Erikson 1968; Marcia 1980, 1987).

5.2.1 Individual-Contexts Interplay in Human Development

The interplay between individual and contexts in human development is a foundational issue in psychology (Bronfenbrenner 1979; Ford and Lerner 1992; Vygotsky 1978). Both in social and developmental psychology, children are conceived of as agents in the very social and psychological processes that shape their being and becoming. In these disciplines, the differentiation between self and others emerges as a process of construction of an *agentic self*.

The psychological conceptualization of agency has been largely influenced by Bandura's theorization, who elaborated a "psychology of human agency" founded on the notion of *self-efficacy*. Self-efficacy concerns the *belief* to have the power to influence and change life circumstances (Bandura 1997). Identity is created through the development of a sense of agentic continuity, that is, the development and maintenance of autonomy and control over time and situations. The role of sociocultural contexts (families, schools, society technological changes, etc.) in such developmental process is acknowledged but it is conceptualized in terms of environmental forces that influence the development of individual agency, fostering or limiting it to different degrees (Bandura 2006).

As highlighted by Zimmerman and Cleary (2006), the main focus of attention of Bandura's approach is kept on the individual's capacities and motivations to exert control *over* the context. In other words, it is the *belief* of being able to act as competent that will drive the individual to *act* as competent. In this view, the primacy of internal/cognitive dimensions emerges as opposed to the external/contextual dimensions.

A similar dichotomy can be traced in the psychosocial approaches of the last decade that have further developed the notion of agency giving particular attention to contemporary societal and cultural changes: what has been named "structures". According to Côté and Levine (2002) social actors function *in context* and, as such, they are never free from structures. Structures can play a role in either facilitating or impeding the possibility to behave in an agentic manner. Individual agency resides in the ability to utilize and transform these structures (Emirbayer and Mische 1998; Schwartz et al. 2005).

The definition of agency provided by these scholars is not far from Bandura's conceptualizations, as it mainly stresses cognitive dimensions: (a) one's responsibility for one's life course, (b) the belief that one is in control of one's decisions and is responsible for their outcomes, and (c) the confidence that one will be able to overcome obstacles that impede one's progress along one's chosen life course.

In a research study, Côté and Schwartz (2002) built a composite measure of agency, consisting of self-esteem, purpose in life, ego strength, and internal locus of control. They found that these dimensions were positively related to identity achievement and negatively related to identity diffusion. In this definition, agency is considered as the facilitator of the development of a positive and coherent identity.

This brief review highlights that psychological studies on self and identity have developed a progressive interest for the notion of agency. This construct has often been operationalized in terms of cognitive dimensions concerned with self-esteem and locus of control. Contexts are conceived of as structures that may limit or favour agency. In this line, we see that what is theorized, in terms of *interplay* between individual dimensions and external structures, becomes instead operationalized in terms of *dichotomy*.

According to Bamberg (2010) empirical works in the domain of identity research are stalled in the 'agency-dilemma', that is, the contrast between self versus world or internal versus external. As pointed out in a recent and extensive cross-disciplinary review (Eteläpelto et al. 2013), the 'agency-dilemma' has been rarely made central in debates over identity in psychology. In the present paper, we endeavour to focus precisely on the agency-dilemma and provide empirical evidence that suggests how it can be unpacked and overcome.

5.2.2 Adolescence: A Crucial Period for Identity Development

In psychology there is a shared agreement on considering adolescence as a *transitional time* in which intense transformations in children's self and interpersonal relations occur. Family relationships in particular are substantially reorganized during this period: both parents and children participate in finding a new balance in terms of competences, power hierarchy, and interpersonal distances (Holmbeck 1996; Everri et al. 2014). Negotiation becomes an important developmental task: parents' claim to social conventions, adolescents' rejections of those claims, and their appeals to personal jurisdiction form an ongoing dialectic which leads to transformations in parental authority and intimacy (Coleman 2010; Kreppner and Ullrich 1998; Smetana 2011). In these dialectical exchanges, adolescents have the opportunity to explore autonomy and pursue their individuation.

The vast literature on the interaction between parents and adolescents has pointed out that an open and clear communication favours youngsters' identity exploration; parenting styles based on flexible control and protection together with moderate levels of monitoring allow adolescents to experiment with their increased independence while still keeping a connection with their families (Beyers and Grossens 2008; Claes et al. 2011; Everri et al. in press; Hartup and Laursen 1991; Laursen and Collins 1994; Stattin et al. 2011).

A small number of interesting works have analysed identity development as part of a wider family process embedded in specific patterns of family communication (Grotevant and Cooper 1985; Shapiro 1988). These pioneering studies have made the effort to analyse the communicative processes occurring between parents and children and link them with identity development during adolescence. Subsequent empirical works in the disciplinary realm of psychology have rarely pursued this line of investigation.

The *fil-rouge* running through the mainstream psychological literature on family communication and adolescence seems in fact to be characterized by a monolithic description of individuation processes: Adolescents have to "struggle" with parents to affirm their identity; parents from their part exert control and children oppose them. Adolescents can be agentic only when they contrast and transform a structure represented by parental authority and control. Identity development is therefore the result of conflicts, crises, and harsh confrontations with "constraining" adults.

In addition, a dated conception of identity formation as a coherent and stable achievement (Erikson 1968; Marcia 1980, 1987) seems to still underlie the mainstream psychological literature on family communication and adolescence. Undoubtedly, critical theory and feminist perspectives on subjectivity have not penetrated the discipline of psychology as deeply as they have anthropology and sociology. Only in recent papers developmental psychologists (e.g., Arnett et al. 2011; Zittoun 2012) have pointed out how the contemporary societal changes affecting the lives of children and families require a re-conceptualization of identity as a lifelong process based on *uncertainty* and *continual changes*.

In this paper, we draw closer attention to the processes entailed in identity development, to unearth their complexity and situatedness. In other words, we argue that by focusing on the communicative exchanges occurring between parents and children we can discern how multiple identities are contingently performed, invoked, contested and negotiated.

Recent studies (Everri et al. 2014; Molinari et al. 2010) have shown that adolescents make different experiences according to the communicative contexts experienced in their families. In families where all members engage in the exploration of emerging changes asserting new competences, sounding out hierarchies, and oscillating between closeness and distance, adolescents experiment from time to time with ways to oppose, challenge, or acknowledge parental roles. In other families where instead conversations among members are based on the parents' tendency to redefine the boundaries of the family hierarchy by affirming their controlling and normative role and setting the limits of distance and differentiation, adolescents tend to give up and conform to the family hierarchy and to the request for closeness. These different ways of communicating become observable in micro-adaptation processes occurring in everyday family conversations.

Other works on family interactions and conversations have documented that in these everyday and mutually constructed exchanges parents and children socialize with each other (Pontecorvo et al. 2001), negotiate family boundaries (Aronsson and Cekaite 2011), and manage conflicts (Arcidiacono and Bova 2011), family values, and morality (Ochs and Taylor 1992; Sterponi 2014).

Following the above considerations, in the next sections we draw on recent linguistic anthropological reflections on identity and discursive psychologists' theorizing on social positioning. These two approaches will set the theoretical foundations of our argument.

5.3 The Contribution of Linguistic Anthropology to the Study of Agency

Linguistic anthropology provides interesting theoretical insights that put under pressure the agency/structure dichotomy (Ahearn 2001) and nuance our understanding of identity construction processes during adolescence.

The studies carried out in linguistic anthropology have widely elaborated on the notion of agency (Duranti 2004; Mahmood 2001; Ochs 1992; Ortner 1996). Three core aspects can be identified in the anthropological definition of agency: (a) it has a co-constructive and interactive nature, (b) it is the organizing principle of identity processes, and (c) its manifestation occurs in discourses. These three aspects are discussed here with respect to a recent field of inquiry that has built a strict connection between agency and identity.

In particular, linguistic anthropologists Bucholtz and Hall (2005) have provided a comprehensive review of identity studies advocating a concept of identity anchored in interactions; these scholars propose five principles—Emergence, Positionality, Indexicality, Relationality, and Partialness—according to which identity emerges as an "intersubjectively achieved social and cultural phenomenon" (ibid 2005, p. 607). In this conceptualization, identity comprises the different positions that individuals *inhabit and perform* in their discursive interactions. Agency is defined as the organizing principle of social actions through which identity processes are accomplished. Consistently, Bucholtz and Hall (2005) argue that agency cannot be defined in terms of individual skills acquired by and located *within* a rational subject; agency is rather relational and *inter*-subjective in its nature. These scholars expand the "relationality principle" entailed in identity processes, suggesting developing further the idea of a "distributed agency" (Bucholtz and Hall 2005, p. 606) that is, the idea of a process of co-construction that is accomplished *in and through* linguistic interactions (Goodwin 1995; Ochs 1993).

These conceptualizations of identity and agency allow us to better explain that individual and contexts are inseparable and mutually constitutive, just as agency and structures are, in identity processes. According to linguistic anthropologists, sociocultural structures emerge and are transformed in the unfolding of social interaction. Structure and agency are therefore inseparable: agency implies a certain degree of control on the part of the subjects but this control is always constructed, enacted, and transformed in and through linguistic interactions. Language is the figurative site where the intertwinement of agency and structures becomes observable.

The focus on linguistic interactions suits well our interest in the study of identity co-construction during adolescence. In this line, we can redefine identity as an *interactional process emerging from discursive encounters* in which adolescents participate and through which they can claim, contest and reconstruct their agency and autonomy in relation to those of the others.

5.4 The Contribution of Discursive Psychology to the Study of Identity

The conceptualization of identity as an interactively constructed and constantly in motion process requires the adoption of an analytical approach to grasp what happens at a micro-level of interaction (Norris 2007). Interesting conceptual and methodological insights can be found in *social positioning theory* developed in the field of discursive psychology.

Discursive psychology is situated at the crossroad of social psychology and conversation analysis studies. Davies and Harré (1990) have pioneered this field, developing a line of studies grounded in the notion of social positioning. This construct refers to a discursive process through which social and psychological phenomena interpenetrate one another and through which individuals produce a diversity of selves (Harré and van Langenhove 1999). In discursive encounters participants take, resist, negotiate and assign positions by locating themselves and others with respect to different social categories or specific topics. Entailed in this conceptualization is the idea that multiple identities can be enacted and that such any particular identity is responsive to contextual conditions. These "discontinuities" in the production of selves are explained with reference to the fact that "multiple and contradictory discursive practices and the interpretations of those practices can be brought into being by speakers and hearers as they engage in conversations" (Davies and Harré 1990, p. 63).

The possibility to track the different positioning processes as parents and adolescents engage in conversations offers a productive methodological framework to grasp the ways in which their identities are co-constructed, interrelated and negotiated.

5.5 Data Corpus and Analytical Procedures

For the purpose of this paper, we selected two cases from a corpus of 40 video-recorded family interviews conducted by the first author. The data corpus pertained to a three-year research project aiming to study different aspects of family development during the adolescence transition of children aged 13–16 years (Everri 2010).

The researcher and the 40 families participating were upper-middle class Caucasians living in cities in a small region of northern Italy. Most families were traditional nuclear families (N = 34), while the others were either separated (N = 4) or step-parent families (N = 2).

The families were interviewed in their homes by two researchers: One conducted the interview, and the other dealt with the video recording. Prior to data collection, parents' informed consent and children's assent were obtained. Following the ethical norms defined by the APA (American Psychological Association), family members were informed of their right to stop the interview and videotaping at any time if they felt uncomfortable or tired.

The technique of the family interview has been widely illustrated in other works (see Everri 2011; Molinari et al. 2010); however, it is useful to mention here that this technique was partially borrowed from systemic family therapy and followed some principle of circular interviewing (Selvini Palazzoli et al. 1980; Tomm 1988): At the beginning of the interview, a series of questions were directed to the adolescent, who was asked to talk about his or her developmental changes (5–15 min). Then the interviewer involved all members in a conversation about the adolescent's and corresponding family's changes. In this phase of the interview (lasting about 30–40 min), each member was called upon to react to the others' points of view, thus developing a circular conversation on the topics raised by all members. Family conversations covered a range of issues pertaining to both individual participants (e.g., going to the disco, claiming more privacy, concerns on going out at night, etc.) and the family as a whole (negotiating holiday plans, defining a monthly allowance, setting the time to get back home at night, etc.). The average duration of family interviews was 57 min and the mean number of the conversational turns was 475.5.

For reason of space, we selected the cases and the excerpts that were indicative of the material as a whole. Three criteria were also taken into consideration when selecting the family cases: (a) The household composition: we selected families having more than one child, so that we could show more complex interactive dynamics; (b) The gender of the adolescent child: we chose two male adolescents presenting rather different characteristics; (c) The intelligibility of the discussed content: we selected cases in which family members talked about everyday issues, devoid of overly specific cultural references, so that the content was transparent to an international audience.

The selected cases were analysed adopting a microanalytical approach based on social positioning principles. Exemplar conversational extracts were identified according to the moments of the interview in which all family members were involved. These extracts will show how all participants in the interview—i.e., parents, adolescents, siblings, and the interviewer—contribute to creating discursive opportunities for the expression of adolescents' agency, and at times to foreclosing such opportunities. Transcript conventions are reported in the Appendix to this chapter.

5.6 The Family Cases

5.6.1 The Rossetti Family

The Rossetti family is composed of five members: mother, father, Giacomo, 15 years old, and two older brothers: Paolo, 30 years old, and Simone, 28 years old. Simone did not participate in the interview because he had moved out to cohabit with his partner.

The interview with this family was particularly long (84 min; 504 conversational turns), unfolding through lively discussions among parents, brothers and the adolescent, in addition to the exchanges with the interviewer.

The extract below (Transcript 5.1) corresponds to the initial segment of the interview after the presentations. The interviewer has just asked the adolescent Giacomo to talk about the changes he experienced in the last two years in terms of interests and aspirations; this question sparked a choral discussion among all family members present.

In this segment several interesting discursive phenomena enact a rather tense negotiation around the adolescent's identity and positionality within the family as well as the ongoing event of the interview. While the interviewer always addresses her questions to the adolescent, both parents contribute to the answer. It is worth

Transcript 5.1 Mother, Father, Giacomo, Interviewer (INT)

		English translation	Italian original version
1.	INT	when did this happen? (0.2) like last year? Two years ago?	e questo quando è capitato tipo l'anno scorso due anni fa?
2.	Giacomo	at the end of the middle school	fine delle scuole medie
3.	Father	no this year *((looks at the adolescent))*	no quest'anno *((guarda l'adolescente))*
4.	Giacomo	first year of high school	prima superiore
5.	Father	practically now *((looks at the adolescent)*	in pratica adesso *((guarda l'adolescente))*
6.	Mother	it's one year ago = one year	è un anno = è un anno
7.	Father	it started with this school year	da questo anno scolastico
8.	Mother	on Saturday	il sabato eh
9.	INT	so what do you do now? do you go out?	quindi adesso cosa fai? esci?
10.	Father	not to the disco! They go out to have a pizza	non in discoteca esce che vanno in pizzeria
11.	Giacomo	<u>unfortunately</u> not to the disco!	purtroppo non in discoteca
12.	Father	maybe to go out it seems to go out to be free! *((looks at the adolescent))*	magari uscire sembra uscire per essere liberi *((guarda l'adolescente))*
13.	Mother	to go out with friends *((looks at the adolescent))*	andare in compagnia *((guarda l'adolescente))*
14.	Giacomo	to have a pizza on Saturday night	mangiare una pizza il sabato sera
15.	Mother	and brum = brum *((makes a gesture as to accelerate on a motorbike and looks at the adolescent))*	e brum = brum *((fa un gesto come accelerare sulla moto e guarda l'adolescente))*
16.	INT	what was mom referring to?	cos'è quello che diceva la mamma?
17.	GIACOMO	the passion for motorbikes	la passione per i motori
18.	FATHER	exaggerated!	esagerata!
19.	INT	did you always have this-?	ma l'hai sempre avuta questa-?
20.	Giacomo	I got it from my older brother *((looks at his brother))*	l'ho presa dal fratello maggiore *((guarda il fratello))*

(continued)

Transcript 5.1 (continued)

		English translation	Italian original version
21.	Father	[it's a virus = a virus	[è un virus = è un virus!
22.	Mother	[this is an obsession! *((looks at the adolescent))*	[questa malattia *((guarda l'adolescente))*
23.	INT	what does it mean this interest? is it something new or something you had since you were a child?	cosa vuol dire questo interesse si è scatenato ad un certo punto o ce l'hai avuto fin da piccolo?
24.	Giacomo	well maybe it is something I had since I was a child. when I was only 3 I used to take my bike brakes apart	ma forse ce l'ho avuto fin da piccolo già a tre anni smontavo i freni della bicicletta
25.	Mother	well you were even younger you were not 3! he used to have a small bicycle and he used to turn it upside down and then he would take his bike brakes apart and then reassemble them again. He was a very little child	ma eri più piccolo forse non li avevi tre anni la prima biciclettina la capovolgeva e poi smontava i freni davanti li aveva solo davanti la prima biciclettina li toglieva poi li rimetteva e faceva così piccolissimo
26.	INT	now do you have a scooter? did they buy you one early?	ce l'hai il motorino adesso te l'hanno comprato subito?
27.	Giacomo	yes = yes my brother Simone bought it for me	si = sì me l'ha preso il fratello Simone

Giacomo's changes

noticing that they do so (1) with no dispreference marking, that is, without framing their interventions as shifting the participation framework. In a sense, they operate as if it is legitimate that they respond to queries pertaining and addressed to their adolescent son; (2) with providing information that delegitimizes the content of the adolescent's answer. The adolescent marks his individual characteristics or achievements as family traits, which were passed to him by his older siblings. In a sense, while presenting himself as having defined preferences and aspirations, the adolescent is framing them as belonging to the family or at least as being shared with his siblings. The inheritance is reframed in negative terms by the father as a virus and by the mother as an obsession.

In other parts of the interview, the same dynamics is observable. The next extract (Transcript 5.2) revolves around the Giacomo' s restrictions for going out with friends.

From the analysis of this second extract, a sequence of discursive moves can be observable through which the adolescent is positioned as the "child of the family". From the beginning, the mother directs Giacomo on what he should tell the

Transcript 5.2 Mother, Father, Giacomo, Interviewer (INT)

		English translation	Italian original version
1.	Mother	*((looks at the adolescent))* tell her that your friends used to have more freedom as they have younger parents. [this was an issue	*((guarda l'adolescente))* perché digli anche che i tuoi amici avevano più libertà con i genitori più giovani. c'è stata [questa cosa qua
2.	Father	[he came that we were old	[eh è arrivato un po' tardi
3.	Mother	[we were over forty	[è arrivato che avevamo over quaranta
4.	Giacomo	my parents are <u>too old</u>	i genitori sono rimasti più <u>indietro</u>
5.	Mother	hey! no!	opplà! no! eh?
6.	Father	we actually felt more experienced we already knew what happened in the discos	ci sentivamo più esperti sapevamo gia' cosa capita nelle discoteche
7.	Mother	we had more experience because of the other kids. Giacomo's friends used to go out when they were younger than him, they used to come here and pick him up 'cause they did not have this problem	avevamo più esperienza per via degli altri figli. Invece gli amici della stessa età della sua scuola hanno incominciato ad uscire prima venivano loro a prenderlo perche' loro non avevano questo problema
8.	Giacomo	freedom! *((whispering))*	la liberta'! *((sospirando))*
9.	Mother	he could not say yes I come with you because we wanted them to come here to pick him up	non poteva dire sì esco vengo anch'io noi volevamo che venissero qui per prenderlo
10.	Giacomo	they at least tried to come to take me out *((in a low voice))*	ci provavano a venire per portarmi fuori! *((a bassa voce))*
11.	MOTHER	it's different when you are a young parent	per i genitori più giovani e' diverso
12.	INT	and you Giacomo, how did you feel?	e tu Giacomo come ti sentivi?
13.	Mother	well, it's not that prohibitions ruled (0.3)	non e' che c'era il proibizionismo, eh? (0.3)
14.	INT	do you agree Giacomo?	sei d'accordo Giacomo?

(continued)

Transcript 5.2 (continued)

		English translation	Italian original version
15.	Father	no was never presented as a definitive NO! It was suggested to him to go out with a little of-	no e' mai stato visto come un NO assoluto! si consigliava di uscire con un pochino di-
16.	MOTHER	yeah, we wanted to know with whom he was going out as we were a bit worried and advised him to be careful	ma si volevamo sapere con chi andava perche' eravamo un po' preoccupati e gli dicevamo di stare attento

Giacomo's restrictions

interviewer (turn 1). Giacomo takes the floor (turn 4) but does not follow his mother's prompt. Nevertheless he aligns with his parents with a provocative confirmation of their assessment regarding their age. Both mother and father react by taking over the lead of the conversation, as to ward off the threat of Giacomo's intervention: the mother rejects Giacomo's assessment and the father rephrases this challenge as being "more experienced" instead of old, which is further elaborated by the mother. Afterward, Giacomo interjects with an emphatic plea for freedom (turn 8) but once more his voice goes unheard: while the parents are reporting their reflective stance with respect to decisions regarding Giacomo and their attempts to involve Giacomo in those decisions, in the present unfolding of the interview Giacomo's voice is not given much space or legitimacy. Even the interviewer's attempts (turns 12 and 14) to grasp the adolescent's opinion are displaced by parents' responses.

These analyses reveal that the adolescent's identity is entangled in a tight matrix of relational expectations. The parents display a sense of entitlement to speak *about* the adolescent and *for* the adolescent. They do so often through oppositional stances that further negate the rights of the adolescent to speak for himself. The adolescent's sense of self, on the other hand, in fact relatedly perhaps, seems very much dependent on his being part of a family, with proclivities and passions that are transmitted from generation to generation and become a family trait.

5.6.2 The Follini Family

The Follini family is composed of four members: mother, father, Roberto, 14 years old, and Chiara, 8 years old. This family interview was concise in terms of conversational turns (367) but still long in terms of duration (74 min) as long pauses segmented the discursive exchanges.

The extract presented below (Transcript 5.3) refers to the central part of the interview, when the researchers involve all family members in the discussion to activate circular reflections on the issues brought up by the adolescent. In this segment, the adolescent's increasingly introverted behaviour is discussed.

Transcript 5.3 Mother, Father, Roberto, Interviewer (INT)

		English translation	*Italian original version*
1.	INT	*((towards the mother))* do you feel the same as before?	*((verso la madre))* lei si sente più uguale a prima?
2.	Mother	absolutely (0.2) I mean I have the feeling (0.3) I mean we manage to have good interactions (0.2) the fact is that sometimes he displays this stubborn silence and it bothers me 'cause I can't access it and I can't make him move away from it	assolutamente (0.2) cioè ho feeling cioè io (0.3) riusciamo ad interagire bene ecco (0.2) è che alle volte lui ha questo mutismo ed io non riesco ad entrare proprio lui e mi disturba perché non riesco a smuoverlo
3.	Roberto	well we are two different persons anyway (0.2) aren't we? *((looks at his mother))*	siamo comunque due persone diverse (0.2) eh? *((guarda la madre))*
4.	Mother	mother and son yes but actually each one has his own qualities and identity	mamma e figlio è però giustamente ognuno ha le sue qualità e la sua identità
5.	Roberto	besides, you know everything about me	a parte che sai tutto tu di me
6.	Mother	no I don't want to know everything about you	no non voglio sapere tutto
7.	Father	well she wants to know everything you want to do also when you are out of home	ah lei vuole sapere anche quello che vuoi fare anche quando sei fuori casa
8.	Mother	that's not true (0.3) but you don't ever discuss with me if you have either sad or cheerful moments	non è vero (0.3) però se tu hai dei momenti di sconforto o di gioia non me ne parli
9.	Roberto	well I do not always know how one thing connects to the other or the reason why I am sad (0.2)	ma non so sempre una cosa a cosa è legato o il motivo per cui sono sconfortato (0.2)
10.	Mother	*((nods))*	*((annuisce))*

Roberto's introverted behaviour

In this segment, personal difficulties and unfulfilled desires are expressed by both parents and the adolescent. Each family member in this exchange acknowledges the other's difficulties as legitimate by offering a response to their expression. The mother initially appeals to her difficulty in knowing more from her son thus letting emerge her concern for losing the mother-son relationship. Afterwards she modifies her position: she first acknowledges and legitimates the increasing mother-son differences and then justifies her worries. The adolescent uses a tag question for gaining agreement, responds by providing argumentations for his "stubborn silence", and appeals to a secure familial relation when he uses the expression "besides, you know me", thus stressing that the mother already has all the information she needs. Also in the last turn, Roberto provides an explanation for his silence, reconfirming the differentiation from his mother. The adolescent therefore characterizes what the mother wants from him as a casual explanation for his mood of silence. The interactive sequence ends with the mother legitimizing Roberto's stance and account through a nonverbal expression of agreement (nodding).

The father and sister keep a peripheral position in these exchanges however, in other parts of the interview, they intervene in the collective negotiation of the adolescent's identity. Despite the young age (8 years), the sister intervenes actively to punctuate some issues about her older brother, as shown in the next excerpt (Transcript 5.4).

The segment presented below is still centred on the adolescents' changes, specifically his silence and isolation from the rest of the family.

Here, the mother re-proposes the issue of her son's isolation, amplified by the little sister who portrays her brother as the one threatening the family unity. The father aligns with the mother in positioning Roberto as a typical adolescent, but he also acknowledges a similarity between his own behaviour and attitudes and the ones manifested by his son lately (turn 6). Similarly, the mother stresses her resemblance with Roberto's characteristics however she anchors them in the past, namely to her own experience as an adolescent (turn 7). The different positions articulated by the parents offer the adolescent multiple opportunities for meanings and interpretations in the process of structuring his identity. Roberto retains his agency through systematic accounts of his criticized behaviours: his responses justify the conduct that was portrayed as problematic, i.e. the adolescent's introversion and isolation from the family. As such they constitute acts of individual affirmation and self-determination.

All together, these extracts show a family in which members affirm their subjectivity and stances and each position is regarded as legitimate, hence respected, even if it is sometimes in conflict with positions, desires and expectations of other family members.

Transcript 5.4 Mother, Father, Roberto, Sister, Interviewer (INT)

		English translation	Italian original version
1.	Mother	I noticed that he tends to be more isolated lastly I mean he goes in his bedroom to listen music (0.3) I mean I think he needs more privacy than before	io ho notato che ha l'esigenza cioè tende ad isolarsi rispetto a prima cioè non so va nella stanzetta ascolta la musica (0.3) cioè ha bisogno più di suoi spazi che ho notato rispetto a prima
2.	Sister	it's true because when we all together in the kitchen he goes in his bedroom with his headphones	si è vero perché molto spesso quando noi tutti siamo in cucina lui va nella sua stanza con le cuffie
3.	Mother	yes he tends to be more isolated (0.3) maybe this is only my feelings so it's not like that	si tende magari un po' di più ad isolarsi (0.3) ma magari è una mia sensazione magari non è così
4.	Father	yes it's true	si è vero
5.	Roberto	well this is your idea!	mah se lo dite voi!
6.	Father	maybe we also do that and we are not aware of that	ma magari anche noi facciamo così e non ce ne accorgiamo
7.	mother	I actually used to do that too	in effetti se ci penso lo facevo anch'io
8.	Father	right we also used to be like you	guarda infatti che anche noi eravamo così
9.	Mother	it's also true that he doesn't speak a lot lately	è vero che di suo dice un po' poco adesso
10.	Roberto	don't I speak? Well (0.2) I don't have big secrets or things to hide though	non dico niente? mah (0.2) non ho d'altronde dei grossi segreti da nascondere per ciò
11.	Mother	I don't want to know your secrets though	no ma non sono i segreti che io voglio sapere anzi!
12.	Sister	actually you are not very open!	te non sei molto aperto!
13.	Mother	well besides this I think that maybe this is right (0.2) it's typical for his age	no ma al di la' di tutto io penso che sia anche giusto così (0.2) è anche legato all'età
14.	Father	then some feelings are sometimes difficult to tell to your parents	e poi ci sono ci sono certe emozioni che difficilmente riesci a raccontare con i genitori alle volte

Roberto's silence and isolation

5.7 Discussion and Conclusions

Our analysis has shown that the adolescent's agency and autonomy emerge as interactional outcomes—neither developing solely from within the individual nor being entirely infused into the growing family member by the adults. Identity processes are always interpersonally stipulated and negotiated. Indeed, the co-construction of adolescent agency and autonomy is not a linear process, devoid of tension and ambivalence. In the examples presented in this chapter, parents and children positioned themselves and each other through opposing and challenging stances. The interactive processes, in which family members engaged, however, drove them toward the construction of two quite different interactional configurations.

In the Rossetti family, we observed an interactive process that we named *foreclosure*: the adolescent's autonomy and agency emerged as a collective process in which everybody (including the adolescent) converged on the idea that Giacomo was not ready to be acknowledged as autonomous and independent. Similarly, the parents were not ready to 'let him go', as indicated by the repeated manoeuvres of positioning themselves as protective and controlling caregivers.

In the Follini family, on the other hand, the adolescent's agency and autonomy were invoked and legitimated. While providing a *figurative space* for the mutual acknowledgment of different positions in the unfolding interaction, the adolescent had the opportunity to contest the way he was positioned without being 'foreclosed'. The legitimacy of Roberto's autonomy was in fact negotiated: the mother initially expressed concern for the adolescent's increasing introversion; when the adolescent provided accounts for it, she stepped back and acknowledged Roberto's need to differentiate from his parents.

In conclusion, our analyses illuminate the dynamic coming into being of individual identity and the intertwinement of subjectivities in family relationships. Deeply situated in interaction, mobilized strategically to align or differentiate personal positioning and stances, agency and autonomy are always an interpersonal matter. By unearthing the highly contingent and ephemeral nature of these constructs, this paper has offered empirical illustration to critical theorists' insights on the performative and fragmented constitution of identity (Bucholtz and Hall 2010; Butler 1990).

We hope that our study has also provided a compelling illustration of the value of bridging different disciplinary perspectives on human development, particularly by deploying discourse analytic methods in developmental research on adolescence and family processes.

Appendix

Transcript Conventions

(0.3)	Pause in seconds
.	A full stop indicates a pause longer than 0.3 s
unfortunately	An underlined word means emphasis on that word
Yes [I think [but I	Simultaneous talk (overlap)
–	Truncated word or interruption
((looks at his brother))	Double parentheses indicate non verbal behavior
=	No break or delay between the words connected

References

Ahearn, L. (2001). Language and agency. *Annual Review of Anthro-Pology, 30*, 109–37.

Arcidiacono, F., & Bova, A. (2011). Argumentative strategies for conflict management and resolution in Italian and Swiss families. *Procedia-Social and Behavioral Sciences, 30,* 1385–1389.

Arnett, J., Kloep, M., Hendry, L. B., & Tanner, J. L. (2011). Debating emerging adulthood. Stage or process? Oxford: Oxford University Press.

Aronsson, K., & Cekaite, A. (2011). Activity contracts and directives in everyday family politics. *Discourse & Society, 2,* 1–18.

Bamberg, M. (2010). Who am I? Narration and its contribution to self and identity. *Theory and Psychology, 21,* 1–22.

Bandura, A. (1997). *Self-efficacy: The exercise of control.* New York: Freeman.

Bandura, A. (2006). Toward a psychology of human agency. *Perspectives on Psychological Science, 1,* 164–180.

Beyers, W., & Grossens, L. (2008). Dynamics of perceived parenting and identity formation in late adolescence. *Journal of Adolescence, 31,* 165–184.

Bronfenbrenner, U. (1979). *The ecology of human development.* Cambridge: Harvard University Press.

Bucholtz, M., & Hall, K. (2005). Identity and interactions: A sociocultural linguistic approach. *Discourse Studies, 7,* 585–614.

Bucholtz, M., & Hall, K. (2010). Locating identity in language. In C. Llamas & D. Watt (Eds.), *Language and identities* (pp. 18–28). Edinburgh: Edinburgh University Press.

Butler, J. (1990). *Gender trouble: Feminism and the subversion of identity.* London: Routledge.

Claes, M., Perchec, C., Miranda, D., Benoit, A., Bariaud, F., Lanz, M., et al. (2011). Adolescents' perceptions of parental practices: A cross-national comparison of Canada, France, and Italy. *Journal of Adolescence, 34,* 225–238.

Coleman, J. (2010). *The nature of adolescence* (IVth ed.). New York: Routledge.

Côté, J. E., & Levine, C. G. (2002). *Identity formation, agency, and culture: A social psychological synthesis.* Mahwah, NJ: Lawrence Erlbaum.

Côté, J. E., & Schwartz, S. J. (2002). Comparing psychological and sociological approaches to identity: Identity status, identity capital, and the individualization process. *Journal of Adolescence, 25,* 571–586.

Davies, B., & Harré, R. (1990). Positioning: The discursive production of selves. *Journal for the Theory of Social Behaviour, 20,* 44–63.
Duranti. (2004). Agency in language. In: A. Duranti (Ed.), *A companion in linguistic anthropology* (pp. 451–473). Blackwell, Malden, MA.
Emirbayer, M., & Mische, A. (1998). What is agency? *The American Journal of Sociology, 103,* 962–1023.
Erikson, E. H. (1968). *Identity: Youth and crisis*. New York: Norton.
Eteläpelto, A., Vähäsantanen, K., Hökkä, P., & Paloniemi, S. (2013). What is agency? Conceptualizing professional agency at work. *Educational Research Review, 10,* 45–65.
Everri, M. (2010). *Families under the microscope. Observing interactional processes in family mictrotransition.* Doctoral thesis, Dspace, http://hdl.handle.net/1889/1457. Accessed 1 April 2016.
Everri, M. (2011). Le microtransizioni nelle famiglie con figli adolescenti. Un gioco di equilibri. Nucleo monotematico: Uno sguardo triadico alla video-analisi dei processi interattivi. Teorie, metodi e linee di ricerca. Giornale Italiano di Psicologia dello Sviluppo [The mictrotransitions in families with adolescent children: A game of balance. Special issue: A triadic look at the video-analysis of interactive processes. Theory, methods, and research lines. *Italian Journal of Developmental Psychology*] *99*, 91–99.
Everri, M., Fruggeri, L., & Molinari, L. (2014). Microtransitions and the dynamics of family functioning. *Integrative Psychological and Behavioral Science, 48,* 61–78.
Everri, M., Mancini, T., & Fruggeri, L. (in press). Disentangling parental monitoring: The role of family communication in achieving parental knowledge. Psicologia Sociale.
Ford, D. L., & Lerner, R. M. (1992). *Developmental systems theory: An integrative approach.* Newbury Park, CA: Sage.
Goodwin, C. (1995). Co-Constructing meaning in conversations with an aphasic man. *Research on Language in Social Interaction, 28*, 233–60.
Grotevant, H. D., & Cooper, C. R. (1985). Patterns of interaction in family relationships and the development of identity exploration in adolescence. *Child Development, 56,* 415–428.
Harré, R., & van Langenhove, L. (1999). *Positioning theory*. Oxford: Blackwood.
Hartup, W. W., & Laursen, B. (1991). Relationships as developmental contexts. In R. Cohen, & A. W. Siegel (Eds.), *Context and development* (pp. 253–279). NJ: Erlbaum Hillsdale.
Holmbeck, N. G. (1996). A model of family relational transformations during the transition to adolescence: Parent-adolescent conflict and adaptation. In J. A. Graber, J. Brooks-Gunn, & A. C. Petersen (Eds.), *Transitions through adolescence. Interpersonal domains and context* (pp. 36–65). Mahwah, NJ: Erlbaum.
Kreppner, K., & Ullrich, M. (1998). Talk to mom and dad, and listen to what is in between. In M. Hofer, P. Noack, & J. Youniss (Eds.), *Verbal interaction and development in families with adolescents* (pp. 83–108). Greenwich, CT: Ablex.
Laursen, B., & Collins, W. A. (1994). Interpersonal conflict during adolescence. *Psychological Bulletin, 115,* 197–209.
Mahmood, S. (2001). Feminist theory, embodiment, and the docile agent: Some reflections on the Egyptian Islamic revival. *Cultural Anthropology, 16,* 202–236.
Marcia, J. E. (1980). Identity in adolescence. In J. Andelson (Ed.), *Handbook of adolescent psychology* (pp. 159–187). New York: Wiley.
Marcia, J. E. (1987). The identity status approach to the study of ego identity development. In T. Honess & K. Yardley (Eds.), *Self and identity: Perspectives across the lifespan*. New York: Routledge.
Molinari, L., Everri, M., & Fruggeri, L. (2010). Family micro-transitions: Observing the process of change in families with adolescent children. *Family Process, 49,* 236–250.
Norris, S. (2007). The micropolitics of personal national and ethnicity identity. *Discourse & Society, 18,* 653–674.
Ochs, E. (1992). Indexing gender. In A. Duranti & C. Goodwin (Eds.), *Rethinking context: Language as an interactive phenomenon* (pp. 335–358). Cambridge: Cambridge University Press.

Ochs, E. (1993). Constructing social identity: A language socialization perspective. *Research on Language and Social Interaction, 26,* 287–306.
Ochs, E., & Taylor, C. (1992). Family narrative as political activity. *Discourse & Society, 3,* 301–340.
Ortner, S. B. (1996). *Making gender: The politics and erotics of culture.* Boston: Beacon Press.
Pontecorvo, C., Fasulo, A., & Sterponi, L. (2001). Mutual apprentices: The making of parenthood and childhood in family dinner conversations. *Human Development, 44,* 340–361.
Schwartz, S. J., Côté, J. E., & Arnett, J. J. (2005). Identity and agency in emerging adulthood: Two developmental routes in the individualization process. *Youth & Society, 37,* 201–229.
Selvini Palazzoli, M., Boscolo, L., Cecchin, G., & Prata, G. (1980). Hypothesizing—Circularity—Neutrality: Three guidelines for the conductor of the session. *Family Process, 19,* 3–12.
Shapiro, E. R. (1988). Individual change and family development: Individuation as a family process. In C. J. Falicov (Ed.), *Family transitions. Continuity and change over the life cycle* (pp. 159–180). New York: The Guilford Press.
Smetana, J. G. (2011). *Adolescents, families, and social development: How adolescents construct their worlds.* West Sussex, England: Wiley.
Stattin, H., Persson, S., Burk, W., & Kerr, M. (2011). Adolescents' perceptions of the democratic functioning in their families. *European Psychologist, 16,* 32–42.
Sterponi, L. (2014). Caught red-handed: How Italian parents engage children in moral discourse and action. In C. Wainryb & H. Recchia (Eds.), *Talking about right and wrong: Parent-child conversations as contexts for moral development* (pp. 122–143). Cambridge: Cambridge University Press.
Tomm, K. (1988). Interventive interviewing: Part III. Intending to ask lineal, circular, strategic, or reflexive questions? *Family Process, 27,* 1–15.
Vygotsky, L. S. (1978). *Mind in society: The development of higher psychological processes.* Cambridge: Harvard University Press.
Zimmerman, B. J., & Cleary, T. J. (2006). Adolescents' development of personal agency: The role of self-efficacy beliefs and self-regulatory skill. In F. Pajares & T. Urdan (Eds.), *Self-efficacy beliefs of adolescents* (pp. 45–70). Greenwich, CT: Information Age Publishing.
Zittoun, T. (2012). On the emergence of the subject. *Integrative Psychological and Behavioral Science, 46,* 259–273.

Author Biographies

Marina Everri is *Marie Curie Research Fellow at the Department of Psychological and Behavioural Science, London School of Economics*. Her research studies focus on the interactive processes of families when dealing with adolescents' changes. Pursuing her interest in transdisciplinary approaches, she is currently working on the analysis of communicative practices in families with adolescent children considering the mediating role of Information and Communication Technologies (ICTs). She is also a systemic family therapist.

Laura Sterponi is Associate Professor of *Language Literacy and Culture at the Graduate School of Education, University of California, Berkeley*. Merging her training in developmental psychology and applied linguistics, she has developed a research program on the role of language and literacy practices in children's education and development. Her studies have examined communicative practices in both typical and atypical children (children with autism). She publishes extensively in language, development, and education journals.

Chapter 6
Rethinking Identity in Adult Language Learning Classrooms

Jenny Rosén

6.1 Introduction

Transcript 6.1: (A—Ahmed, T—Teacher)

1	A:	hola hola cómo estás señorita hon kan ö[ö	hola hola cómo estás señorita she can u[uh
2	T:	[hola sta	[hola sta
3	A:	nää hola cómo estás	no hola cómo estás
4	T:	hola cómo estás å vilket språk ä de [ä de pakistanska	hola cómo estás and which language is that [is it Pakistanish
5	A:	[spanska nä spanska	[Spanish no Spanish
6	T:	ä de spanska[vilken tur	is it Spanish [how lucky
7	A:	[ja hon kan spanska ja	[yes she knows Spanish yes
8	T:	hon kan [spanska	she knows [Spanish
9	A:	[ja	[yes
10	T:	å du kan spanska också	and you know Spanish too
11	A:	ah	ah
12	T:	hola estás	hola estás

The interaction between a teacher, Vincent, and a student, Ahmed, displayed in Transcript 6.1, illustrates how participants in a Swedish language learning classroom use their (trans)linguistic resources to construct meaning about the world and who they are in it. The talk-in-interaction between the teacher and Ahmed took place in one of five classrooms included in an ethnographic study of an adult Swedish language learning program called SFI (Swedish For Immigrants). From an ethnographic and a sociocultural point of view, the aim of the study presented here is to examine the doing of identity positions in these language-focused classrooms. As noted by Pavlenko and Lantolf, language learning can be seen as "a struggle of concrete socially constituted and always situated beings to participate in the sym-

J. Rosén (✉)
Department of Language Education, Stockholm University,
Dalarna University, Falun, Sweden
e-mail: jenny.rosen@isd.su.se

S. Bagga-Gupta et al. (eds.), *Identity Revisited and Reimagined*,
DOI 10.1007/978-3-319-58056-2_6

bolically mediated lifeworld [...] of another culture" (2000: 155). Thus, language learning involves the investment of one's identity (Norton 2000) as well as a transformation of that identity, as students negotiate their position in relation to the community of practice in which they seek to participate (Kanno and Norton 2003). In other words, learning a new language involves a transformation of identities, since people negotiate not only who they are, but also who they have been and who they become.

Hence, the following paper builds upon the "boom of publications linking identity and SLA" (Second Language Acquisition) during the last two decades, as identified by Block (2007b: 864). The fluidity of identity as socially constructed and/or performed through language has been highlighted by many researchers as part of a "linguistic turn" in social science and humanities (Block 2007a; Butler [1990]1999, 1997; Weedon 2004). A number of studies have highlighted the importance of identity work with regard to social categories such as gender, ethnicity and age in language-learning processes (e.g. Norton 2000; Pavlenko et al. 2001). Using a post-structuralist approach, these researchers have highlighted the agency of learners in the processes of learning a new language and thus the doing of identities in new communities of practice. However, Block (2014: 18) argues that there is "a tendency to prime agency over structure in research on language and identity, relating this tendency to the rise of individualization as an all-pervasive concept in late modern societies". Hence, the aim of this paper is to explore how participants in a Swedish language-learning program use their (multi)linguistic resources in the negotiation of identity in general and gender and national belonging in particular through a multi-scaled approach (Bagga-Gupta 2014b; Hult 2010; Scollon and Scollon 2004), first zooming into the national policy of the SFI program and, later on, into interaction in one SFI classroom.

In the Swedish context, several ethnographic studies have involved women with a limited educational background, addressing the specific challenges of this social category in SLL (Carlson 2002; Lundgren 2005). Yet, treating both the social category of women and the target language (Swedish) as rather stable, these studies have not addressed how gender, sexuality and national belonging intersect and how the participants use their linguistic resources in order to negotiate these categorizations. Language education as well as language planning is performative (Butler [1990]1999; 1997; Milani 2004), producing categories (i.e. second language learner, native speaker, Spanish speaker) through which individuals organize their "ways of being" in the world. Moreover, languages are not separated as either "mother tongue" or "target language", since participants in the language learning classroom use the linguistic resources available to them, often in an integrated manner, in translanguaging practices (Canagarajah 2011; García 2009; García and Wei 2014).

The present study combines a sociocultural framework emphasizing the relation between learning, participation and identity (Wenger 1998) with a post-structural and intersectional understanding of identity (Butler 1997; Weedon 2004; McCall 2005; Lykke 2003, 2005).

In the following section, the empirical material of the study will be presented. It is followed by the theoretical framework, as different approaches towards the doing of identity are brought forward and discussed. The analysis and the findings of the study are presented in two sections. In the first section, national policy of the SFI program during the period 1986–2012 is analyzed. In the second section, the interaction from an SFI classroom is analyzed. Finally, concluding remarks are presented.

6.2 Empirical Data

The study presented here draws upon empirical data from the project entitled Categorization of Identities and Communication (CIC).[1] Project CIC targets the social practices and discourses that frame a language-learning course designed for adult immigrants in Sweden. Heller points out that the "power of ethnographic sociolinguistics is precisely its ability to follow social processes across time and space, and to see how agency and structure engage each other under specific political economic conditions" (2011: 10). In order to illuminate social processes across time and space, the project includes a wide range of empirical data, including historical text material such as curricula, commission reports, public inquiries, laws, teacher manuals from 1965 to 2011, and approximately 95 h of audio and video material and ethnographic field notes. The audio and video material, as well as the field notes, were created during observations in a learning center for the SFI program.[2]

The interactional data analyzed in the study was created during a ten-week ethnographic field study at a learning center for SFI located in Sweden. The researcher participated in the different activities both inside and outside of the classrooms, and data was created mainly by audio recordings and field notes. The study draws upon material from one of the five classrooms included in the CIC project. The classroom from which the material has been chosen differs from the other four classrooms, since both teacher and students used a number of linguistic varieties in the classroom. While teachers in the four other classrooms tried to implement a "Swedish-only policy" to various degrees, the teacher in the fifth classroom (analyzed in this paper) not only tolerated other language varieties in the classroom but also used them himself (Rosén and Bagga-Gupta 2015).

Members in the typical SFI classroom include 10–20 people categorized as adult immigrants with diverse language experiences and cultural backgrounds. The students in the classroom studied came from Iraq, Somalia, Thailand, and Serbia, and had a limited educational background. They had been studying at the learning center for a period of time ranging from a few weeks to a year and participated in the lower level language course (Course B). Every class had one teacher who taught the students until they were ready to move up to the next level.

---

[1]See www.ju.se/ccd.

[2]See Rosén (2013) for more on the empirical data.

6.3 Theoretical Framework

6.3.1 From Being to Doing Identity

For many people, (post)modern life is an existence filled with complexity, fluidity and instability, since boundaries regarding place and time are continuously being challenged. In a globalized world, people cross geographical borders of nation states legally or illegally, and by doing so, they not only navigate geographical spaces, but also become positioned by specific discourses into certain categories, such as *criminals*, *immigrants*, *asylum seekers*, *foreigners*, or *second language speakers*. Puzzlingly, in an era marked by globalization, societies continue to be dominated by the mindset of the nation-state constructing boundaries between insiders and outsiders, especially in the Global North where national identity is seen as constructed around one language.

A central and shared assumption in the different theoretical approaches applied in this paper is the notion that it is through language and in it that meaning about the world and who we are in it is constructed (Berger and Luckman 1966; Linell 1998, 2009; Säljö 2000; Wertsch 1998). Davies and Harré use the term *positioning* in order to highlight how identities are constructed in discourse. They argue that (Davies and Harré 1990: 47):

> We wish to defend the adoption of 'position' as the appropriate expression with which to talk about the discursive production of a diversity of selves.

The linguistic turn in social and educational sciences has stressed the importance of language and language use in relation to identity. Taking a social constructivist and post-structuralist point of departure, Pavlenko and Blackledge argue that (2004: 14):

> We see identity options as constructed, validated and offered through discourses available to individuals at a particular point in time and place.

In line with Pavlenko and Blackledge, the focus of the analysis presented in this paper is how individuals make meaning about the world and who they are in it, through the linguistic resources available. Language (as in specific discourses) constructs the means through which we constitute and negotiate our identities and is also essential in terms of language ideologies for how individuals values their and others' language resources. In other words, linguistic belonging is a category in relations to which we form our identities, such as bilingual or Arabic speaker. But it is also through languaging that identities are constituted and performed.

Research concerned with studying human action through interaction is rooted in both the work of Goffman (2009) as well as in ethnomethodology (Garfinkel 1984). Although Goffman highlighted the way in which individuals perform themselves in every-day life, his work is hardly ever mentioned in later theories on performativity. The work of Butler ([1990]1999, 1997) has brought attention to how individuals do gender through language. Butler (1997: 7) argues that language is thought of "mostly as agency—an act with consequences". Inspired by Butler's work, Pennycook (2004) argues for a shift in linguistic research from a postcolonial perception of language as fixed and systematic towards embracing performativity as a "ground for considering languages themselves from an anti-foundationalist perspective, whereby language use is an act of identity that calls that language into being" (Pennycook 2004: 17).

A need for intersectional analysis has been stressed by several feminist and postcolonial scholars, emphasizing how social categories such as gender, ethnicity, class, age and disability intersect (e.g., Crenshaw 1989, 1991; Lykke 2003, 2005, 2011; Marx Ferree 2011; Yuval-Davis 2011a, b; de los Reyes et al. 2005; de los Reyes and Mulinari 2005; Mohanty 2004). Thus, an intersectional perspective on identity is more than just adding identity categories to the analyses, since the core focus is on how identity categories intersect and co-construct one another. In using an intra-category approach (McCall 2005), the present study does not aim to deconstruct identity categories, but rather to examine how people negotiate meaning through categorizations in a specific educational context. By scrutinizing how people negotiate identity positions in social interactions, the construction of identities by the participants in the language-learning classroom is highlighted.

To conclude, identities can be perceived as a socially constructed, continuous narrative that individuals perform, interpret and express in acts, body look and language, but also limited in relation to which identity positions are available in the dominating discourse. Identity processes are both locally situated and distributed across time and space (Bagga-Gupta 2013, 2014a, b). The doing of identities concerns the fixation of an individual on one of the available identity positions, creating a shared understanding about who the individual "is". Identity work is made in the intersection between past, present and future, as individuals construct who they are in the present in relation to who they were in the past, while simultaneously reconstructing their social histories. Hence, identity work is about ongoing processes that traverse different spaces as well as time.

6.3.2 *Belonging*

Taking a sociocultural perspective as a point of departure, language, learning and identity are intertwined. Learning involves identity work, as individuals participate in different social practices, and therefore includes both action and belonging. Wenger argues that "participation shapes not only what we do, but also who we are and how we interpret what we do" and thus identity is "a way of talking about how learning changes who we are and creates histories of becoming in the context of our communities" (Wenger 1998: 4–5). Learning takes place through participation in social practices as we negotiate the meaning of our actions and who we are in relation to them. Hence, learning in the SFI program is not merely about acquisition of the Swedish language but also about participation in the SFI classroom and thus being positioned as an SFI-student, an immigrant, etc. (Rosén and Bagga-Gupta 2013).

From a dialogical perspective, in which the present is always in relation to the past and the future, participation is not just about which communities of practices one participates in right now but also the communities in which we imagine ourselves to participate, in both the past and the future. Kanno and Norton (2003), Norton (2001) highlight that learning is not only about participation in available communities of practice in the present but also about the imagined communities that the learner could think him/herself as belonging. They suggest that (Kanno and Norton 2003: 242):

> [...] these imagined communities are no less real than the ones in which learners have daily engagement and might even have a stronger impact on their current actions and investment.

Hence, the imagined communities that an individual sees him/herself as participating in make certain identity positions available. In relation to language learning, Norton argues that the investment in the target language of the learner needs to be seen in relation to imagined identities in the imagined communities of practices. The identity positions made available are not restricted to participation in the here and now. In other words, a language learner could be assumed to belong to a community of practice of language learners in the school setting, but also imagine him/herself to belong to a community of practice of bakers as soon as he/she finishes the language program.

Moreover, a dialogical approach to language (Bakhtin 1981; Linell 1998, 2009) stresses that meaning, including identity, is made in the interaction *between* participants, rather than expressed by them. From a dialogical approach, it is in language practices that meaning about who are we (our identity positions) are constituted, negotiated and transformed. Linell emphasizes the indispensable interplay between situated interactions and sociocultural resources and practices, finding that there is a form of "double dialogicality", as participants in a communicative activity are engaged both in the situated interaction and in sociocultural (trans-situational) praxis (Linell 2009: 52).

6.4 Findings and Analysis

6.4.1 The SFI Program—Zooming into National Policy

In his analysis of Swedish language policy, Milani (2004), using Butler's work on performativity, shows how national identity is produced in the emerging discourses of immigrants in Sweden during the 1970s. A number of institutions, including the SFI program, emerged as part of this discourse (Hyltenstam and Milani 2012; Rosén 2013; Rosén and Bagga-Gupta 2013) in order to "adjust" immigrants to the new language and Swedish society.

The SFI program has been an established educational form in Sweden since 1965 and is free of charge to people classified as immigrants. Classes are arranged on a municipal level, either through the adult education system run by a municipality or through private agencies. The overall aim of the program is described in the 2009 syllabus as follows: "Swedish Tuition for Immigrants is advanced language instruction aiming to give adult immigrants basic knowledge of the Swedish language. Students with a mother tongue other than Swedish should learn and develop a functioning second language. The education should provide language tools for communication and active participation in daily, societal and working life" (Skolverket 2012).

Although the SFI program is presented as an "advanced language instruction", the national curricula of the program serves as an essential artefact in which discourses about immigrant-ness and Swedish-ness are constructed. A number of researchers have examined how certain understandings of gender equality (between men and women) and a feminist consciousness are constructed as a central part of Swedish (and Nordic) national identity (de los Reyes et al. 2005; Honkanen 2008; Keskinen 2009; Magnusson et al. 2008; Towns 2002; Tuori 2007).

The analysis of the national curricula of the SFI program shows how such discourses are reproduced in describing the goals and aims of language learning. Table 6.1 shows the aims and goals related to norms and values in all curricula from 1986 (where a common national curriculum for the program was published) until 2012. In the first three curricula, norms and values specified as Swedish are explicitly stated as an important part of the instruction. Thus, certain values and norms are perceived as specifically Swedish, tied to the geopolitical space of Sweden. Furthermore, certain *values* are identified in the curricula, such as democracy, gender equality, gender roles, children's rights, law and juridical rights. Since these values are given specific attention in the curricula, they could be seen as a core of an imagined Swedish national identity and essentially different from the values and norms of the Other, the immigrant student. From 2002 onwards, no specific values and norms are stated in the curricula, which should be seen as a shift of the program towards a "pure language education", and in 2006 municipalities were given the responsibility for providing civic education to immigrants enrolled in integration programs.[3] The new program, which was separated from the language learning in SFI, was supposed to guarantee all participants an introduction to such fundamental values as democracy and individual equality; what it means to live in Swedish society; gender equality; and respect for the privacy of young people (Arbetsmarknadsdepartementet 2009a, 2010). In the suggested curriculum, students study a topic called "Creating a family in Sweden", which includes individual and collective perspectives on the family, the idea and development of the welfare state, including the idea behind separate taxes, preschool, and parental insurance, as well as laws concerning marriage and common law marriage, laws concerning LGBT (Lesbian, Gay, Bisexual, Transgender/Transsexual) -rights, gender equality in the constitution, international conventions, law, and in daily life (Arbetsmarknadsdepartementet 2010).

[3]In December 2010 the organization of the introduction program for newcomers in Sweden was reformed (Arbetsmarknadsdepartementet 2009b) and responsibility for it was transferred from the municipalities to the Swedish Public Employment Service.

Table 6.1 Values and norms in SFI curricula(SKOLFS 1994, 2002, 2009; Skolverket 2012; Skolöverstyrelsen 1986,1991)

1986	In the SFI program, people with different apprehensions and values come together. This can refer to philosophy of life, politics, social values or morality. It can also refer to a view of man and way of life. Teachers in the SFI program should be open for different values and opinions but at the same time explain the view on democracy in Swedish society. Teachers should also clarify the view on gender equality and gender roles in Swedish society	The instruction should include: labor market, work life and unions, education and career orientation, education programs and the educational system, gender equality, gender roles and social life
1991	In the SFI program, people with different apprehensions and values come together. This can refer to philosophy of life, politics, social values or morality. It can also refer to a view of man and way of life. The teacher should be open for different values and opinions but at the same time clarify the norms and values that are central in the Swedish culture and in the Swedish society and which importance these norms and values have in the labor market e.g. the work of institutions and in private life. The teacher should also clarify the view on democracy, children's rights, and equality between women and men in Swedish society	Thus, the instruction should include: labor market, work life and unions, education and career orientation, education programs and the educational system, law and juridical rights, children's rights, questions that concerns equality between women and men, social life as well as the norms and values that are central in the Swedish society
1994	To have in-depth knowledge about the Swedish society, law and juridical rights e.g. children's rights, about equality between men and women and about norms and values that are central in the Swedish society	
2002	Develop knowledge about democratic principles and work models and the value system in the Swedish society	
2006	Selection of material for studies of texts, conversations and discussion should be based on the course level and bring into focus topics that concern knowledge and understanding of the surrounding society	
2009	Students should also develop their intercultural competence by reflecting over their own cultural experiences, and comparing these with phenomena in daily, societal and working life in Sweden	
2012	Students should also develop their intercultural competence by reflecting over their own cultural experiences, and comparing these with phenomena in daily, societal and working life in Sweden	

6.4.2 Zooming in on the Language SFI Classroom

In the following section, an analysis of interaction in one of the five classrooms included in the project will be presented. The interaction will be displayed in transcript form both in the original language varieties and translated into English. In order to capture the complexity of the language use among participants as interrelated and cooperative rather than distinct and separated, shifts between language varieties are not marked in the transcript.

The interaction displayed in Transcript 6.2 took place during scheduled classroom activities. Teacher and students had been talking about a new teacher replacing the regular teacher in the coming days. The teacher and two students, Ahmed and Huwaida, are active in the conversation, although the rest of the class is listening and participating through gazes and body language.

Transcript 6.2: (A—Ahmed, H—Huwaida, T—Teacher)

1	A:	hola hola cómo estás señorita hon kan ö[ö	hola hola cómo estás señorita she can u[uh
2	T:	[hola sta	[hola sta
3	A:	nää hola cómo estás	no hola cómo estás
4	T:	hola cómo estás å vilket språk ä de [ä de pakistanska	hola cómo estás and which language is that [is it Pakistanish
5	A:	[spanska nä spanska	[Spanish no Spanish
6	T:	ä de spanska[vilken tur	is it Spanish [how lucky
7	A:	[ja hon kan spanska ja	[yes she knows Spanish yes
8	T:	hon kan [spanska	she knows [Spanish
9	A:	[ja	[yes
10	T:	å du kan spanska också	and you know Spanish too
11	A:	ah	ah
12	T:	hola estás	hola estás
13	A:	hola cómo estás	hola cómo estás
14	T:	hola cómo estás och hur mår ni frök[en	hola cómo estás and how are you mi[ss
15	A:	[ja ja	[yes yes
16	T:	inte fröken va ä señorita	not miss what is señorita
17	A:	señorita ööö betyder ö[h	señorita uhh means u[h
18	T:	[kvinna	[woman
19	A:	kvinna	woman
20	T:	mm å va betyde va betyde flicka då	mm but what means what means girl then
21	A:	señorita också	señorita also
22	T:	señorita [señorita	señorita [señorita
23	A:	[ja	[yes
24	T:	nej ja tro spanien dom ha spa[nskan spanska har ordet flicka	no I think in Spain they have Spa[nish Spanish has the word girl
25	A:	[dom åla senior många señora	[they hola señor many señora
26	T:	señor	señor
27	A:	ja señor	yes señor
28	T:	señor är en man[men	señor is a man [but
29	A:	[man señorita är i till flicka eller kvinna till säger man	[man señorita is for girl or woman to you say
30	T:	åååå ja tro att dom har ett speciellt namn för kvinna å ett	oohh I think they have a special name for woman and a
31		speciellt namn för flicka	special name for girl
32	A:	ah ja vet inte	ah I don't know
33	T:	de e samma so[m	it is the same a[s
34	A:	[ja ä inte som du (xxx)	[I am not like you (xxx)
35	T:	på arabiska↑ (.) finns de på arabiska inte en skillnad	in Arabic ↑ (.) is there in Arabic not a difference
36		→ mellan flicka å kvinna↑	→ between girl and woman↑
37	A:	a vet inte faktiskt (.) fråga d[om	ah don't know really (.) ask th[em
38	T:	[okej då måste ja ja måste använda min tolk	[ok then I need I need to use my interpreter
39	A:	ja	yes
40	H:	[hihihi	[hihihi
41	T:	*[eh excuse me Huwaida (.) can you please tell me (.) is there a*	*[eh excuse me Huwaida (.) can you please tell me (.) is there a*
42		→ *difference between girl and women in Arabic*	→ *difference between girl and women in Arabic*
43	H:	ja *that's right*	yes *that's right*
44	T:	va hete kvinna på arabiska	what is woman in Arabic
45	H:	ö sayyida	uh sayyida
46	T:	sayyida va hete (.) va hete flicka på arabiska	sayyida what is (.) what is girl in Arabic
47	H:	flicka bint	girl bint
48	T:	bint du ser [du kan inte säga inte säga till en flicka (.)	bint you see [you cannot say not say to a girl (.)
49	A:	[ja	[yes
49		→ goddag min kära kvinna (.) de blir [så ((gör en örfil i luften))	→ hello my dear woman (.) it becomes [like ((slaps in the air))
50	A:	[hahahhaha	[hahahhaha
51	T:	eller hur	right
52	A:	ja	yes

In line 1, Ahmed introduces the phrase “hola señorita, como estás” (hello miss, how are you), a phrase whose meaning is then negotiated by him and the teacher. The teacher does not recognize what Ahmed is saying, which results in a repair by Ahmed in line 3. The teacher now understands Ahmed is using a language variety not familiar to him and asks if he is speaking “Pakistanish”. The question about “Pakistanish” expresses an assumption on the teacher’s part grounded in a nationalistic and monolingual understanding of the world, where language, geographical space and national belonging go hand in hand. Swedes live in Sweden and speak Swedish, hence Pakistanis speak Pakistanish and live in Pakistan. Therefore, the question in line 3 “is it Pakistanish” positions Ahmed as a Pakistani and presumes he should be using Pakistanish as a language variety. Ahmed answers in an overlap that he is speaking Spanish. In the next lines, the teacher and Ahmed work out who knows Spanish, which both the substitute teacher and Ahmed do. Even though the language variety used by Ahmed has been identified, the teacher repeats the phrase “hola cómo estás” (hello how are you), while also suggesting a translation in line 14. Ahmed agrees to the translation, but the teacher corrects his previous translation, questioning the meaning of the word “señorita” (miss). Ahmed is uncertain about this, shown by his hesitation (“uhh”). The teacher suggests a new meaning of “señorita” (miss) with the Swedish word “kvinna” (woman). Ahmed agrees to this as well, but the teacher addresses a new question about the Spanish word for girl. Ahmed answers that girls can also be called “señorita” (miss). The teacher then rejects the possibility that “señorita” (miss) could be used for both girls and women, and suggests that there need to be different words for girl and women in Spanish. In line 24, the teacher once again ties language to geographical spaces as he positions Spanish in Spain. Ahmed answers by first positioning himself as non-Spanish, adding “they say” referring to Spanish speakers in Spain saying “hola señor många señorita” (hello mister many miss) in line 25. The teacher corrects Ahmed, arguing that “señor” (mister) is used for a man. Ahmed then again states that “señorita” (miss) can be used for all females, both girls and women. The teacher insists that there need to be different words for woman and girl, which makes him turn to Arabic in lines 35–36. Through the question, Ahmed is positioned by the teacher as a person knowing Arabic, a position which he opposes in line 37 saying “ah I don’t know really, ask them”. Thus, Ahmed positions himself as somebody who does not know Arabic and thereby does not belong to “them”, the Arabic speakers in the classroom. We can see how Ahmed opposes the two linguistic identities, “Pakistanish” speaker and Arabic speaker, which the teacher used in order to define who Ahmed is. As Ahmed does not identify with the Arabic speakers, the teacher turns to Huwaida, who he refers to as his “interpreter”. The giggling by Huwaida in line 40 can be understood as an acceptance of the position of both Arabic speaker and interpreter. However, turning to Huwaida in line 41, the teacher shifts to English. Through the expression “Excuse me Huwaida, can you please tell me…”, the teacher, again, orients towards Huwaida’s position as an interpreter or expert rather than a student in the classroom. In line 43, Huwaida replies with “ja that is right” (yes that is right), which confirms the distinction made by the teacher between woman and girl. The teacher then switches back to a

Swedish language variety asking Huwaida for the translation of girl and then woman to Arabic. Huwaida answers by giving the teacher the word in Arabic for girl and woman. In the final turn, the teacher starts out by "you see", directed at Ahmed (who, again, suggested women and girls can be both called "señorita" (miss)), that such confusion may cause a bad reaction, even a slap in the face. Ahmed confirms this by a yes, without any further argument.

Ahmed, Huwida and the teacher are engaged in translanguaging using different language varieties in order to construct meaning and in the identity work. Ahmed uses a language variety identified as Spanish to talk about a substitute teacher coming to class the next day. What kind of work does a shift to Spanish do in the interaction? Ahmed positions himself as a speaker of several languages which is knowledge that gives him certain capital in the classroom. Spanish is a European language, studied by students in Swedish schools, as well as a language known by the substitute teacher. Ahmed never claims an identity position as Spanish or even a Spanish speaker as he talks about "them" rather than "we" (line 25). Ahmed also rejects the positions of "Pakistanish" speaker and Arabic speaker in which the teacher put him. His knowledge of Spanish is however questioned by the teacher in lines 10, 16, 20, 22, 24, 26, and 30. The high number of questionings and doubts about Ahmed's skills in Spanish needs to be viewed through the intersection between linguistic identities (who has the right to speak which language) and institutional identities of student and teacher (see the next section). The negotiation of knowledge of Spanish is done in Swedish, which is the target language of the program in which Ahmed participates. However, the teacher does not question Ahmed's position as a Swedish speaker, but rather expects him to engage in the conversation in Swedish.

Huwaida is positioned as the interpreter by the teacher, which she confirms by her giggling in line 40. The teacher's shift to English in line 41 positions Huwaida not only as the interpreter for the Arabic speaker but as a speaker of English. Huwaida confirms this and also answers the teacher in English. After this invitation of Huwaida into the conversation, the teacher shifts back to Swedish, as he turns to ask her about translation. Huwaida is expected to translate between English and Arabic, thus positioning her as a person with good knowledge of English, Swedish and Arabic.

In the conversation, different linguistic varieties are used by all the participants in order to make meaning concerning the conversation regarding the proper way to address women and girls in Spanish, but also in order to make certain identity positions in the classroom. Ahmed positions himself as a multilingual individual who speaks Spanish and Swedish, but gets positioned as a "Pakistanish", Arabic and Swedish speaker by the teacher. The teacher also positions himself as a multilingual person claiming knowledge of Spanish as well as using different language varieties in the conversation.

The linguistic identity positions intersect with positions of national belonging but also with institutional identities of teacher and student as well as gender and sexuality. Institutional interaction in classroom settings is characterized by IRE-sequences (Heritage and Clayman 2010; MacBeth 2004). Although it is

Ahmed who introduces the phrase "hola cómo estás", the teacher orients towards a teacher position by initiating questions to Ahmed and then evaluating his answers. In lines 4–6, the teacher asks which language Ahmed is speaking and later evaluates the reply with "it is Spanish, what a luck". The teacher then asks several more questions (lines 8, 10, 16, 20, 35–36, 41–42, 44, 46) of Ahmed and Huwaida. Both Ahmed and Huwaida confirm the identity position of students by replying to the questions initiated by the teacher. In performing a teacher identity, the teacher claims his knowledge of the topic discussed. Although he does not recognize the language variety spoken by Ahmed at first (line 4), he later asserts knowledge about the language by presenting what he claims to be a correct translation of "señorita" (miss) (line 18), as well as knowledge regarding Spanish vocabulary (lines 24, 30–31). Ahmed's knowledge of and about Spanish is questioned by the teacher, thus positioning him both as a student with less knowledge than the teacher, and as a non-Spanish speaker. Furthermore, through the interaction concerning how to address women, Ahmed and the teacher are performing a male heterosexual identity position. Through male bonding and mentorship, the teacher is mentoring Ahmed about how to be with women.

The mentorship performed in the interaction between the teacher and Ahmed is not entirely present in the interaction with Huwaida, who is approached by the teacher as his "interpreter", positioning her as an expert able to translate between English, Swedish and Arabic. However, the interactional order between the teacher and Huwaida in lines 44–48 can be described in terms of IRE sequences, typical of teacher and student exchanges. Moreover, the invitation directed at Huwaida by the teacher in line 41 may also be in gendered terms, as the teacher is performing a male position and the "way to address women", positioning Huwaida as a woman. The formal and polite tone of the teacher may be interpreted as a way of positioning Huwaida as an expert but also as a woman and himself as a gentleman addressing her in a polite manner.

6.5 Conclusion

The point of departure in the analysis of classroom interaction is the way individuals constitute and negotiate meaning about the world and who they are through (trans)languaging. As discussed in the theoretical framework, learning involves identity work for participants in language-learning classrooms where identities are often mediated in the target language. In five classrooms included in the CIC project, Swedish was the dominant language in the classroom during classes as the object of the learning activities as well as the medium through which meaning about the practice, the participants and the world outside of the classroom was negotiated. The use of Swedish as the dominant language enforced the unequal distribution of power between teacher and students, since the teacher, having the most advanced skills in Swedish, could express himself with more ease in the classroom. Since meaning-making in the interaction between participants was mainly done in

Swedish, the discourses available for the students were limited. In other words, the linguistic order and the institutional identities in the classroom intersect and enforce the unequal distribution of power.

However, as shown in the analyses of transcript, participants in the classroom used different language varieties in the interaction. The interactional order in the classroom analyzed in this chapter was, compared to the four other classrooms included in the CIC project, characterized by an open attitude towards the use of language varieties other than Swedish (Rosén and Bagga-Gupta 2015). The interaction displayed in the transcript was just one of many examples in which both teacher and students used not only Swedish but also the language resources available to them in their meaning-making. Students, but also the teacher, used different language varieties in order to perform certain identity positions in the classroom. By tolerating as well as using different language varieties, the teacher positioned himself as a multilingual person rather than a monolingual Swede, and thus allied himself with the students. Allying with the students, the teacher challenged his belonging to a Swedish monolingual and monocultural community. The belonging to certain linguistic communities was also negotiated by Ahmed, who did not agree with belonging to "them", the Arabic speakers. The argument "I am not like you" (line 34) was directed towards the teacher but it is unclear which differences Ahmed was referring to.

The interplay between linguistic and institutional identities in the intersection of identity positions in the classroom highlights the importance of applying an intersectional perspective in the analysis. In the interaction between Ahmed and the teacher, as well as between Huwaida and the teacher, the doing of gender identities in relation to institutional and linguistic identities is at play. Huwaida is approached as the expert, "the interpreter", but also positioned as a woman, while the teacher is performing a position of the "polite man". Gender is also relevant in the identity work between Ahmed and the teacher, performing male heterosexual identity positions. In the last part of the conversation (lines 48–52), the teacher tells Ahmed he cannot call a woman a girl. The lecturing manner of the teacher can be understood as part of an institutional teacher identity but also as a man instructing a younger man on how to behave towards women. Hence, age, gender and institutional identities intersect.

Finally, the interaction between the teacher, Ahmed and Huwaida is embedded in an institutional practice regulated by a national curriculum. As illuminated in the sociohistorical analysis of the national curricula of SFI, the language-learning program is constructed in and reproduces an imagined national identity where certain values and norms are perceived as Swedish, thus upholding boundaries between the Swede and the Other. These postcolonial boundaries are also evoked through positioning certain bodies in different geopolitical spaces and linguistic communities. As the examples in this chapter show, such boundaries are at play in the everyday interaction of the language learning classroom. The chapter highlights the complexity of language in identity work and how participants engage in such processes through (trans)languaging. Finally, combining an intersectional perspective on identity with a sociocultural framework on language learning creates possibilities to grasp such complexities.

Transcription key

regular	original utterance in Swedish
italics	original utterance in English
((points at))	non-verbal action
[look]	overlapping utterances
(.)	pause
↓	indicates falling intonation
↑	indicates rising intonation
→	indicates continuation of turn.

References

Arbetsmarknadsdepartementet [Ministry of Employment.] (2009a). Samhällsorientering för nyanlända invandrare. [Civic education for newly arrived immigrants] Dir. 209, 101. http://www.regeringen.se/contentassets/30001a44fdfe4f25962b2cc9914ab9f4/samhallsorientering-for-nyanlanda-invandrare-dir.-2009101. Accessed 20 May 2016.

Arbetsmarknadsdepartementet [Ministry of Employment.] (2009b). Nyanlända invandrares arbetsmarknadsetablering – egenansvar med professionellt stöd [Newly arrived immigrants' establishment in the workforce–personal responsibility with professional support]. Prop. 2009/10:60. http://data.riksdagen.se/fil/0D18E02F-DCD6-4C51-98D1-7626444B7C28. Accessed 2 April 2016.

Arbetsmarknadsdepartementet [Ministry of Employment.] (2010). Sverige för nyanlända. Värden, välfärdsstat, vardagsliv. [Sweden for newly arrived. Values, welfare state, every-day life].SOU 2010:16. http://www.regeringen.se/contentassets/4c6969b7b04746d6ade9eaa6d6ce4ede/sverige-for-nyanlanda—varden-valfardsstat-vardagsliv-sou-201016. Accessed 3 April 2016.

Bagga-Gupta, S. (2013). The boundary turn. (Re)locating culture, identity and language through the epistemological lenses of time, space and social interactions. In I. Hasnain, S. Bagga-Gupta, S. Mohan (Eds.), *Alternative voices: (Re)searching language, culture, identity...*(pp. 28–49). England: Cambridge Scholars Publishing.

Bagga-Gupta, S. (2014a). Languaging: Ways-of-being-with-words across disciplinary boundaries and empirical sites. In H. Paulasto, H. Riionheimo, L. Meriläinen, & M. Kok (Eds.), *Language contacts at the crossroads of disciplines* (pp. 89–130). Newcastle-upon-Tyne: Cambridge Scholars Publishing.

Bagga-Gupta, S. (2014b). Performing and accounting language and identity: Agency as actors-in-(inter)action-with-tools. In P. Deters, X. Gao, E. Miller, & G. Vitanova-Haralampiev (Eds.), *Theorizing and analyzing agency in second language learning: Interdisciplinary approaches* (pp. 113–132). Bristol: Multilingual Matters.

Bakhtin, M. (1981). *The dialogic imagination: Four essays*. Austin and London: University of Texas Press.

Berger, P., & Luckman, T. (1966). *The social construction of reality: A treatise in the sociology of knowledge*. London: Penguin.

Block, D. (2007a). *Second language identities*. London: Continuum.

Block, D. (2007b). The rise of identity in SLA research, post Firth and Wagner. *The Modern Language Journal, 91*(1), 863–876.

Block, D. (2014). Structure, agency, individualization and the critical realist challenge. In P. Deters, X, Gao, E, Miller, G. Vitanova-Haralampiev (Eds.), *Theorizing and analyzing agency in second language learning: interdisciplinary approaches* (pp. 17–36). Bristol: Multilingual Matters.

Butler, J. ([1990]1999). *Gender trouble: Feminism and the subversion of identity*. New York: Routledge.

Butler, J. (1997). *Excitable speech: A politics of the performative*. New York: Routledge.

Canagarajah, S. (2011). Codemeshing in academic writing: Identifying teachable strategies of translanguaging. *The Modern Language Journal, 95*(3), 401–417.

Carlson, M. (2002). Svenska för invandrare-brygga eller gräns?: syn på kunskap och lärande inom sfi-undervisningen [Swedish Language Courses for Immigrants (SFI)—Bridge or Border? On Views of Knowledge and Learning in SFI Education]. Departmet of Sociology, University *of* Gothenburg.

Crenshaw, K. (1989). Demarginalizing the intersection of race and sex: A black feminist critique of antidiscrimination doctrine, feminist theory and antiracist politics. *University of Chicago Legal Forum,* 138–67.

Crenshaw, K. (1991). Mapping the margins: Intersectionality, identity politics, and violence against women of color. *Stanford Law Review, 43*(6), 1241–1299.

Davies, B., & Harré, R. (1990). Positioning: The discursive production of selves. *Journal for the Theory of Social Behaviour, 20*(1), 43–63.

de los Reyes, P., Molina, I., Mulinari, D. (2005). Introduktion – makten (o)lika förklädnader [Introduction—the different disguises of power]. In P. de los Reyes, I. Molina, D. Mulinari (Eds.), *Maktens (o)lika förklädnader. Kön, klass & etnicitet i det postkoloniala Sverige* [*The different disguises of power: Gender, class & ethnicity in post-colonial Sweden*] (pp. 11–30). Stockholm: Atlas.

de los Reyes, P., & Mulinari, D. (2005). *Intersektionalitet: kritiska reflektioner över (o) jämlikhetens landskap.* [*Intersectionality: Critical reflections about (in)equality landscapes*]. Malmö: Liber.

García, O. (2009). *Bilingual education in the 21st century: A global perspective*. Malden, MA: Blackwell.

García, O., & Wei, L. (2014). *Translanguaging: Language, bilingualism and education*. Basingstoke, UK: Palgrave Macmillan.

Garfinkel, H. (1984). *Studies in ethnomethodology*. Cambridge: Polity.

Goffman, E. (2009). *Jaget och maskerna: en studie i vardagslivets dramatik.* Falun: Norstedts. English edition: Goffman, E. (1959). *The presentation of self in everyday life* (S. Bergström, Trans.). New York: Doubleday.

Heller, M. (2011). *Paths to post-nationalism: A critical ethnography of language and identity*. New York: Oxford University Press.

Heritage, J., & Clayman, S. (2010). *Talk in action. Interactions, identities, and institutions*. Chichester: Wiley-Blackwell.

Honkanen, K. (2008). Equality politics out of the subaltern. In E. Magnusson, M. Rönnblom, H. Silius (Eds.), *Critical studies of gender equalities. Nordic dislocations, dilemmas and contradictions* (pp. 205–219). Göteborg: Makadam.

Hult, F. (2010). Analysis of language policy discourses across the scales of space and time. *International Journal of the Sociology of Language, 2010*(202), 7–24.

Hyltenstam, K., & Milani, T. (2012). Flerspråkighetens sociopolitiska och sociokulturella ramar [The sociopolitical and sociocultural framing of multilingualism] In K. Hyltenstam, M. Axelsson, I. Lindberg (Eds.). *Flerspråkighet – en forskningsöversikt* [*Multilingualims—A reserach review*] (pp. 17–152). Stockholm: Vetenskapsrådet.

Kanno, Y., & Norton, B. (2003). Imagined communities and educational possibilities: Introduction. *Journal of Language, Identity & Education, 2*(4), 241–249.

Keskinen, S. (Ed.). (2009). *Complying with colonialism: Gender, race and ethnicity in the Nordic region*. Farnham: Ashgate Publishing Ltd.

Linell, P. (1998). *Approaching dialogue: Talk, interaction and contexts in dialogical perspectives*. Amsterdam: John Benjamin.
Linell, P. (2009). *Rethinking language, mind, and world dialogically: Interactional and contextual theories of human sense-making*. Charlotte, NC: Information Age.
Lundgren, B. (2005). *Skolan i livet - livet i skolan: några illitterata invandrarkvinnor lär sig tala, läsa och skriva på svenska som andraspråk* [School as part of life—Life as part of school. Five illiterate women learn to speak, read and write Swedish as a second language]. Department of Swedish and Social Sciences, Umeå University.
Lykke, N. (2003). Intersektionalitet – ett användbart begrepp för genusforskningen [Intersectionality—A useful concept for gender reserach]. *Kvinnovetenskaplig tidskrift [Journal of Women Studies], 1*(3), 47–56.
Lykke, N. (2005). Nya perspektiv på intersektionalitet. Problem och möjligheter [New perspectives on intersectionality. Problems and possibilities]. *Kvinnovetenskaplig tidskrift* [*Journal of Women Studies*], *2–3*(5), 7–17.
Lykke, N. (2011). Intersectional analysis: Black box or useful critical feminist thinking technology? In H. Lutz, M. Herrera Vivar, L. Supik (Eds.), *Framing intersectionality. Debates on a multi-faceted concept in gender studies* (pp. 207–221). Farnham: Ashgate.
Macbeth, D. (2004). The relevance of repair for classroom correction. *Language in Society, 33*(5), 703–736.
Magnusson, E., Rönnblom, M., & Silius, H. (2008). *Critical studies of gender equalities. Nordic dislocations, dilemmas and contradictions*. Göteborg: Makadam.
Marx Ferree, M. (2011). The discoursive politics of feminist intersectionality. In H. Lutz, M. Herrera Vivar, & L. Supik (Eds.), *Framing intersectionality. Debates on a multi-faceted concept in gender studies* (pp. 55–68). Farnham: Ashgate.
McCall, L. (2005). The complexity of intersectionality. *Signs: Journal of Women in Culture and Society*, *3*(3), 1771–1800.
Milani, T. (2004). Om performativitet – ett postmodernistiskt angreppssätt på språkpolitik och språkplanering [About performativity—a postmodern perspective on language politics and language planning]. In B. De Geer, A. Malmbjer (Eds.), Språk på tvärs: rapport från ASLA: s höstsymposium [Language across: Report from the autumn symposium of ASLA] (pp. 23–38). Södertörn, 11-12 November 2004. Uppsala: Association Suédoise de Linguistique Appliqueé.
Mohanty, C. (2004). Feminism without borders: Decolonizing theory, practicing solidarity. Durham: Duke University Press.
Norton, B. (2000). *Identity and language learning: Gender, ethnicity and educational change*. Harlow: Longman.
Norton, B. (2001). Non-participation, imagined communities and the language classroom. In M. Breen (Ed.), *Learner contributions to language learning: New directions in research* (pp. 159–171). London: Pearson Education.
Pavlenko, A., & Lantolf, J. (2000). Second language learning as participation and the (re)construction of selves. In J. Lantolf (Ed.), *Sociocultural theory and second language learning* (pp. 155–177). Oxford: Oxford University.
Pavlenko, A., Blackledge, A., Piller, I., & Teutsch-Dwyer, M. (Eds.). (2001). *Multilingualism, second language learning and gender*. Berlin: Mouton de Gruyter.
Pennycook, A. (2004). Performativity and language studies. *Critical Inquiry in Language Studies, 1*(1), 1–19.
Rosén, J., & Bagga-Gupta, S. (2013). Shifting identity positions in the development of language education for immigrants: An analysis of discourses associated with 'Swedish for immigrants'. *Language, Culture and Curriculum, 26*(1), 68–88.
Rosén, J., & Bagga-Gupta, S. (2015). Prata svenska, vi är i Sverige! [Talk Swedish, we are in Sweden!] A study of practiced language policy in adult language learning. *Linguistics and Education, 31*, 59–73.
Rosén, J. (2013). *Svenska för invandrarskap? Språk, kategorisering och identitetskapande inom utbildningsformen Svenska för invandrare (Sfi) [Swedish for immigrantness? Language,*

categorizations and construction of identities in the education Swedish for immigrants (Sfi)]. Örebro: Örebro University.

Scollon, R., & Scollon, S. (2004). *Nexus analysis: Discourse and the emerging internet*. London: Routledge.

SKOLFS. (1994). Förordning om kursplan för svenskundervisning för invandrare [Decree regarding the syllabus for swedish education for immigrants]. http://www.skolverket.se/skolfs?id=111. Accessed 2 April 2016.

SKOLFS. (2002). Förordning om ändring i förordningen (SKOLFS 1994:28) om kursplan för svenskundervisning för invandrare. [Decree regarding changes in the decree regarding the syllabus for swedish education for immigrants]. http://www.skolverket.se/skolfs?id=1054. Accessed 2 April 2016.

SKOLFS. (2009). Förordning om kursplan för svenskundervisning för invandrare. [Decree regarding the syllabus for swedish education for immigrants]. http://www.skolverket.se/skolfs?id=1491. Accessed 2 April 2016.

Skolöverstyrelsen [Swedish National Agency for Education.] (1986). *Lgrund-sfi-86. Allmän del*. Läroplaner 1986:11 [Curriculum in Swedish for Adult Immigrants, 1. General Part]. Stockholm: Liber Utbildningsförl.

Skolöverstyrelsen [Swedish National Agency for Education] (1991). *Läroplan för grundläggande svenskundervisning för vuxna invandrare. Lsfi-91* [Curriculum in Swedish for adult immigrants Lsfi-91]. Stockholm: Liber Utbildningsförl.

Skolverket [Swedish National Agency for Education.] (2012). Syllabus for Swedish tuition for immigrants. Swedish National Agency for Education. http://www.skolverket.se/publikationer?id=2910. Accessed 2 April 2016.

Säljö, R. (2000). *Lärande i praktiken* [Learning in practice]. Stockholm: Prisma.

Towns, A. (2002). Paradoxes of (in)equality. Something is rotten in the gender equal state of Sweden. *Cooperation and Conflict, 37*(2), 157–179.

Tuori, S. (2007). Cooking nation gender equality and multiculturalism as nation-building discourses. *European Journal of Women's Studies, 14*(1), 21–35.

Weedon, C. (2004). *Identity and culture: Narratives of difference and belonging*. Maidenhead: Open University Press.

Wenger, E. (1998). *Communities of practice: Learning, meaning and identity*. Cambridge: Cambridge University Press.

Wertsch, J. (1998). *Mind as action*. New York: Oxford University Press.

Yuval-Davis, N. (2011a). *The politics of belonging: intersectional contestations*. Los Angeles: Sage.

Yuval-Davis, N. (2011b). Beyond the recognition and re-distribution dichotomy: intersectionality and stratification. In H. Lutz, M. Herrera Vivar, & L. Supik (Eds.), *Framing intersectionality. Debates on a multi-faceted concept in gender studies* (pp. 155–169). Farnham: Ashgate.

Author Biography

Jenny Rosén is Assistant Professor of Swedish as a Second language at the Department of Language Education at Stockholm University and holds a postdoctoral position in Educational Work at Dalarna University, Sweden. Her research focuses on multilingualism, learning, diversity and identity mainly in educational settings, working with sociocultural and decolonial perspectives.

Chapter 7
The Passage of Time as a Narrative Resource in Constructing a Better Self

Julia Sacher

7.1 Introduction

In most cases, the passing of time is something we only observe when it becomes a problematic event for us—for instance, when we miss a train or realize that we just spent three hours surfing the internet instead of cleaning the house or grading students' writing assignments.

Most of the time we do not notice how actual events and experiences change us over time. In narrative discourse however, these changes become retrospectively accessible and can therefore become an essential topic. Conversation and discourse analysis have shown that storytelling is a highly complex activity where narrators are confronted with different conversational tasks, such as providing the recipient with a coherent story—that means with a conversational structure that encompasses a certain stretch of time, reconstructs it and explains more or less implicitly and more or less logically how the course of events unfolded (cf. Jefferson 1978; Quasthoff 1980; Sacks 1986; Gülich and Hausendorf 2000). Through narrative actions like these the change of a person's actions and attitudes becomes reflexively accessible to the narrator.

As Brockmeier (2009) shows, time is a cultural construction that can be conceptualized differently—even within one culture. As an example he refers to the "Newtonian view" of time on the one hand—the idea that there is one absolute timeline onto which every event can be mapped—and to "narrative time" on the other hand. The latter is a symbolic construction that is accomplished linguistically and is closely connected to the construction of autobiographical narratives. Narrative time does not necessarily proceed linearly; the linguistic construction of "autobiographical time" (Brockmeier 2000) allows time to be presented in a circular, a cyclical, a spiral, a static or a fragmentary fashion. More often than not

J. Sacher (✉)
University of Cologne, Cologne, Germany
e-mail: julia.sacher@uni-koeln.de

S. Bagga-Gupta et al. (eds.), *Identity Revisited and Reimagined*,
DOI 10.1007/978-3-319-58056-2_7

these different constructions of individual time take the shape of narratives: each culture has its own canon of narrative forms and models to shape the reconstructions of the self in the context of past events. Autobiographical narratives thus can be regarded as documents of past versions of the self—and as such they are a form of discoursive identity construction. For Bruner (2004: 692) narrative is the only form by which "lived time" can be described, and it always involves the construction of the narrator's identity.

Conceptualizing narrative as a conversational mode for the construction of both the self and the world it is located in is a characteristic trait of the narrative turn in the Humanities and the Social Sciences in which narratives are seen not only as "a privileged site for identity analysis" (Bamberg 2009: 133) but as much more: "self-making" and "world-making" (Bruner 2001) are basically regarded as the same, because they are both assumed to happen narratively.

The impact culturally different concepts of time, narrative and self have can be shown by cross-cultural comparisons of autobiographic narratives: Brockmeier (2003) demonstrates that narrative identity construction differs depending on the cultural background of a narrator.[1] He refers to Western and Eastern narratives about earliest childhood memories and finds that these narratives differ significantly: while the Western narrator tells a story about herself as a 3-year-old girl that does mischief at a family celebration, the Eastern narrator tells a story about her father teaching her traditional poems and explaining their meaning to her. While the Western story is characterized by a self that appears independent and agentive, the Eastern storyteller describes herself as related to another person. She subordinates her narrated self to her father, who in turn appears as the main protagonist of the story.

The two narratives that will be analyzed in this chapter are told by Western narrators. What is striking in them is that the passage of time is used as a narrative means to indicate change within the storytellers' selves.

Drawing on the analytic traditions of conversation and discourse analysis, I want to introduce a type of stories I call *Before-and-After stories*. These stories have a particular structure: They consist of three phases—a *Before* and an *After*, linked by a *Turning Point*—in which narrators present two different facets of their selves. Temporality plays an important role in the structure of these stories, as the passage of time is narratively used to establish evaluative contrasts between the two presented facets of the narrators' selves. In telling stories with such a structure, the presented facets of the selves are evaluated in such a way that the chronologically more recent facet is (more or less implicitly) presented as the better (or improved) one. In doing so, narrators can tell their recipients a story about individual development. Consequently, identity construction is a prominent feature of these narratives.

[1]See also Keating (in this volume) on cultural differences as a cause for misunderstandings in a job-related environment.

First I will give a brief overview of my data and the analytic methods and concepts I used. All methods and concepts can be subscribed to the constructivist paradigm and are employed to examine how speakers construct social reality by means of conversational interaction. Telling a story and constructing identity are examples of reality being conversationally constructed. After that, I will explain how time, narrative and identity are connected. I will then analyze two narratives with a Before-and-After structure. In these two narratives, two teachers talk about difficult situations they faced in their career. In the discussion, I will finally point out that in Before-and-After stories the passage of time is used as a means of face-work.

7.2 Identity Construction in the Interview—Concepts and Methods

The data presented in this article are part of a corpus of nine interviews that were conducted in the context of an interdisciplinary project about communication in the classroom (Trautmann and Sacher 2010). Teachers were interviewed about their motivation to take part in the research project, about their teaching style, their experience with being videotaped during teaching, their expectations about their own participation in the project and about the effects they hoped their participation might have on their future teaching. During these interviews, narrative accounts of professional self-conceptions and sequences of job-related biographical narratives were produced frequently.[2]

In order to be able to describe how identity construction takes place in the interviews, a social constructivist perspective on the data is adopted. I will first explain the methods used and then show how different theoretical concepts can be integrated to reconstruct what happens in the interview data with the speakers' construction of interactional reality as a starting point for analysis.

7.2.1 Discourse Analysis and Interview Interaction

Discourse analysis focuses on the micro level of interactions, i.e. on the sequential level of conversation. It can be traced back to the Schützean phenomenology, Garfinkel's ethnomethodology and Sacks's conversation analysis. Discourse analysis makes the following basic assumptions about conversational interaction

[2]Some of these narratives were used as data for a PhD project on conversational repertoires of identity construction and self-presentation (Sacher 2012). All teachers gave their permission for their interviews to be used in different research contexts.

(cf. e.g. Sacks et al. 1974; Sacks 1984; Bergmann 1994; Silverman 1998; Ten Have 2007; Deppermann 2008; Gülich et al. 2008).

Social reality is something that is constructed in everyday interaction. During interaction, each participant has individual interactional goals and intentions. These goals and intentions can conflict and lead to local problems that need solving. To construct social reality and solve emerging interactional problems, speakers use a wide array of conversational methods (in the sense of ethnomethods, Garfinkel 1967) to mutually make sense of their actions. Those methods are multimodal ones —it is not only important what is said but also how it is said, how gaze is organized, how body posture and orientation contribute to the utterance, etc.

Necessary for analyses are detailed transcripts of naturally occurring conversations—i.e. interactions that have not been arranged experimentally in order to analyze them or data that consist of exemplary made-up sentences. In the transcripts, small and seemingly irrelevant phenomena like pauses, breaks, reformulations, overlap etc. are important because they help the analyst to reconstruct how the process of meaning-making happens sequentially. One basic assumption is that there is "order at all points" (Sacks 1984: 21): each utterance serves the analyst as a document of how a previous utterance has been understood by its speaker—each utterance is a document of the speaker's understanding of what just happened. Analytic reconstruction of conversational interaction requires the analyst to "bracket" (Schütz 1972) his/her own interpretation of the data in order to adopt the speaker's perspective. Important are only the speakers' analytical categories, not the analysts'—because only the speakers' ethnomethods and relevance structures are of interest within conversation and discourse analysis. Analytical interpretations cannot reach inside the speakers' heads but stop literally in front of those heads. Research is data-driven insofar as it leads to hypotheses instead of presuming a priori what the relevant analytic focus could/should be—analytical statements and interpretations typically come "from the data themselves" (Schegloff and Sacks 1973: 291).

In this understanding of verbal interaction, the significance of interview data differs from their use in social scientific research contexts: interview data are not analytically framed as the instrument to generate theoretical categories or codes but serve as genuine data—the interview situation is regarded as a specific interactional setting with specific conversational characteristics (Baker 2002). From such a discourse analytic perspective it is interesting to investigate how the speakers manage to switch from everyday interaction to interview specific conversation, i.e. how they "do" the interview and actively adopt the situational roles of interviewee and interviewer (Uhmann 1989).

These two situational roles cause an interactional asymmetry, which is also characteristic for interview interaction: the interviewer's main activity consists in asking questions and producing backchannel signals (Heritage 1998). S/he behaves interactively abstinent (Sacher et al. 2015) and thus leaves the room for the interviewee, whose main activities consequently consist in producing autobiographic narratives and other accounts of his/her self. Holmes (2006: 168) observes that "individuals draw on different aspects of their social and personal identities in different interactions […].” This is especially true for the scientific interview: the interviewee participates and speaks as expert on a specific topic or at least as a member of a certain category (e.g. as a member of the category “teacher”, cf. also Johnson 2006), so the narratives s/he produces are concordant to the expert role s/he is ascribed. Baker (2002: 781) consequentially points out that from an ethnomethodological point of view, everything that is told within an interview has to be seen as the interviewee’s account, i.e. as sense-making work through which participants [i.e. interviewees, J.S.] engage in explaining, attributing, justifying, describing and otherwise finding possible sense or orderliness in the various events, people, places, and courses of action they talk about.

It is important to point out that these processes of sense-making happen on two different levels in the interview: One level is what I will call *actual interview interaction*, i.e. the interaction between the interviewer and the interviewee, where questions are asked and answered and the interview as a special kind of interactive setting is accomplished. The other level can be described as *interview narrative*.

But what does actually happen when someone produces a narrative? In everyday discourse, the beginning of a story is jointly accomplished by all participants of a situation (Jefferson 1978): the speaker gets the floor by announcing that s/he is about to tell a story, and gets the permission to do exactly that. In most cases these “story prefaces” (ibid.) happen rather implicitly, e.g. by indicating that something extraordinary has happened to the narrator-to-be. A story can also be elicited by recipients who explicitly ask an interactant to tell a specific story. By whatever means a story is introduced into a conversation, the way in which all interactants engage in conversation changes in comparison to non-narrative talk: the storyteller gets the privileged right to produce a series of consecutive utterances (i.e. the actual narration), and the recipients react to the story in progress by producing mostly “backchannel signals” (Schegloff 1982) or engaging in “byplay” (Goodwin 1997). This also means that once the format of narration is successfully established, the speaker is granted a certain interactive space in which s/he can unfold his/her interpretation of events, introduce relevant protagonists, place them in a certain light, equip them (and him-/herself as well!) with specific characteristics etc. to his/her own liking.

As Quasthoff (1980) points out, it is important not to confuse the original event with the story that is made of it. The original event is not accessible to the recipients; they are witnesses to a subjective construct of one of the narrator’s experiences. The communicative operations that take place in constructing a story can be described as follows: according to Lucius-Hoene and Deppermann (2004: 21), narrating a story requires a segmentation of the stream of events. Single elements from these events are selected and linearized verbally in consecutive utterances. Meaning is constructed by the choice of events, the choice of narrative genre (heroic story, tragedy, romantic story, bildungsroman, …) and their narrative presentation.

Bamberg (2011) groups the discursive practices to accomplish this telling of lifetime in situ as “identity navigation”. He identifies three dimensions of relevant navigational processes: (1) agency, (2) sameness versus difference and (3) constancy and change across time. The narrative activities on these three dimensions construct different kinds of boundaries around the self—against other people by demonstrating differences between the self and others, against the world by demonstrating how oneself acts as an agentive subject, and in a certain way also against oneself, by demonstrating how oneself has become the person one is at a certain moment in time (i.e. a moment in time at which an autobiographical story is told). The last point is crucial for my own data, because in my analyses of Before-and-After stories I will argue that speakers use the passing of time as a narrative resource for implicitly influencing other people's impression of themselves. The dimensions *sameness versus difference* and *constancy and change across time* are central here. From a discourse analytic perspective, analyzing narrative identity means to focus on the question of how to use narrative structures to reconstruct past experiences and to make them meaningful.

Compared to everyday interaction, the right to narrate something is easier to obtain in an interview. As I have explained above, the interviewees' interactional task consists in producing accounts of themselves, and narratives are a very common format for such accounts. The narrative level of the interview is embedded in the level of actual interview interaction and at the same time caused by it: On this level, the interviewee produces answers, and these answers often consist of narratives. Both levels offer the interviewee different opportunities for identity construction, i.e. the interviewees use different methods to construct their selves which must be conceptualized accordingly. As the activities on both levels are closely intertwined, it is promising to combine the discourse analytic take on interview interaction with a positioning analytic perspective, as narratives and the individual positions established in them serve as positioning devices for the narrator in the situation where the story is told. In the next two sections I will introduce positioning analysis and Goffman's concept of interactional face (Goffman 1967) as additional methodical tools that in combination with my discourse analytic approach help to reconstruct activities of identity construction in the interview.

7.2.2 Positioning Analysis

Positioning analysis has its origin in discourse psychology (e.g. Davies and Harré 1990; van Langenhove and Harré 1999) and is closely connected to identity reconstruction (e.g. Bamberg 1997). From a discourse analytic perspective, the important question is how social positions are constructed verbally and how they serve as a conversational instrument to convey a speaker's sense of self. As Hausendorf and Bora (2006: 87) put it:

> Social positioning is not made for us analysts – to help us in our jobs – but it is done by the participants themselves since they themselves have to display to each other how their being this or that is to be considered a relevant social item in the on-going social interaction, at whatever implicit level such positioning can occur.

With this view on positioning activities, their interactional impact on a conversation can be described and the mutual negotiation of social positions can be made explicit. The basic structure of positioning sequences consists of three steps (ibid.: 90ff.): (1) Social positions have to be assigned, (2) the associated categories have to be ascribed and (3) finally be evaluated. All three steps can be completed interactionally by the speaker him-/herself (self-positioning) or by another person (other-positioning). As Wolf (1999) points out, the positioning of self and others open up specific scopes of action and can therefore be described as rhetoric strategies. With them, speakers can make several interactional moves to legitimize their own perspective, such as emphasizing their role membership and the knowledge that goes along with it or making their individual perspective on interactionally negotiated topics relevant. Additionally, positioning analyses serve to explain how activities on the situational level can influence activities on the narrative level and vice versa.

In the next section I will come back to interview interaction and explain how the discourse analytic take on storytelling and positioning analysis can be complemented by Goffman's notion of "face" (Goffman 1967). The combination of these concepts and methods allows for the analytical reconstruction of Before-and-After stories on a structural level. It also helps to describe how their structural characteristics relate to identity construction.

7.2.3 Identity Construction in the Interview

Like producing narrations, identity construction is a frequent interactional task in everyday interactions. The works of Erving Goffman focus on the question of how a person manages to provide his/her interactional counterpart with an idea of how s/he sees him-/herself. It is important to stress that Goffman sees social interaction as a quintessentially semiotic activity: qua socialization the individual acquires knowledge about different semiotic codes to convey information about him-/herself. This knowledge is not individual but culturally shared and assumed to be common possession of every member of a society. Mutual knowledge of the semiotic inventory of a culture is key in Goffman's theory of interactional identity construction. The notion of face is a key concept in answering the question of how an individual provides others with an idea of who s/he is. According to Goffman (1967: 5), face can be defined as "the positive social value a person effectively claims for himself by the line others assume he has taken during a particular contact."

Face thus combines self-image with public image: the individual can only confirm his/her self-image by interactional validation of the other, i.e. if the other interprets him/her the way s/he wants to be interpreted. The interactional counterpart thus has the function of a social mirror: only if s/he reflects the image that a speaker wants to convey about him-/herself, that image has an accepted social meaning. As face is something that every person possesses, mutual face-protection is an important aspect of interactions: Goffman calls the various interactional techniques we use to manage our own and our counterpart's face-protection „face-work"(ibid.). He also states that face-work has an essential function for everyday interaction: it keeps the "expressive order" (Goffman 1967) and the "ritual balance" (ibid.) of an encounter and ensures that interaction per se can take place. Individuals learn mutual face-protection during socialization; the techniques Goffman describes are everyday politeness routines like avoiding conversation lapses, ensuring that conversational topics suit everyone, etc. This is in line with the sociolinguistic understanding of identity as a local product of interaction that Bucholtz and Hall (2005) describe: speakers use different linguistic means to show what they subjectively regard as important aspects of their own self.

Here, too, discourse analysis can be used to gain further insight into the conversational mechanisms of face-work: Schenkein (1978) shows how interactionally constructed facets of self can be the object of interactional negotiation or modification (Schenkein 1978)—the speaker provides its counterpart with an "identity-rich puzzle" (ibd.: 66) that includes hints at the speaker's self-understanding. In a similar way, Antaki (1998: 1) uses the notion "identity-in-interaction" and defines it as "[…] something that is used in talk: something that is part and parcel of the routines of everyday life, brought off in the fine details of everyday interaction."

However, as stated above, the interview situation differs significantly from the everyday mechanisms of identity negotiation: for long periods, the interviewer remains relatively passive. Therefore, the interviewee does not really know to what extent his/her interactional face-work succeeds, i.e. whether the interviewer understands him-/herself the way s/he wants to be understood. From this perspective, the amount of (narrative) accounts interviewees produce can not only be seen as role-related activities, but also as an interactional method used to make sure that the interviewer gets a chance to understand the way the interviewee sees him-/herself.

In the next section, I will bring together the discussed topics and concepts. I will analyze two interview narratives about difficult situations in the narrators' work history. I will show that these stories have a very similar structure: they are Before-and-After stories in which the two narrators use the passage of time as a central feature to show the interviewer how their identities have changed. Thus, both stories are examples for narrative face-work.

7.3 Before-and-After Stories: Data Analyses

The two sequences I want to discuss are taken from the abovementioned corpus of interviews. Both sequences have structural characteristics in common, which I will refer to by using the concept of Before-and-After stories. It refers to narrations that consist of three phases in which different states of the self are described: A *Before* phase in which the narrator faces a difficult situation, a *Turning Point* at which a transformation of the self with regard to these difficulties is described, and an *After* phase in which the narrator presents him-/herself as having overcome the difficulties.

I will give a brief overview of each sequence before I go into greater detail. In both cases the German original can be found in the Appendix; here I will refer to the English translation, which tries to reflect the conversational properties of the German original to facilitate reading. The concept of Before-and-After stories has been developed using the German data. Both stories have been transcribed using the German transcription system GAT (Selting et al. 1998).

7.3.1 *"Catastrophe"*

Liza is a teacher who works for a university at the time the interview was recorded. During the interview, she remembers her own beginnings as a teacher and reflects on her first two years at school: she experienced those first years as a "catastrophe" that made her seriously doubt her own capability as a teacher. In retrospect, she is able to explain that her doubts were the result of a teacher training that in fact had not much to do with her everyday work life, as it only focused on content-related aspects and not on individual and/or social factors. The whole narrative is organized in the structure of a Before-and-After format. Concerning Liza's story, it is interesting to focus on the way she presents (or in Bamberg's terms "navigates") her own professional development.

Transcript 7.1 Catastrophe

0455	Li:	well (-) at the beglnning of one's professional llfe (-)
0456		one is vEry much concerned with (--) fActual accUracy (.)
0457		and with that every (-) Other factor (-)
0458		gets pushed asIde (-) a bIt?
0459		[<<acc> or even> downwards. it just doesn't work.
0460	I:	[<<p> mh=hm?>
0461	Li:	but Once you start (-) let's say to feel a lot safer (--)
0462		concerning factual [Aspects? .hh then (-)
0463	I:	[<<p> mh=hm?>
0464	Li:	at least that's what I realized (.) you can open up a lOt mOre
0465		for those Other thIngs? [(---) a::nd in: (-)
0466	I:	[<<p> mh=hm?>
0467	Li:	<<acc> well when=I look at that> retrospectively (--)
0468		I would say my fIrst two years (-)
0469		they were a catAstrophe? (-)
0470		I=was on the verge of chucking everything [UP?
0471	I:	[oh;
0472	Li:	because=I thought (1.25) you are not ABLE (-)
0473		to teach properly? [(--) yea:h (.)
0474	I:	[oh; (.) mh=hm?
0475	Li:	I=was li:ke (.) a real creative crisis?=
0476	I:	=oh my;

(1.0)
Li: a:nd um:; (---) then (--) thank God I got
<<laughing> my act together>? ((laughs)) you know and the- (-)
the crucial thing was (.) that I was trained um:; (-)
to (-) convey a lot of (-) of that
factual knowledge? (.) but (-) I ha' (.)
no one told me (-) that there is something like
group dynamics;
I: <<p> mh=hm>
Li: no one told me (.) that there are good (--)
and wEA:k (.) and mediOcre [pupils
I: [mh=hm?
Li: and what that in turn means for my own prepa[ration; (--)
I: [mh=hm?
Li: no one told me:; (-) um:; (--)
that the time of the dAy; er; (-) the day of the wEEk; (-)
the rhythm of one SCHOOL year; (.) um [plays a rOle; (.)
I: [<<p> mh=hm?>
Li: I ALways used to relate everything that did not wOrk [to mE
I: [<<p> mh=hm?>
Li: and to what I DID; [(-)
I: [<<p> mh=hm?>
Li: and THAT was what let me become like very exasperate during
that um:; (-) ((clicks tongue)) first time?

Liza begins her narration with a generalized statement about first-time teachers and their main objective ("factual accuracy", 455–456). She claims that this main objective is so important that it suppresses every other kind of objective (457–459), and that the shift in a job novice's attention does not take place until s/he gains more confidence in teaching (461–462). After that brief exposition she turns to a more personal level and connects her initial observations to her own autobiographical experience. Crucial for that narrative is its twofold structure: it consists of the rather dramatic description of a prior first state and a succeeding second state where the dramatic impact of the initial phase is resolved. Both narrative self-positions are connected by a turning point where Liza as the protagonist of her story gains experience. This experience serves as the catalyst that helps her narrated self to transform into the facet of self that is presented in the second state of the narration. The presented narrative can be structurally described as consisting of three parts: a Before, a Turning Point, and an After.

In the Before phase of the story (467–477), Liza drastically depicts the consequences of her first years of being a teacher with "extreme case formulations" (Pomerantz 1986): "I was on the verge of chucking everything up" (470). Additionally, she blames her (supposed lack of) professional competence for being unable to change a situation she perceives as unbearable. This description culminates as she wraps up the climax of the situation as a "creative crisis" (475), upon which the interviewer responds sympathetically and thus acknowledges her account (476). The first part of the story is designed to establish a certain evaluative stance towards her narrated self "back then". Through this stance, Liza shows her interactive counterpart how she assesses her past actions from her present perspective: she self-positions herself as a, by now, experienced teacher, whose experience allows her to put her past crisis into perspective.

The very moment when that relativization was made possible is reconstructable in the Turning Point of the story, which Liza herself introduces by saying "then I got my act together" (478–493). She lists several factors that contributed to a relativization of her initial self-assessment: her sense of failure was not the result of her personal incapability as a teacher but an effect of a more theory-driven academic education.

Once this new perspective on her job is established within the story (and at the same time established as a reconstructed phase in her life), the interviewer is, as a result, implicitly able to conclude how the present Liza (as narrating self) has to be characterized—he can other-position Liza the narrator. In this case, the After phase of the narrative consists in Liza's professional development from the Turning Point on. Liza does not characterize herself explicitly in any way, but through the narrative contrasting of the two stages of professional development she self-positions herself in a way that leads to the conclusion that the later Liza (i.e. that facet of herself that resulted from the transformation process) is a "better" self insofar as it is able to distinguish between contextual and individual determinants of everyday work situations. In relation to the short exposition in 455–466, the benefits of the first two years consist of the ability to see the bigger picture instead of focusing only on singular aspects.

The change Liza traces here encompasses a period of roughly two years—it is apparent that this is a time frame where narratives about individual change are highly expectable. But the narrative format of Before-and-After stories can also encompass a shorter period of time. I will now give a second example of such a story where a change within one single lesson is presented. The overall structure is the same as in Transcript 7.1, but in contrast to "catastrophe", the narrator of the second story elaborates in greater detail on the comparison between the older and the more recent facet of his self.

7.3.2 *"Belly up"*

By the time the interview was conducted, Chris, the narrator of the second example, was a teacher in training who had the opportunity to teach at a school. The story I chose to analyze is about one lesson that did not go as planned in at least two respects: Chris originally wanted to discuss a homework assignment that none of his pupils had done, and the resulting improvised lesson was once again on the verge of collapsing when a student asked a question with potential for discussion—which Chris perceived as another threat to his schedule. But this second challenge turned out to be less threatening than suspected: Chris was able to transform the rest of the lesson into a discussion that he perceived as productive. According to him, that turn of events contributed to an improved classroom atmosphere and a better mutual understanding.

Transcript 7.2 «Belly up»

0725 Ch: <<decr> and then; (-) there are gOOd lessons? (.)
0726 and- (--) um; (-)
0727 a kind of lesson can emErge- where I was; (-)
0728 um; that was something I was really hAppy abou' (-)
0729 well; (.) where at fIrst you think- (-)
0730 oh (-) what am I going to DO now (-)
0731 that we; (--) err:: (1.0)
0732 <<p> um::> (--) well it was (.)
0733 it happened in a DIFferent (.)
0734 you know in a class from lAst TERM (.) and um (.)
0735 NO one had done his HOMEwork (-)
0736 a real clAssic so to speak [(.) exActly (--)
0737 IN: [<<pp> (xxx)>
0738 Ch: and you think (-) crAp (-)
0739 the whole currIculum goes belly-UP?
0740 IN: m=hm?
0741 Ch: u::m::; (.)
0742 and then: (--) err I didn't know for sUre;
0743 <<quickly> then I said well okAY-> (.)
0744 we'll do it NOW? (-)
0745 not the smartest thing pedagogically speaking (.)
0746 [I guess (.)
0747 IN: [((chuckles))
0748 Ch: but- (--) there was no other WAY. [I mean you could have'
0749 IN: [<<p> m=hm?>
0750 Ch: there wouldn't have been ANY progress otherwise?
0751 IN: <<p> m=hm?>
0752 Ch: and then it was like preparAtion phase?
0753 and then::- (-) <<p> um:;> (-)
0754 out of the BLUE (.) JUST before class was over
0755 ONE pupil um: (.) put his hand up (-)
0756 <<quickly> or not really put his hand up- (.)
0757 well> (.) so one pupil just SAID- (1.25)
0758 who::- (.) <<p> um:;> usually just likes (.)
0759 to tEAse a lot; [(.)
0760 IN: [m=hm?
0761 Ch: and <<p> m:; (.) m: (.) um:; m::>
0762 and likes to contribute silly jOkes
0763 and so on (-) and um:; (-)
0764 <<p> um;> (-) he said? (-) um::
0765 he would like to address a SErious issue now.
0766 and I was like ya=ah? (-)
0767 whAt in fAct does happen after DEATH. (1.5)
0768 an::d [u::m;
0769 IN: [<<p> well that certainly IS something.
0770 [((chuckles))>
0771 Ch: [that in fact IS sOmething? and um: (.)
0772 I remember in thIs vEry sEcond (.) it (.)
0772 it crossed my mInd

0773		whAt will you DO now? (-)
0774		the whole curricu' (.)
0775		if you start to- (-)
0776		if you start to elaborate on thAt
0777		the curriculum is DONE for?
0778		[u::m: (--)
0779	IN:	[<<p> m=hm>
0780	Ch:	and thEn at the sAme time I thought (.)
0781		well that's the VERY occasion; (-) um; (--)
0782		to get into a conversAtion with one another? [(-)
0783	IN:	[m=hm?
0784	Ch:	and- (-) um; (-) the resUlt was? (--)
0785		um; (1.25)
0786		with the whOle clAss; (.)
0787		all of a sudden they were ALL involved; (.)
0788		<<quicker> and the Actual task was (-)
0789		no longer impOrtant>
0790		and that was a gOOd thing- (--) um; (--)
0791		for thrEE-quarters of an hour or so;
0792		a conversation about these kinds of questions. [(-)
0793	IN:	[<<p> m=hm?>
0794	Ch:	then it was somehow about (.)
0795		about euthanasia- [(.) and (-) essEntial questions- and- (-)
0796	IN:	[<<p> m=hm?>
0797	Ch:	and so ON and so fOrth. [(.)
0798	IN:	[<<p> m=hm?>
0799	Ch:	and it All went in a direction- (--)
0800		mh:: (2.0)
0801		where I thought (.)
0802		THAT is (-) where I (.) where we; (.)
0803		well where I thInk (.)
0804		the pupils too noticed and
0805		where especially !I! noticed (--)
0806		that I (-)
0807		that (.) I am not the one who provides the answers
0808		and they are not the ones who ask the quEstions [(-)
0809	IN:	[<<p> m=hm?>
0810	Ch:	but we are on this quest toGEther.
0811	IN:	<<p> m=hm?>
0812	Ch:	and um; (-)
0813		we can mutually offer each other questions and answers?
0814	IN:	<<p> m=hm?>
0815	Ch:	and um; (1.75) YEAH; (-)
0816		allOW for things like that.
0817	IN:	<<p> m=hm?>
0818	Ch:	and um; (-)
0819		allOw for a lesson to evolve in- [(---)
0820	IN:	[<<p> m=hm?>
0821	Ch:	a dIfferent direction than the one actually planned at home
0822		at one's working desk. (---) yah.

In the analysis I will again focus on structural aspects of the story. Similar to the story told in Transcript 7.1, Chris initiates the narration with a generalized introduction in which he anticipates the positive outcome of the story he is about to tell. The following narrative contains two unexpected events; there are two Before phases that lead up to each other. I will call them Before (1) and Before (2).

In Before (1), Chris depicts a classroom situation that did not go as planned because "no one had done his homework" (735). Similar to the Before phase in Liza's story, he uses extreme case formulations ("crap", "the whole curriculum goes belly-up"), and thus establishes an evaluative stance towards the narrated events. In addition to that, he gives the interviewer the chance to get a glimpse at his thoughts: Chris stages his internal monologue during the narrated situation and provides the interviewer with an exclusive perspective on the difference between Chris's actual behavior in the classroom and what he thought about it at the same time. He self-positions himself as a bit helpless and unsure about how to act in the face of unforeseen events.

Even if Chris decides to "do it [i.e. the homework] now" (744), his lesson was not saved yet. The events in Before (2) are dominated by another threat to Chris's quickly improvised plan: "a serious issue" (765) gets addressed. The protagonist of that second Before phase is one pupil who "put his hand up" (755) or "just said" (757) something, respectively. After the introduction of that pupil occurred rather en passant, the following exchange between Chris and his pupil is restaged in dialogic form. The narrative climax of that second Before phase consists in an unforeseen topic that comes up (752–765) and seems to put Chris's lesson in danger again. This second Before phase, too, is given a negative evaluation and serves to position Chris as a teacher who has to work hard to stick to the schedule of his lesson. This time, the evaluation does not take the form of extreme case formulations but as narrative "atomization" (Quasthoff 1980) of the crucial decision-making moments, including staging of internal dialogue (772–779). With this restaging another effect of immediacy is achieved: the interviewer becomes a witness to the unfolding of events. That the implicit evaluation and the possible consequences in terms of the lesson's progression are anticipated by the interviewer as well can be seen in 769 where the interviewer reacts by saying "well that certainly IS something" and thus demonstrates that he interpreted Chris's narrative presentation accordingly.

After the initial shock, the second threat to Chris's lesson proved to be "a good thing" (790). The Turning Point of his story consists in Chris being able to regard the events as a chance and, at the same time, being able to take that chance ("well that's the VERY occasion; (-) um; (–) to get into a conversAtion with one another?"; 780f.). He was able to steer the class into a discussion about the topic of life after death (784ff.), which turned out to be so productive that all previous activities were abandoned (788ff.).

Again, the evaluation of the After phase differs significantly from the previous evaluation of events. Chris describes the effect of the unforeseen discussion as a new orientation towards classroom atmosphere: "we are on this quest together" (810) is the metaphor he uses. He evaluates the turn of events explicitly as positive

(790) and incorporates it into the bigger context of classroom atmosphere and the understanding of one's role (801–813). Similar to Liza's story (Transcript 7.1), a relativization takes place. This relativization is verbalized in his last utterances: events that at first sight seem to be a problem can lead to a good outcome and personal growth. In addition to that explicit change in evaluations and interpretations of the situation, it is interesting to note that Chris the narrator distances himself from his narrated former facet of self by using the impersonal German pronoun "man" ("one"). As Yates and Hiles (2010) show, the use of pronouns is an important analytic aspect in order to reconstruct positioning activities and identity construction. They discuss the use of impersonal pronouns as a conversational means speakers use in narrative accounts of events in which they experience certain restrictions and limitations: "Such limitations are potentially threatening to a presentation of oneself as a self-expressing and active agent." (ibd.: 549). Like Liza in Transcript 7.1, Chris uses his narrative to self-position himself on the level of the interview interaction as "more professional" compared to the narrated version of himself that had to face the difficult situation in his classroom.

7.3.3 Before-and-After Stories: Characteristics

The analyses show that the following aspects are characteristic for the three phases of the discussed Before-and-After stories.

The *Before phase* is about different events in the past that, in general, create a difficult situation for the narrated self. These events are evaluated negatively in different ways: the use of extreme case formulations, restaging of dialogues and atomization of events are the techniques that could be observed in the examples. These evaluations serve a double purpose: on the level of the interview situation, they provide the counterpart/the interviewer with a more or less explicit specification of the subjective quality of experience in the narrated event and serve as narrative means to create immediacy. On the level of the interview narrations, a complex stage for narrative positions is created: through the negative evaluation of the narrated events, the narrator constructs a past facet of self with certain attitudes towards the event and other people involved in it. These other-positionings in turn influence the indirect self-positioning of the narrated past self.

This past facet of self changes throughout the narrated course of events. In the *After phase*, different or even opposite evaluative stances towards the immediately prior constructed facet of self are described. On the structural level of the narrative, this change is made possible through the introduction of a *Turning Point*, which serves as a link between the two states of the narrative format: in the retrospective view of the interview situation, the narrator describes how a change of judgement and/or a change of perspectives was triggered by sudden events, an individual insight, or other things that the narrated self in the past situation was not able to anticipate. The narrator's reaction on these unforeseen events causes the change of his/her self—a change that is presented narratively in the After phase of the story.

From this new self's perspective, the events in the Before phase are assessed differently than from the older self's perspective.

7.4 The Passage of Time as a Narrative Resource in Constructing a "Better" Self

Crucial for Before-and-After stories are their Turning Points, because they serve as a link between the two phases of the narration in which different facets of self are described, contrasted and positioned. Turning points, however, are not a new concept for the study of narrative interaction. According to Bruner (2001: 32f.), they

> mark off the narrator's consciousness from the protagonist's and begin closing the gap between the two at the same time. [...] Turning points are a step towards narratorial consciousness.

In contrast to the discussed data, Bruner's definition of turning points is connected to "big" events in life—his concept of turning points encompasses events like college graduation, marriage, etc. [see also the concept of the "springboard effect" as described in Pals (2006)]. Obviously, no one got married or graduated in my data—the turning points here had nothing to do with such "big" events. Instead, they seemed to mark individual stages of knowledge acquisition and to offer the recipient a narrative snapshot of the moment where an individual gain in knowledge has happened—and where the passage of time and the narrators' reactions to difficult situations during that time lead to a change in the narrators' self-concepts. The two facets of self that are constructed during the two phases of the narration differ regarding the narrated self's knowledge. The problematic quality of the narrator's Before state is narratively enacted through staged internal monologue, atomization of events and explicit negative evaluation. In contrast, the After phase (and thus, the narrators' state in that phase) is evaluated positively and the self seems to emerge from the problematic situation with new insights. The recipient is presented with a narrative performance where s/he witnesses the narrator's change over time—where a new facet of identity emerges. Before-and-After stories thus establish a temporal contrast between two facets of the narrator's self: an "older" facet that was confronted with a situation almost too difficult to handle, and a "newer", more grown facet that has overcome these difficulties through learning and a more agentive stance towards the narrated events. The two key mechanisms which facilitate this kind of face-work consist in (1) using contrastive evaluations of these two facets of self and (2) their presentation in narrative format.

7.4.1 Contrastivity as a Means of Identity Construction

Establishing contrastivity seems to be one central mechanism of identity construction. In most cases other people serve as a narrative resource to show the interactional partner on various levels of interaction to what extent a person is unique—i.e., where s/he differs from comparable others or is similar to them (and in which respects). These "Alter-Ego-Positions" (Sacher 2012) create the proverbial "rough edges" that shape a person and provide the interactional counterpart with an idea of who s/he is dealing with. However, this contrastivity need not specifically consist of contrasts to other people—with the narrative format of Before-and-After stories the speaker can redefine a former facet of his/her own self to an internalized Alter position and thus demonstrate to his/her counterpart how exactly change has happened, what caused this change and how exactly the narrator dealt with the requirements of the situation. By "charging" the first phase of the narrative with negatively connoted meaning and thus establishing a narrative position contrastive to the one in the After phase, the narrator at the same time depreciates the older facet of his/her self—both Liza and Chris present a Before self that was almost overstrained with the situation it found itself in. By evaluating the second phase of the narrative positively, the new facet of self, too, is evaluated positively without the narrator needing to make this self-assessment explicit.

7.4.2 Creating a "Better" Self—The Construction of Temporal Contrastivity

Even if the construction of an agentive and individual self is very common in Western narratives (see Brockmeier as cited above), there are constraints that can be attributed to the status of self-praise in Western societies and the avoidance of it. Pomerantz (1978) has described the everyday dilemma one faces when dealing with self-praise from a conversation analyst's perspective: Even if the presentation of an agentive self seems to be typical for Western narratives (see above), praising oneself is a clearly dispreferred activity in Western societies that can be sanctioned by others (by teasing or by openly criticizing the speaker for bragging). Pomerantz points out that when receiving a compliment, speakers face a complicated situation: on the one hand, affirmation and acknowledgement are preferred reactions towards assessments. On the other hand, to react affirmatively can easily be interpreted as self-praise. She observes that in order to avoid being potentially regarded as vain or arrogant, speakers use a number of conversational techniques to acknowledge initial praise and at the same time avoid the interactional danger of self-praise ("Oh thank you, but the dress is second-hand", "Thank you, but my husband prepared that dinner", etc.). As the analyses of Transcripts 7.1 and 7.2 have shown, there seem to be other, narratively based versions of self-praise avoidance: With Before-and-After stories, the speaker can implicitly suggest a positive evaluation of a facet of his/her own self and trace the way this facet of self came into existence. Additionally, by explaining the situational circumstances that caused the narrator to act the way s/he acted, the danger of being regarded as a braggart is prevented. Therefore, the passage of time is not only an analytical concept to describe central functions of narrative discourse. It is also a means for the speakers to deal with culturally specific demands of interactions—they can provide their counterpart with an idea of how they want to be seen without violating sensitive norms of conduct. Before-and-After stories thus serve as a means of implicit narrative face-work.

The presented study can be seen in the tradition of other work which shows that construction and modification of identity does not necessarily happen in "big" stories (i.e. Georgakopoulou 2007; Bamberg 2009). Drawing on theories and concepts from conversation, discourse, positioning and interaction analysis, I reconstructed two stories in which not only the content served as means for the narrators' identity construction but also the specific structure of the stories (therefore named Before-and-After stories). Analytical questions to pursue for future research are in line with Bagga-Gupta et al.'s claim that identity can be seen as action (in this volume): Are there other types of narratives where the narrative structure is a crucial mechanism in identity construction? If so, do they differ with regard to the situation in which they are told—e.g. in the classroom or in challenging situations like a job interview? Does the content of the story influence how narrators position themselves?

Questions like these could give a better insight into the intricate mechanisms used for identity construction as a means of everyday action—not only on the level of a story's content, but also on a structural level.

Appendix

Transcription Symbols

The data was transcribed according to the transcription system GAT (Selting et al. 1998) (Table 7.1).

Table 7.1 Transcription key

[but i think [like i said	Overlap
=	Quick succession of turns or units
(.)	Micropause
(-), (–), (—)	Short, middle and longer pauses (0.25-0.75 s)
(1.75)	Estimated length of pauses from 1 s on
and = uh	Slurring
:, ::, :::	Stretchings
ehm, um	Hesitationssignals
becau’	Glottal stops
tha(h)at	Laughter within units
hehehe	Laughter
hm = hm, ye = ah	Backchannel signals
((clears throat))	Para- and extra verbal actions und events
≪clears throat≫	Speech accompanying para- and extraverbal actions and events with information about their scope
≪amused≫	Interpreting comments with information about their scope
(xxx)	Incomprehensible utterance
(such)	Assumed wording
(such/much)	Possible alternatives
EMphasis/emphAsis	Emphasis
!EM!phasis	Strong emphasis
?	Rising pitch at the end of a unit
–	Constant pitch at the end of a unit
;	Falling pitch at the end of a unit
↑, ↓	Differences in the pitch (higher or lower)
≪p≫	= piano, quiet
≪pp≫	= pianissimo, very quiet
≪f≫	= forte, loud
≪acc≫	= accelerando, getting faster
≪rit≫	= ritardando, getting slower
≪cresc≫	= crescendo, getting louder
≪decr≫	= decrescendo, getting more quiet
.h, .hh, .hhh	Intake of breath
h, hh, hhh	Breathing out

German Data

"Katastrophe"

Transcript 7.3 Katastrophe (German original)

0455 Li: also man (-) Is in der ANfangsphase seiner berUfstätigkeit; (-)
0456 sEhr auf die fAchliche rIchtigkeit; (--) konzentriert (.)
0457 und damit fallen erst mal so alle (-) ANderen faktOren (-)
0458 son bIsschen (--) an die sEIte?
0459 [<<acc> oder sogar> hinten rUnter. das GEHT gar nich.
0460 IN: [<<p> mh=hm?>
0461 Li: aber wEnn man (-) sozusagen ANfängt sich im fAchlichen (--)
0462 SIcherer zu [fühlen? .hh dann (-)
0463 IN: [<<p> mh=hm?>
0464 Li: hab Ich jedenfalls gemerkt (.) kAnn man sich auch mehr für
0465 diese ANderen dInge öffnen? [(--) u::nd im: (-)
0466 IN: [<<p> mh=hm?>
0467 Li: <<acc> so wenn=ich das jetzt> rÜckblickend betrachte- (--)
0468 würd=ich sagen meine ERsten zwei jahre- (-)
0469 waren ne katastrOphe? (-)
0470 da war=ich auch kurz davor alles hInzuschmei[ßen?
0471 IN: [oh;
0472 Li: weil=ich gedAcht hab (1.25) du KANNST (-) nicht gut
0473 unterrichten? [(--) ja: (.)
0474 IN: [oh; (.) mh=hm?
0475 Li: da war=ich so: rIchtige schAffenskrise?=
0476 IN: =ohje;
0477 (1.0)
0478 Li: u::nd ä::hm:; (---) dAnn (--) hab=ich aber gOtt sei dank die
0479 kUrve <<lachend> bekOhommen>? ((lacht)) jA; und der- (-)
0480 und der pUnkt war eben (.) dass ich AUCH so ausgebildet äh:;
0481 (-) wUrde (.) dass=ich eben ganz VIEL (-) von diesem
0482 FAKtenwissen? (.) transportieren sollte- aber- (--) ich ha' (.)
0483 bIn nIch drauf vOrbereitet worden- (-) dAss es ne
0484 grUppendynAmik; [(.) gibt. (--)
0485 IN: [<<p> mh=hm>
0486 Li: ich bin nicht drauf vorbereitet worden- (.) dass es stArke (--)
0487 und schwAche:; (.) und mIttlere schüler [gibt;
0488 IN: [mh=hm?
0489 Li: und was das für die planu[ng bedeutet; (--)
0490 IN: [mh=hm?
0491 Li: ich bin nIcht drauf vorbereitet wo:rden:; (-) äh:; (--)
0492 dass tAgeszeiten; äh:; (-) WOchentage; (.)
0493 ein SCHULjahresrhythmus; (.) äh [ne rOlle spielt; (.)
0494 IN: [<<p> mh=hm?>
0495 Li: ich hab IMmer alles was nich funktionIErte auf mIch [bezogen;
0496 IN: [<<p> mh=hm?>
0497 Li: und mein TUN; [(-)
0498 IN: [<<p> mh=hm?>
0499 Li: und DAS hat mich sozusagen in der ERsten zeit sehr; ähm:; (-)
0500 ((schnalzt)) verzwEIfeln lassen?

"Inne Dutten"

Transcript 7.4 Inne Dutten (German original)

0725	Ch:	<<decr> und dann; (-) gibt=s gUte stUnden? (.) und- (--)
0726		ähm; (-)> dann entstEht auch mal so ne stUnde- da wAr=ich; (-)
0727		ähm; hab=ich=mich sEhr gefrEUt drü' (-)
0728		also; (.) man in der Ersten sekunde gedacht hat- (-)
0729		oh (-) was mAchste jetzt- (-) dass wir; (--) ähm:::; (1.0)
0730		<<p> ähm::;> (--) das war also (.) war in nem ANdern; (.)
0731		also im kurs vom lEtzten seMEster- (.) und äh (.)
0732		KEIner hatte die hAUsaufgaben gemAcht- (-)
0733		der klAssiker [sozusagen- (.) genAU- (--)
0734	IN:	[<<pp> (xxx)>
0735	Ch:	und man dEnkt sich- (-) schEIße- (-) die gAnze
0736		Unterrichtsplanung geht inne dUtten? [(-) Ä::hm:::; (.)
0737	IN:	[m=hm?
0738	Ch:	und dann: (--) ö wUsst=ich aUch erst nicht so genAU;
0739		<<schnell> dann hab=ich gesagt ja okAY-> (.)
0740		mAchen wir das jetzt im KURS? (-)
0741		p' pädagogisch auch nicht das klÜgste; (.) [glAUb=ich- (.)
0742	IN:	[((schmunzelt))
0743	Ch:	aber- (--) GING nicht anders. [also man hätte'
0744	IN:	[<<p> m=hm?>
0745	Ch:	sonst wär=mer ja NIE: wohIn gekOmmen?
0746	IN:	<<p> m=hm?>
0747	Ch:	und dann war irgendwie erArbeitungsphAse? und dann::- (-)
0748		<<p> ähm::;> (-) aUs hEIterem hImmel (.) ↑kUrz vor Ende
0749		mEldet sich ähm: (.) EIN- (-) <<schnell> was heißt mEldet- (.)
0750		also::> (.) sagt sozusagen eIn schÜler- (1.25) de::r- (-)
0751		<<p> ähm:;> sOnst auch VIEL so:; (.) Eher so frOtzelEIen; [(.)
0752	IN:	[m=hm?
0753	Ch:	und <<p> m:; (.) m: (.) ähm:; m::> mal so=n blÖden spruch von
0754		lInks (.) und so; (-) also so eInbringt- (-) und äh:; (-)
0755		<<p> ähm;> (-) sAgt? (-) äh:: er hÄtte jetzt mal ne ERNste
0756		frAge. und ich so ja=a? (-)
0757		wAs kOmmt eigentlich nach dem tOd. (1.5) un::d [ä::h;
0758	IN:	[<<p> das is ja
0759		dirEkt n klOpper. [((schmunzelt))>
0760	Ch:	[dAs ist dirEkt ein klOpfer? und äh: (.)
0761		in dEr sekUnde wusst=ich noch (.) geht mir (.)
0762		ging mir also durch den kOpf was mAchst du jEtzt? (-)
0763		die ganze stUndenpla' (.) wenn du jEtzt- (-)
0764		wenn du jEtzt noch drauf eIngehst ist die ganze stundenplanung
0765		sowieso HIN? [(--) ä::hm; (--)
0766	IN:	[<<p> m=hm>
0767	Ch:	und ich hab dAnn <<cresc> gleichzeitig gedAcht> (.)
0768		aber es ist DIE gelegenheit; (-) ähm; (--)
0769		mIteinander ins ge[sprÄch zu kommen? (-)
0770	IN:	[m=hm?

Ch:	und (-) ähm; (-) es ergAb sich dann? (--) ähm; (1.25)
	mIt dem geSAMten kUrs; (.) da warn dann plötzlich alle dAbei;
	(.) <<schneller> und die aUfgabe war dann auch; (-) von der
	eInen sekUnde auf die ANdere auch UNwichtig-> (-)
	das war auch gUt so- (--) ähm; (--)
	ne drEIviertelstUnde oder so was; n gespRÄCH über solche
	frAgen. [(.)
IN:	[<<p> m=hm?>
Ch:	dann gings irgendwie um (.) über stErbehilfe- [(.) und (-)
IN:	[<<p> m=hm?>
Ch:	sInnfrAgen- und- (-) und so wEIter [und so fOrt. (.)
IN:	[<<p> m=hm?>
Ch:	und gIng so=n bIsschen so in die rIchtung- (--) mh:: (2.0)
	und wo=ich gedAcht hab (.) das IS (-) was wo i' (.) wo wir; (.)
	also wo ich glAUbe (.) auch die schüler gemErkt haben und
	wo Ich das auch noch mal besonders gemerkt habe (--)
	dass ich (-) dass (.) Ich n' nicht der mit den ANTworten
	und sie die mit den frAgen sind- [(-)
IN:	[<<p> m=hm?>
Ch:	sondern dass wir gemEInsam auf dieser sUche sind. [(-)
IN:	[<<p> m=hm?>
Ch:	und ähm; (-) uns gemeinsam fragen und antworten anbieten
	können? [(-)
IN:	[<<p> m=hm?>
Ch:	und ähm; (1.75) JA; (-) und so was eben dann auch zUlassen.[(-)
IN:	[<<p> m=hm?>
Ch:	und ähm; (-) zUlassen auch dass ne stUnde dann mal- [(--)
IN:	[<<p> m=hm?>
Ch:	ANders läuft als man sich das zu hause am schreIbtisch geplant
	hat. (---) (ja.)

References

Antaki, C. (1998). Identity as an achievement and as a tool. In C. Antaki & S. Widdicombe (Eds.), *Identities in talk* (pp. 1–14). London: Sage.

Baker, C. D. (2002). Ethnomethodological analyses of interviews. In J. F. Gubrium & J. A. Holstein (Eds.), *Handbook of interview research: Context and methods* (pp. 777–796). Thousand Oaks: Sage.

Bamberg, M. G. (1997). Positioning between structure and performance. *Journal of Narrative and Life History, 7*(1–4), 335–342.

Bamberg, M. (2009). Identity and narration. In P. Hühn, J. Pier, W. Schmid, & J. Schönert (Eds.), *Handbook of narratology* (pp. 132–143). Berlin, Boston: De Gruyter.

Bamberg, M. (2011). Narrative practice and identity investigation. In J. A. Holstein & J. F. Gubrium (Eds.), *Varieties of narrative analysis* (pp. 99–124). Thousand Oaks: Sage.

Bergmann, J. R. (1994). Ethnomethodologische Konversationsanalyse. [Ethnomethodological conversation analysis]. In G. Fritz & F. Hundsnurscher (Eds.), *Handbuch der Dialoganalyse* (pp. 3–16). [*Handbook of dialogue analysis*]. Berlin: Walter de Gruyter.

Brockmeier, J. (2000). Autobiographical time. *Narrative Inquiry, 10*(1), 51–73.
Brockmeier, J. (2003). Die Zeit meines Lebens. [The time of my life]. *Journal for Psychology, 11* (1), 4–32.
Brockmeier, J. (2009). Stories to remember. Narrative and the time of memory. *Journal of Narrative Studies, 1,* 115–132.
Bruner, J. (2001). Self-making and world-making. In J. Brockmeier & D. A. Carbaugh (Eds.), *Narrative and identity: Studies in autobiography, self, and culture* (pp. 25–37). Toronto, Berlin: John Benjamins.
Bruner, J. (2004). Life as narrative. *Social Research, 71*(3), 691–710.
Bucholtz, M., & Hall, K. (2005). Identity and interaction: A sociocultural linguistic approach. *Discourse Studies, 7*(4–5), 585–641.
Davies, B., & Harré, R. (1990). Positioning: The discursive production of selves. *Journal for the Theorie of Social Behaviour, 20*(1), 43–63.
Deppermann, A. (2008). *Gespräche analysieren: Eine Einführung. [Analyzing conversation: An introduction]* (3rd ed.). Wiesbaden: VS.
Garfinkel, H. (1967). *Studies in ethnomethodology.* New Jersey: Englewood Cliffs.
Georgakopoulou, A. (2007). *Small stories, identity and interaction.* Amsterdam, Philadelphia: John Benjamins.
Goffman, E. (1967). *Interaction ritual.* New York: Anchor Books.
Goodwin, M. H. (1997). Byplay: negotiating evaluation in storytelling. In G. R. Guy, C. Feagin, D. Schiffrin, J. Baugh (Eds.), *Towards a social science of language. Papers in Honor of William Labov. Vol 2: Social interaction and discourse structures* (pp. 77–102). Amsterdam, Philadelphia: John Benjamins.
Gülich, E., Hausendorf, H. (2000). Vertextungsmuster: Narration. [Narrative as a model for creating texts]. In K. Brinker, G. Antos, W. Heinemann, S.F. Sager (Eds.), *Text- und Gesprächslinguistik: Ein internationales Handbuch zeitgenössischer Forschung. 2. Halbband: Gesprächslinguistik* (pp. 1086–1094). [*Linguistic of texts and dialogues: an international handbook of contemporary research. 2. Volume: Discourse linguistics*]. Berlin: De Gruyter.
Gülich, E., Mondada, L., Furchner, I. (2008). *Konversationsanalyse. Eine Einführung am Beispiel des Französischen.* [*Conversation analysis. An introduction using the example of French*]. Tübingen: Niemeyer.
Hausendorf, H., & Bora, A. (2006). Reconstructing social positioning in discourse. Methodological basics and their implementation from a conversation analyst perspective. In H. Hausendorf, A. Bora (Eds.), *Analysing citizenship talk. Social positioning in political and legal decision-making processes* (pp. 85–97). Berlin: John Benjamins.
Heritage, J. (1998). Conversation analysis and institutional talk: Analyzing distinctive turn-taking-systems. In S. Cmejrková, O. Hoffmannová Müllerová, J. Svetlá (Eds.), *Proceedings of the 6th International Congress of IADA (International Association for Dialogue Analysis)* (pp. 3–17). Tübingen: Niemeyer.
Holmes, J. (2006). Workplace narratives, professional identity and relational practice. In A. deFina, D. Schiffrin, M. Bamberg (Eds.), *Discourse and identity* (pp. 166–187). Cambridge: University Press.
Jefferson, G. (1978). Sequential aspects of storytelling in conversation. In J. Schenkein (Ed.), *Studies in the organization of conversational interaction* (pp. 219–248). New York: Academic Press.
Johnson, G. C. (2006). The discursive construction of teacher identities in a research interview. In A. deFina, D. Schiffrin, M. Bamberg (Eds.), *Discourse and Identity* (pp. 213–232). Cambridge: University Press.
Lucius-Hoene, G., & Deppermann, A. (2004). *Rekonstruktion narrativer Identität.* [*Reconstructing narrative identity*]. Opladen: Leske + Budrich.
Pals, J. L. (2006). Constructing the "springboard effect": Causal connections, self-making and growth within the life story. In D. P. McAdams, R. Josselson, & A. Lieblich (Eds.), *Identity and story: Creating life in narrative* (pp. 175–199). Washington: APA.

Pomerantz, A. (1978). Compliment responses: Notes on the co-operation of multiple constraints. In J. Schenkein (Ed.), *Studies in the organization of conversational interaction* (pp. 79–112). New York: Academic Press.
Pomerantz, A. (1986). Extreme case formulations: A way of legitimizing claims. *Human Studies, 9* (2–3), 219–229.
Quasthoff, U. M. (1980). *Erzählen in Gesprächen: Linguistische Untersuchungen zu Strukturen und Funktionen am Beispiel einer Kommunikationsform des Alltags*. [*Narrating in dialogue: linguistic investigations of stuctures and functions of an everyday conversational form*]. Tübingen: Narr.
Sacher, J. (2012). *Sprechen über sich selbst als kontrastives Verfahren: Die Etablierung von Alter-Ego-Positionen, Identitätskonstruktion und Selbstdarstellung im Interview*. [*Talking about oneself as contrastive method: The establishment of Alter-Ego-Positions, identity construction and self presentation in the interview*]. Mannheim: Verlag für Gesprächsforschung.
Sacher, J., Lingnau, B., & Knerich, H. (2015). (Ko?)-Konstruktion in institutionellen Settings. [(Co-?) Construction in institutional settings]. In U. Dausendschön-Gay, E. Gülich, & U. Krafft (Eds.), *Ko-Konstruktionen in der Interaktion. Die gemeinsame Arbeit an Äußerungen und anderen sozialen Ereignissen* (pp. 349–372). [*Co-Constructions in interaction. The joint production of utterances and other social events*]. Bielefeld: Transcript.
Sacks, H. (1984). Notes on methodology. In J. M. Atkinson & J. Heritage (Eds.), *Structures of social action: Studies in conversation analysis* (pp. 21–27). Cambridge: University Press.
Sacks, H. (1986). Some considerations of a story. *Poetics, 15*(1986), 127–138.
Sacks, H., Schegloff, E. A., & Jefferson, G. (1974). A simplest systematics for the organization of turn-taking for conversation. *Language, 50*(4/1), 696–735.
Schegloff, E. A. (1982). Discourse as interactional achievement: Some uses of 'uhhuh' and other things that come between sentences. In D. Tannen (Ed.), *Analyzing discourse: Text and talk* (pp. 71–83). Washington: Georgetown University Press.
Schegloff, E. A., & Sacks, H. (1973). Opening up closings. *Semiotica, 8*(4), 289–327.
Schenkein, J. (1978). Identity Negotiations in conversation. In J. Schenkein (Ed.), *Studies in the organization of conversational interaction* (pp. 57–78). New York: Academic Press.
Schütz, A. (1972). Einige Grundbegriffe der Phänomenologie. [Some fundamental terms of phenomenology]. In A. Schütz (Ed.), *Gesammelte Aufsätze, Teil II: Phänomenologie und die Sozialwissenschaften* (pp. 113–115). [*Collected essays, part II: Phenomenology and the social sciences*]. Berlin: Springer.
Selting, M., Auer, P., Barden, B., Bergmann, J., Couper-Kuhlen, E., et al. (1998). Gesprächsanalytisches Transkriptionssystem (GAT). [The discourse analytic transcription system GAT]. *Linguistische Berichte, 173*, 91–123.
Silverman, D. (1998). *Harvey sacks: Social science and conversation analysis*. Cambridge, Oxford: Polity Press.
Ten Have, P. (2007). *Doing conversation analysis*. London: Sage.
Trautmann, M., & Sacher, J. (Eds.) (2010). *Unterrichtsentwicklung durch Videofeedback. Besser kommunizieren lernen.* [*Classroom development through videofeedback: Learning to communicate better*]. Göttingen: Vandenhoeck & Ruprecht.
Uhmann, S. (1989). Interviewstil. Konversationelle Eigenschaften eines sozialwissenschaftlichen Erhebungsinstrumentes. [Interview style. Conversational features of a socio-scientific survey method]. In V. Hinnenkamp, M. Selting (Eds.), *Stil und Stilisierung* (pp. 125–165). [*Style and stylization*]. Berlin: Walter de Gruyter.
van Langenhove, L., & Harré, R. (1999). Introducing positioning theory. In R. Harré, L. van Langenhove (Eds.), *Positioning theory. Moral contexts of intentional action* (pp. 14–31). Oxford: Blackwell Publishers.

Wolf, R. (1999). Soziale Positionierung im Gespräch. [*Social positioning in dialogue*]. *Deutsche Sprache, 27*(1), 69–94.
Yates, S., & Hiles, D. (2010). 'You can't' but 'I do': Rules, ethics and the significance of shifts in pronominal forms for self-positioning in talk. *Discourse Studies, 12*(4), 535–551.

Author Biography

Julia Sacher is a linguist who specializes in the analysis of discourse. She has received her Ph.D. from the University of Bielefeld, Germany. Her interdisciplinary research interests center on the analysis of (narrative) discourse, identity research, and the analysis of the development of professional behavior. She is currently working at the University of Cologne, Germany, focusing on the development and implementation of research classes for master students.

Part III
Politically Framed Identities in Embodied Interaction

Part III of the volume "*Identity Revisited and Reimagined. Empirical and Theoretical Contributions Across Time and Space*" brings together three chapters that, in different ways, explore identity construction in political/public contexts.

In the opening chapter of Part III, Chap. 8 titled "From Political to National Identity in Zanzibar. Narratives on Changes in Social Practices", Sigrun Marie Moss argues that people sort other people into categories, and define themselves into groups they feel part of and distance themselves from groups they do not belong to. She also highlights that identity constellations influence emotions, cognitions and behavior towards in-group members and out-group members, and shifts in group identity are accompanied by changes in social practices that express these identities. Taking anthropological tenants as points of departure, Moss describes how a shift from polarized political identities to a shared nation-state identity is mirrored in changes in social practices on the semi-autonomous archipelago Zanzibar, off the coast of the geopolitical spaces of Tanzania. She makes the case that there is a dearth of research on such processes in intergroup conflict, and that uniting under a shared overarching identity has been emphasised as a way of overcoming intergroup conflict. Moss also builds on the premise that given that people increasingly see themselves as members of a singular (national) identity, this influences emotions and behaviours towards (and evaluations of) former outgroup members. The analysis builds upon extensive fieldwork and interviews with members of the population including political leaders in the community. The chapter illustrates how people talk about the reconciliation processes in relation to the conflict and how these shape social practices in the community.

Ellen Andenæs discusses embodiment related to professional identity in Chap. 9, "'She Didn't Know I'm Black, You See'—Practices, Body Signs, and Professional Identity". Andenæs contrasts the common conceptualization of professional identity as the image people build up based on the way an individual performs a job, related to particular kinds of knowledge and competencies that are shared with colleagues, with identity as being embodied. She discusses the latter in terms of complex relationships between competencies and bodies. This second chapter in section three presents research based upon an interactionist, practice based approach to professional identity. The research focuses Norwegian nursing homes where the employees were ethnically diverse and were represented by an unusually high proportion of males on the one hand, and residents were overwhelmingly white ethnic Norwegians. Thus, how the bodies of nurses are perceived by the patients, and how such interpretations figure in negotiations of nurse's professional identity positions are center-staged in the chapter. Issues related to identity conflict are reported to be common in that it was not unusual that some residents rejected nurses whom they disliked or distrusted. Andenæs discusses this by taking Dorte Marie Søndergaard's work on 'body signs' relating it to the nurses' appearance i.e. their skin colour, accents, and markers of gender. The chapter focuses on how nurses account for such situations in research interviews, and on the nature of identity work their accounts accomplish.

The final chapter in Part III, Chap. 10 "The Complexities of Deaf Identities", addresses the dynamic processes of deaf identity formation. Irene W. Leigh theorizes identity by deploying intersectionality and identifies gaps in research on deaf identity formation. She notes the importance of recognizing the fluid and dynamic nature of identities that are shaped through biology, cognition, sociohistorical contexts and language choices. Leigh's point is that knowledge of the fact that an individual cannot hear does not automatically confer a deaf identity to the individual. In contrast to stereotypical perceptions of deaf people as a homogenous group, she calls for the acknowledgement of the existence of different groups of deaf individuals, all of whom can and do claim different deaf identities. Life experiences, including those related to parent influences, school environments, exposure to deaf people, attitudes about deaf people, and cultural environments shape the specific deaf identity that deaf individuals have the possibility to become part of. The chapter also focuses identities related to ethnic background, sexual orientation, and additional disability status among other individual characteristics—none of which exist in isolation. These multiple layers intersect with one another and with deaf identities in unique dynamic, rather than static, ways, argues Leigh.

Chapter 8
From Political to National Identity in Zanzibar. Narratives on Changes in Social Practices

Sigrun Marie Moss

8.1 Zanzibaris Together

Uniting under a common identity has been emphasised as a way of overcoming intergroup bias. If people increasingly see themselves as members of a shared overarching identity, this should foster pro-social behaviours, cognitions and emotions. Little is known, however, of such processes in actual intergroup conflict.

Zanzibar—a semi-autonomous archipelago off the coast of Tanzania – has been the scene of conflict between the ruling party *Chama Cha Mapinduzi* (the party of the Revolution, CCM) and the equally large opposition party Civic United Front (CUF) since 1992. This political conflict has been especially intense during election periods, as the opposition party claims to have been robbed of every election victory. The social structures of Zanzibar were highly influenced by the political conflict. The political identities were salient, with people often putting their political belonging above their shared Zanzibariness, which was habitually pushed to the background in troubled times. In November 2009, a fourth reconciliation process was initiated (called *Maridhiano* in swahili), which resulted in a Government of National Unity (GNU) with both parties represented. Intergroup relations underwent changes that were observable in daily interactions and in general social practices.

The present study covers the period from 2010 to 2013. Based on in-depth interviews conducted with 79 Zanzibaris at four separate intervals, I here explore how these respondents account for changes in intergroup social practices following the reconciliation. Most respondents did say that there had been changes in group identification in Zanzibar after the reconciliation, emphasising the idea of a common Zanzibari identity. One thing is the experienced salience of an identity; another is how identity changes impact on social practices, making it important to explore how potential changes in identities are spoken of as visible in people's daily lives.

S.M. Moss (✉)
Department of Psychology, University of Oslo, Oslo, Norway
e-mail: s.m.moss@psykologi.uio.no

S. Bagga-Gupta et al. (eds.), *Identity Revisited and Reimagined*,
DOI 10.1007/978-3-319-58056-2_8

This chapter attempts to map out how people say the changed identity manifests itself in people's daily lives through social practices.

8.2 "The Bad Times" and the Identity Process

Before commencing with the theory presentation, I will introduce two aspects from the material which serve as important contextual information for the study (for more details on Zanzibar, see the appendix). First, I briefly present participants' sentiments on social practices *before* the reconciliation process. Second, a short backdrop on the process of identity alterations in Zanzibar is included.

8.2.1 Sentiments on the Social Practices Before the Maridhiano

Most participants speak of the social practices before the *Maridhiano* as different to social practices after the *Maridhiano* took hold. To clarify the contrast, I have included some extracts describing the situation prior to the *Maridhiano.* One local respondent (interview number 16, conducted in 2011) explained:

> At the grass-root level there were many misunderstandings and a lot of problems for a long time. There were several indicators it was becoming worse. You could see from the social interactions that contact between CUF and CCM supporters became more limited. When there were ceremonies, it became more and more rare for members of the opposite party to join in. Both sides became more and more separated.

He here emphasises how the relations were bad and getting worse, and how people were separating more and more into groups of either CUF or CCM supporters in many different realms of life. A teacher (interview number 12, conducted in 2011) focused on the violence, and talked of earlier election periods:

> During the elections in 2005, the situation was very bad. People were fighting each other, burning down each other's houses. At night, a car may come, someone would knock your door, and they would beat you. They may even take you away in their lorry, and beat you and drop you far from your home. We were fighting a lot.

Here the intergroup fighting is in focus, as he describes how "we (Zanzibaris) were fighting a lot". Such violent stretches were typically worse in the build up to elections, but were also reported throughout non-election periods.

8.2.2 Sentiments on the Identity Process

In the interviews, the respondents emphasise the increased focus on their shared Zanzibariness after the *Maridhiano*. The political leadership encouraged this

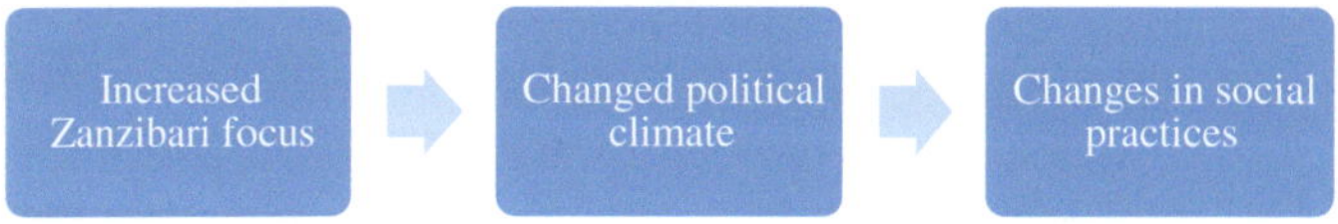

Fig. 8.1 The suggested process of changes in social practices in Zanzibar

common identity and many people slowly came to agree that a sense of national belonging was the better approach (see Moss 2016; Moss and Tronvoll 2015). The majority of the respondents expressed that they increasingly perceived themselves as Zanzibaris rather than polarising their identities in relation to the opposing political parties, and that this in turn contributed to the changed political climate. The political atmosphere is described as having been altered as a result of Zanzibaris coming together under a national identity. One respondent explained:

> There have been some changes here, mainly in the attitudes of the people. They now trust each other. Earlier, before the *Maridhiano,* there was a lot of doubt and mistrust between them. Now CCM and CUF are working together, this is no longer a problem. If you are opposition or not, it is not relevant anymore (22P2011)

The altered attitudes of the people and the establishment of intergroup trust are put forth as important transformational factors. This respondent goes to the length of saying that it is now irrelevant whether one belongs to one party or the other—something that was long considered to be a key identity marker.

In the material, the changed atmosphere is spoken of as contributing to the changes in social practices. Process tracing was not a specific part of the method, but most of the respondents did allude to the increased Zanzibari focus enabling changes in the political climate, which in turn encouraged changes in social practices (Fig. 8.1).

This does not mean that these were not interwoven or cyclical processes, but for example many respondents specifically spoke of the increased sense of Zanzibariness leading to alterations in political climate, which again was deemed necessary for people to feel comfortable being openly friends with people from the opposing party, where, among other aspects, not being seen as a traitor when you visited people from the other party was emphasised. One framework within social psychology has dealt specifically with such alterations in identities, emphasising the positive effects of a shared common identity.

8.3 Common Identities and Social Practices

8.3.1 Common Identities

People sort people into categories, and define themselves *into* groups they feel part of (ingroups) and *out of* groups they feel they do not belong to (outgroups).

This process makes the world more manageable, and according to Allport (1954/1988), p. 20) "ordinary living depends on it". Identity constellations influence emotions, cognitions and behaviour towards ingroup members and outgroup members. This is the starting point for focusing on common ingroup identities as a path to improving intergroup relations, as explored in the Common Ingroup Identity Model (Gaertner and Dovidio 2000). This framework postulates that unifying under a common ingroup identity (also called recategorisation) can extend pro-social emotions; behaviours and cognition to former outgroup members if one begins to consider them fellow ingroup members. This builds on identity hierarchies, where some identities—subordinate identities - are nested within or falls within overarching identities—superordinate identities (e.g. political identities of CUF and CCM within the territorial Zanzibari identity). Research has tested this in a variety of contexts, and found support for the reduction of intergroup bias when uniting under a shared superordinate identity (see Dovidio, Gaertner and Saguy 2009).

The recategorisation literature has focused on two main approaches. First, in *single* recategorisation, subordinate identities are abolished, and the superordinate identity is emphasised. This has been attempted in Rwanda, where the group identities of Hutu, Tutsi and Twa have been abolished to make room for the shared Rwandan identity, as a way of overcoming intergroup conflict (see Moss 2014; Moss and Vollhardt 2015). The single approach has been widely criticised for causing threat to meaningful identities and hindering the need for distinctiveness (Hornsey and Hogg 2000). Second, in a *dual* recategorisation approach, the subordinate identities are retained whilst emphasising a superordinate identity. This fits with the Zanzibari approach: the political identities of CUF and CCM were retained whilst leadership emphasised the shared Zanzibariness. This is a more widely supported identity approach for reducing intergroup prejudice and bias (see González and Brown 2003). However, it can be difficult to achieve, as the subordinate categories—the key to the conflict—are retained. This can then stand in the way of the superordinate identity growing salient (see Gaertner and Dovidio 2000).

The main bulk of this research consists of laboratory studies, and several researchers have questioned whether the approach is realistic outside the laboratory (e.g. Hewstone 1996). Studies using natural groups have found higher resistance to the recategorisation compared to lab-studies (Mullen et al. 1992). As context is often not included as a factor in most studies of recategorisation, the degree to which people identify with the category in question becomes the main go-to explanation for categorization. Thereby salience is put above most other explanations. Following Brubaker's (2004, p. 4) line of argument, where "groupness" is a variable, and should not be seen as a constant, this removal of context is problematic. Similarly, Tajfel (1982) emphasised that group specificity and context-focused analysis need to be at the forefront when studying social phenomena. As Zanzibar clearly demonstrates, identities reflect the social and political landscapes of a specific time and place. Given other circumstances, these categorizations can grow stronger or decline in importance. Looking at how potential alterations in categorization manifest themselves in practices offers an alternative approach to the salience focus when studying recategorisation processes.

8.3.2 Social Practices

In work on common identities, there is a focus on the interconnectedness of categorizations with emotions, cognitions and behaviour. In this perspective, social practices would be embedded in how changes in categorizations impact on emotions, cognitions and behaviours. For example, people tend to react more positively to ingroup members than to outgroup members, demonstrating more pro-social behaviour and retaining more positive information (Dovidio, Gaertner, Saguy, and Halabi 2008). In the Robbers Cave study, with boys at summer camp, categorizations influenced seating patterns, sharing, and other types of intergroup behaviour and distance (see Sherif 1966). In a study on Manchester United supporters, Levine et al. (2005) found that helping behaviour is extended to a larger extent to those perceived as ingroup members rather than outgroup members, and that the perception of others as ingroup members and outgroup members is dynamic. Limited research has looked at this in terms of social practices as defined within sociological writing, however. Within practice theory (see Bourdieu 1990), practices (praktik) represent a "routinized type of behaviour which consists of several elements, interconnected to one other: forms of bodily activities, forms of mental activities, 'things' and their use, a background knowledge in the form of understanding, know-how, states of emotion and motivational knowledge" (Reckwitz 2002, p. 249). These aspects are interconnected, and the practice cannot be reduced to a few of these elements. A practice then consists of many different actions that reproduce the practice. For example, Reckwitz (p. 250) emphasises that "a certain way of consuming goods can be filled out by plenty of actual acts of consumption". Comparing this to social practices in Zanzibar, one could for example see ways of greeting others as a practice, and the many different acts of greeting as individual actions composing the pattern the practice represents.

According to Reckwitz, calling these *social* practices is a tautology, as the practices are socially embedded, and the social is placed in the practices. However, in order to clarify that I am here focusing on practices related to intergroup relations, I have chosen to call these social practices.

8.4 Methodology

I conducted 68 interviews with a total of 79 Zanzibaris. 61 interviews were individual semi-structured interviews. Six of these respondents were interviewed twice or more. This enabled some continuity from one visit to the next, and it was interesting to trace individual narratives over the political processes. Six interviews were spontaneous group interviews, as individuals that I had organised to meet with chose to bring along others to the interview (one-two additional respondents per group interview). One larger group interview was organised. In Zanzibar, men often discuss politics at the "*baraza*", which are stone benches outside houses or open wooden structures in rural areas. I organised a CUF baraza interview in central Unguja (the main island), with 14 CUF members. Attempts to organise such an interview with CCM members was not successful. In both the *baraza* interview and in the other group interviews, the respondents interacted and discussed the topics at hand. They corrected each other, disagreed and agreed, and gave me insights into areas of more and less controversy within the political and social spheres.

The study was conducted over four visits (total of 5.5 months) between October 2010 and January 2013, which included periods of heightened conflict.

8.4.1 Sample

The 79 Zanzibaris were recruited through purposive diversity sampling and snowball sampling. Sixty-six of these were from the general population, whilst the remaining 13 were political leaders. In the recruitment process, diversity was aimed for across age, occupation, gender, socio-economic status, geographical area, and, where possible, party belonging. Ages ranged from 20 to 90, with a mean age of approximately 40. Interviews were held with respondents across a broad range of occupations, and conducted in urban and rural areas across the two islands. Men were generally available for interviews. It was difficult to recruit women on the whole, and only eight women were interviewed. Women frequently referred to politics as a topic for men, not women, to discuss publically. At the time of interviewing, the political and social atmosphere was one of downplaying political differences. Statements such as "*tuko Zanzibari pamoja*" ("we are Zanzibari together") and "*Zanzibar kwanza, siasa badaye*" ("Zanzibar first, politics later") were common. After deliberations with Zanzibari contacts, I decided not to ask people about their political belonging so as not to contribute to political polarisation. This is a limitation in terms of comparing group narratives, but it is crucial to avoid leaving a negative footprint when conducting this type of research, especially in vulnerable conflict contexts. However, about one third of the local respondents either volunteered this information during their interview, or it was known to me ahead of the interviews (local sample: CUF: 35 (including the *baraza* group interview with 14 CUF supporters); CCM: 8; unknown affiliation: 23).

Regarding the leadership sample, I interviewed eleven male and two female leaders, six each in Pemba (the smaller and less developed island) and Unguja (and one in Dar es Salaam). CCM politicians were relatively reluctant to be interviewed, as is often the case with incumbent parties. CUF representatives however, were generally available for interviews. Nine of the thirteen interviewed leaders were CUF leaders—four CCM—and the positions consisted of the following: first vice-president (1), minister (1), members of parliament (2), party secretaries (2), election commission (1), and regional/district leadership (3/3).

8.4.2 Interview Schedule

To the respondents, the research was introduced as being focused on the *Maridhiano* process and Zanzibari relations. Two questions are most essential for this chapter: Have there been any changes in group identification? If so, how are these changes visible in your daily lives? With the help of experienced research assistants, the interviews were conducted in English and Swahili (about 50% each). A common challenge doing interviews in conflict settings is that people do not wish for the interview to be recorded. Only four granted permission. For the rest, I relied on extensive notes. Here I used a coding system which enabled me to write down an approximate 80% of the words (based on the overlap between notes and recordings). When possible, respondents were asked if they wanted to go over the interview transcript and alter this as they wished. It is my impression that this improved openness and trust. The few who did correct the transcript only made minor changes.

8.4.3 Ethical Considerations

Permits to conduct the study were granted from the Norwegian Centre for Research Data (NSD) and the Zanzibar Research Committee. People were given extensive information on the study and its purpose, as well as about the other groups of people who were being interviewed. Especially in conflict settings, this is often essential information for giving informed consent. I had lived in Pemba before, observing voter registration, which in may ways was a great asset for conducting this current study: my extensive network; familiarity with the context and the language. It also had some downsides. Pemba is the opposition island, and having spent a year there I was closer to the opposition narrative. I remained reflexive of this and kept reviewing both what I knew, and how I knew what I knew (in accordance with Bourdieu). Additionally, I conducted more interviews on Unguja. Further, CUF politicians and supporters on Pemba frequently asked me why I would not be sending reports to the international community as the team had done during my posting there. It was difficult to communicate (and at times justify) the more academic goals for my current study.

8.4.4 Analysis

To analyse the material, I used thematic analysis (Braun and Clarke 2006), positioned within constructionism. Basing the study on interviews, I allow room for participants' narratives, and thereby attempt to acquire acceptable social knowledge by "telling it like it was for them" (Fielding 1982, p. 83).

Transcripts were read repeatedly, and all the material was coded. Many people talked about the consequences of the *Maridhiano* on daily interactions. Therefore, for this chapter, I wanted to look at how the changes in categorization were manifested in social practices. Attempting to map out how people say the changed sense of identity manifests itself in social practices, I chose to do a broad analysis. This is thereby a rich description of the data set, rather than a detailed account of one particular aspect. Here, breadth is gained, but some complexity and depth is lost. This approach is often recommended for under-researched areas, or participants whose viewpoints are not known (see Braun and Clarke 2006)—both well-fitting descriptions of this case.

The interview extracts included below are examples of shared sentiments on a topic, or statements demonstrating nuance within a theme. The interview extracts are all marked with interview number, year of interview, and either P for population, L for leadership, CS for civil society or A for academics.

8.5 Changes in Social Practices

Working through the material, I identified three main themes in the responses pertaining to changes in social practices: social changes; ceremonial changes; and political changes (Fig. 8.2).

These are interrelated, and as they all speak to intergroup relations it is difficult to pry them apart completely. Even if all three identified themes are social, it was still necessary to include social changes as something different than, for example, ceremonial changes.

8.5.1 Social Changes

As previously discussed, many respondents described social practices prior to the *Maridhiano* as influenced by the political polarisation and conflict. Many respondents also emphasised that this was not an absolute, as most people saw themselves

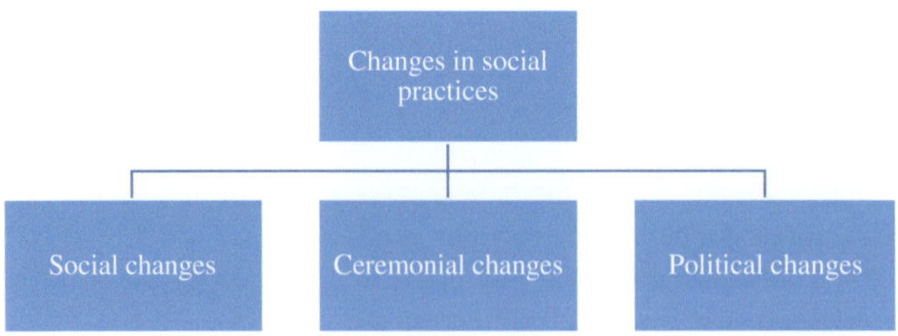

Fig. 8.2 Thematic Map

as Zanzibari together throughout the troubled times as well (see Moss 2016). Either way, most respondents did report changes in social practices in terms of how people from the two parties now interacted. A journalist explained:

> These questions about social relations are very important questions for us. Generally, it is good now. The 2010 elections were peaceful; there was no violence pre-, during or post-election. To us, social relations start with the political situation. We were living in fear and mistrust. The real situation after the *Maridhiano* is very different than before—people did not pray together, they did not attend ceremonies or funerals, they could even put something bad in each other's wells. We reached that stage. It was bad. After the GNU, the situation is good (36CS2012).

This extract indicates a shift in intergroup relations, where the groups are no longer polarised into political identities. Two sub-themes were identified under this theme: first, greetings—a key aspect of Zanzibari social life; and second: friendships, cooperation, and social calls.

8.5.1.1 Greeting People

Greetings are an essential part of Zanzibari social relations, where lengthy exchanges with inquiries about news, health, families, home and work are common. Thereby, not greeting someone is seen as a "bigger deal" than many other places, and it is an important marker of the state of intergroup relations. A civil society representative explained that relations were not completely transformed, but in local situations the differences were noticeable:

> …people are living peacefully together at village and town level. Earlier it was not like this —if you were CUF, and you met someone, and you realized they were CCM, many would stop talking to this person, and walk off. The same thing for the other way around. Now, we even go together to football matches. This is the first and foremost issue: there is now peace in Zanzibar (6CS2011).

Again, the statement indicates improved intergroup relations and changed practices. A man from Pemba agreed: "It was so bad. We even stopped saying hello to each other when we passed in the street. Now it is like we never had that bad time, and we are together again" (15P2011). The timing issue here is interesting, as this is described as a *re*conciliation where people are brought back together. Being "together again" indicates an increase in the shared superordinate Zanzibariness.

Some of the interviewed leaders said that before the *Maridhiano* they would often cross over to the other side of the street when meeting an opposing political leader, as exemplified by the following extract from a CCM politician: "We would often cross to the other side of the road if we saw a CUF leader on our side. Now we are completely together. A few are against it though, but you always have those" (28L2012). He continued, and explained that one of the CUF leaders is closely related to him after marrying into his family:

> Before the *Maridhiano* we were not together. We were real different; we would pass on separate sides of the road, and not greet each other. We are now very close, we greet each other in the street and see each other often. Before the multiparty-system we were also close. It is like Popo Bawa [a bat spirit causing mainly election related harm] got into our heads at that time, and we were like wild animals. We have now spoken about the bad times, as have many others—about how things were bad between us, and now they are good. (28L2012).

He here speaks of the transformation in ingroup and outgroup constellations changing from good (before multiparty-system) to bad, and now back to good, and that this process has manifested itself in social practices such as greetings.

8.5.1.2 Friendships, Cooperation and Social Calls

There was much talk among the respondents about the visible changes in social practices in terms of friendship, cooperation and social calls. Many mentioned that it was now possible to visit each other without the risk of being seen as a traitor. Several people said that in earlier times, political ideology was seen as more fundamental than the normal social structures that would otherwise tie people together. A teacher said:

> The gap or division that was here before was between the political parties. People were always quarrelling and fighting each other, because of politics. Only those of the same party went to funerals, people who belonged to opposite parties did not talk or visit each other, even if they were from the same family. Political ideology was stronger than social bonds and interactions. Now people visit each other, they go to each other's funerals, and talk together—regardless of political affiliation (12P2011).

Political leaders on Pemba mentioned several different ways interactions had changed: "People are now together, they visit each other, and have even formed cooperations together. They are together also in civil society, and community based organisations" (32L2012). Changes were also reported in areas that were traditionally more polarised than others, as here by an academic in Stone town discussing the improved relations between two groups that were formerly very polarized:

> The individual relationships at grassroots level—between people from Pemba and Unguja, and CUF and CCM, have changed. At Kiembe Samaki for instance, where the Nationalist party [ZNP] was established… The people of this area were more or less ostracized during the revolution. There was great animosity then, and people from areas like Kizimkazi looked at these people as traitors. Some people from Kiembe Samaki had to relocate because of their link to ZNP, and many moved to Zanzibar town. Some even lost their lives. Now, people from these two areas are having coffee together! (2A2011)

The respondent seemed genuinely baffled by this change in practices (from animosity to coffee), and he followed up saying again how unlikely this development was. The extract demonstrates the extent of some of the changes in social practices.

This first theme indicates that most respondents appreciated the changes in social practices, and that respondents saw these in their everyday life in Zanzibari society after the *Maridhiano*. Further, the theme also touches on the tension that used to exist between the normal, important rules of social interaction and the political polarisation—as a teacher said: "Political ideology was stronger than social bonds and interactions" (12P2011).

8.5.2 *Ceremonies*

Previously, the political rift was making it difficult for people to attend ceremonies of people belonging to the other party. People would frequently boycott ceremonies held by people from the opposing party, even at times within their own families. As family and social relations are strongly emphasised in Zanzibari society, the boycotting of ceremonies it would otherwise be natural to attend is—similarly to not greeting people—very grave. Also, if they did attend, members of opposing parties could very well be taunted by the participants at the ceremony, and criticized by members of their own party for being traitors. Ceremonial changes was one of the things that came up frequently when people talked about how the changes in categorization were visible in daily lives. I have divided this theme into two subthemes: attending weddings and attending funerals, though the extracts frequently incorporate both.

8.5.2.1 Attending Weddings

Many respondents said that it had been common for people to boycott the ceremonies of opposing political party supporters, or not to welcome members from the other party at ceremonies. According to a CUF leader, however, one *had to* attend weddings if one was family. Attending a CCM wedding, she explained, was often uncomfortable:

> In weddings—where you have to be invited, people would not invite people from other groups. But again, family members needed to be invited. This was often uncomfortable. During the Taarab [traditional music] in the weddings, the other party could be laughing or saying bad words to the opposite party. Now this has changed so much, and it is almost gone; especially so at the weddings. The divide between the two parties could often be difficult to notice in the funerals, but in the weddings it was always very open. Now I can attend the weddings of the families of CCM politicians, without facing any problems. In Taarab we have CUF and CCM songs, but now—not to hurt each other's feelings—we only play neutral songs, songs about love. We feel very comfortable now, very welcomed (30L2012).

Going from alienating or even ridiculing representatives of the other party to playing neutral songs signals a large shift in social practices, where the focus has moved from taunting or excluding the outgroup, to arranging inclusive ceremonies. Several respondents reiterated this shift. One CCM leader in Pemba said: "Many things go okay now—people attend funerals, business and weddings together" (33L2012). In a CUF leadership group interview on Pemba, this was repeated:

"There is no evil here now. People work together for development, without involving any political ideology…. They cooperate fully now, and attend both weddings and funerals" (32L2012).

8.5.2.2 Attending Funerals

Several respondents said that prior to the *Maridhiano*, people avoided the funerals of those of the opposing party, like this CCM leader: "Before, people would not go to each others funerals, even those of relatives, or social gatherings that crossed party lines, but now they are together, and they freely attend each other's ceremonies" (29L2012). A CUF leader in Stonetown supported this sentiment:

> Yes, I believe the social relations here have changed, both in the local population and amongst politicians. Before we came to GNU, we used to be very separated into CUF and CCM, even within families. In some cases, during funerals, some were not happy to attend funerals if the person was from the other political group, even within families. But if the person who passed away was from your family, you had to attend, but then we would sit separately—CUF on one side, CCM on the other (30L2012).

This CUF politician starts talking about a relative who is a senior CCM leader:

> He had to come for our ceremonies, as he is family, and I went there. Once, they had a funeral at his house, and I was there to help, and CUF supporters in Stone Town tried to block me from going, asking me why I should work for CCM and help them. I was very angry, and it was very difficult. Even when people were sick in my house, it was difficult for… [the CCM leader] to come, as he was accused of being CUF. Now things are different. We are together, we talk and we meet. We have talked about the difficult times we had before (30L2012).

The tension between social rules within more general settings (paying respects at funerals or attending weddings) and the more conflict-specific social rules is evident from these extracts. In the first extract, the respondent talks of people now being *free* to attend each other's ceremonies. This may allude to the socially imposed processes involved in the boycotting of ceremonies. Social rules and ways of doing things are embedded in practices, and especially in polarised situations the consequences of breaking these social rules may be difficult.

The ceremonial changes highlighted in this theme portray a powerful picture of how social practices have changed. Several respondents did however paint a somewhat more nuanced scene. A local respondent said that the practices in terms of ceremony attendance had changed, but also emphasised that people had—throughout the hard times—been Zanzibari together, seeing each other as one:

> The politics have changed how we relate to each other here. Most people were separated before, CUF on one side, CCM on the other. They didn't attend each other's funerals or wedding ceremonies. Now they do. But at the same time, we have always been Zanzibari together. It was always there, behind all the conflict. The political leaders manipulated us into fighting, but we still saw ourselves as one people (21P2011).

This speaks to a social complexity, where people were divided, as evident from aspects such as not attending each other's ceremonies, but simultaneously seeing each other as fellow Zanzibaris, alluding to the shared superordinate identity.

In terms of the ceremonies, a few respondents disagreed with this general sentiment, claiming there had been no big changes in social practices when it came to ceremonies due to the *Maridhiano* process, as this CUF leader in a group interview on Pemba: "The situation never got as far as that people stopped attending each other's funerals and weddings because of politics" (32L2012).

8.5.3 Political Changes

Many Zanzibaris were relatively sceptical to the *Maridhiano* when it was initiated. Many referred to earlier failed peace processes, asking how and why it would be any different this time. Zanzibaris often scrutinize their leaders for indications of what to do, how the situation is going, and what the future will bring. Therefore, the social practices among the political leaders themselves, following from the *Maridhiano* were topics brought up time and again by respondents. It was clear that people needed to see changes in how leaders from the two parties interacted before they would believe in the genuineness of the *Maridhiano*. This theme has been divided into two subthemes. The first is seating arrangements in the House of Representatives, and the second is changes in how political discussions proceeded.

8.5.3.1 Seating Arrangements

Most respondents emphasised the changed political environment, and the changes in interparty cooperation at leadership level. Among the grass roots, this seemed to indicate the process was more genuine than earlier reconciliation attempts, which had not manifested themselves as clearly in practice. One concrete, visible social practice that was brought up was the seating arrangements in the House of Representatives restaurant. A civil society representative explained: "Interestingly, when you go to the House of Representatives restaurant, you do not see CUF tables and CCM tables. They all mix so well. What is happening now is amazing; we can't believe it" (35CS2012). A CCM leader brought up the same point:

> CUF and CCM are now mixing in the restaurant of House of Representatives, but not only this: the discussions in the House are now between the cabinet and the backbenchers. There is no more of the: "this is the minister for CCM so we in CCM need to defend him." It is God's blessing that made it work (28L2012).

A CUF leader also discussed the seating pattern, and said: "People who were fighting each other before are now sitting together and finding good points for the union discussion" (30L2012). She further referred to two high-level politicians from opposite parties now sitting together frequently: "they are sitting together, and before they were the worst of enemies". Changes in seating-patterns have been used several times in research to indicate changes in social relations in terms of altered categorization (e.g. see Sherif 1966). Here this has been pointed to as a move towards placing more emphasis on the superordinate over the subordinate identities, which fit with many of the respondents' accounts of these changes.

8.5.3.2 Political Discussions

The social relations between leaders and the way of discussing politics in the House of Representatives were topics that were frequently brought up. It is not uncommon for Zanzibaris to follow the House sessions on TV or radio, so many people are very well-informed about the political atmosphere in the House. An academic explained the changes:

> Before, if something were in the CUF manifesto, CUF would oppose it. This does not have a strong position anymore. If good things are said by CUF, both CUF and CCM agree, and if bad things are said by CUF or CCM, bot CUF and CCM disagree. They both have their chance now, and they focus on good ideas rather than the party (27A2012).

A CUF leader agreed:

> The situation in Zanzibar now is good. Before the new form of government we have now, people were divided into parties. If you were CCM, and someone inside the party did something wrong, you could not say anything. We just quarrelled with the other party. Now you can't differentiate between CUF and CCM in the House of Representatives. We go together. The format helps us come together rather than divide.... In the House of Representatives we have left political interests aside, and focus on national interests now (30L2012).

Many leaders emphasised the same aspect—that when the parties were polarised, the social rules dictated that one needed to support all that ones' own party said and oppose all the other party said. Many, like this respondent, emphasised that the shift towards national focus rather than party focus improved the situation. Again, the emphasis on the subordinate level is largely replaced with the superordinate level. The respondents also frequently discussed this change in political cooperation as an important aspect in the reconciliation, as it demonstrated to people that the process was genuine. A high level CUF leader said:

> ...there is no more political tension. It was good for the public to see ministers from both parties come, and they commented on us working well together. This gives them increased hope in their unity government. I would say something, and my CCM colleague would agree, and the other way around. Earlier we always opposed each other, no matter what (4L2011).

A civil society representative emphasised the magnitude of this change:

> The legislatures from both parties have been doing a good job. The House of Representatives is very active, more so than before. Some of the legislatures are very close friends, rising beyond party belonging for national loyalty. It is unbelievable. CUF and CCM are cooperating very well. If a CUF minister is being bombarded by CUF, CCM try to help him, and the other way around (35CS2012).

Supporters and leaders from both parties reiterated this, saying that there had been substantial changes in social practices with regards to party interaction and cooperation. A few respondents were more sombre, like this CCM leader on Pemba:

> There are still things dividing both parties and individuals. We do not trust CUF that much. We are in government together, but we still do not trust them 100%. We know each other, even if you trust, you still distrust that they will follow up. There is no guarantee (33L2012).

The frequency of this theme on changes in social practises among the top political leadership can be seen as an indication of the emphasis the respondents placed on the social practices among leaders and the importance of this in an unfolding reconciliation process. Many respondents did point out that the earlier peace processes had "only been a lot of talk", and that they now wanted to see more than talk to have faith in the process. Seeing alterations in interparty social practices may then have been much more convincing as to the authenticity of the process, compared to leadership speeches and the likes.

8.5.4 No Changes

Importantly, there were also specific areas of practice people said had not undergone changes, and these were also frequently brought up. An example was employment. A civil society representative explained: "There have been changes here in relations. These are not 100%. There is still unfairness in employment regarding who of CCM and CUF are employed" (6CS2011). Others did think that the situation had improved, also within employment. When asking a group of CUF leaders on Pemba whether social relations had changed, one said: "There is still political discrimination here, for example in terms of vacancies, but not as much as before. The Government of National Unity has somehow managed to change this" (32L2012).

8.6 Social Practices in Zanzibar

As seen from this analysis of respondents' narratives, the former conflict influenced social practices. This is particularly acute in a very socially interwoven context such as Zanzibar, where both tradition and religion dictates that one should be united. Most of the participants did indicate that the changes in how identities were structured (at least publically), i.e. the shift towards focusing more on the Zanzibariness over political party belonging, did manifest itself in changes in social practices. Seeing practice as a 'nexus of doings and sayings' (Schatzki 1996), practices are known and understandable both to those carrying it out but also to others within the same culture. In terms of a world understanding and routinised ways of doing things, some social practices in Zanzibar do seem to have changed for people in the course of the reconciliation process. Looking at social practices enables the exploration of how identity alterations and reconciliation processes influence daily lives, and what people make of the different changes (e.g. respondents from the general population referring to changes in seating arrangements in the House and alterations in the social practices of political discussion as an indication of genuine change, rather than "just talk"). Additionally, it shows the difficult social processes in conflict, where politically steered practices collide with religious or socially expected practices (e.g. the boycotting of ceremonies versus the social and religious obligations to attend and ensure harmony).

Linking the above analysis of social practises to the recategorisation framework, it shows that social practices are an interesting avenue for discussing recategorisation processes in real life. In terms of investigating recategorisation as an approach for reducing intergroup bias and conflict, looking at how respondents speak of it as manifested in social practices speaks to societal consequences that could not be captured by looking at salience alone. The indications that change has occurred in social practices and that respondents often tie this to the changes in Zanzibariness, is a concrete and meaningful approach to studying effects of recategorisation processes. Mapping such changes in daily lives is crucial to gain a better understanding of vulnerable recategorisation processes, which often—as detailed next—deteriorate.

At the time of writing—May 2016—the government of national unity has been dissolved. CUF announced themselves the winners of the 2015 elections (a claim widely supported by election analysts) after which the Zanzibar electoral commission annulled the elections on the counts of fraud and irregularities. In March 2016, CCM organised a rerun election, which CUF boycotted, and all political cooperation was terminated. CCM has now formed a one-party government, and the political situation is tense. So far, the political changes within social practices have been largely reversed, and there are tendencies for grassroots social relations deteriorating, especially in Pemba. General grassroots social relations however do not seem to be worsening significantly, and people are still mostly keeping up the social practices of greetings, visits, praying together, and attending each other's ceremonies. How long this will last, however, is unclear. Whether the recategorisation process has contributed to these continued positive social practices, and if so—whether this is strong enough to withstand increasing political conflict, time will tell.

Appendix: Zanzibari Background

Zanzibar's population is divided between two main islands: Pemba (400,000), and Unguja (900,000). Together with former Tanganyika, Zanzibar makes up the Republic of Tanzania. The Republic and Zanzibar each has a president and parliament, and within this union Zanzibar is semi-autonomous.

The division in Zanzibar is between two relatively equally sized parties: incumbent CCM and opposition party CUF. The latter is strongest on Pemba (which is often referred to as the opposition island), and Pemba has long been economically and politically marginalised (Bakari 2011). The divide can be traced back to turbulent periods in the late 1950s and early 1960s with identity divides influencing politics. There is no significant difference today between the populations of Unguja and Pemba (or CUF and CCM): they share language, culture, religion, and way of life. According to CUF, CCM has stolen every election victory since the reintroduction of multiparty rule in 1992 (with several election observations supporting this claim). Election periods have been especially turbulent.

Three former peace agreements have failed (*Muafaka* I-III). CUF supporters, especially in Pemba, frequently have a harder time registering for the necessary documents to vote (see ILPI 2010), and in July 2009, with the commencement of establishing a permanent voter registry, intergroup relations again deteriorated. In November 2009, however, political leadership from both parties initiated a reconciliation process and called for cooperation and peace (see Moss and Tronvoll 2015). Leaders from both sides emphasised the shared Zanzibari identity, and asked people to focus on their commonalities over their political differences. The general population was sceptical at first, but many came to endorse the situation. This process overlapped with growing anti-union sentiments in Zanzibar, where many Zanzibaris wanted more autonomy for the archipelago. In July 2010, through a referendum, the establishment of a Government of National Unity (GNU) was decided. After non-violent election campaigns and a very peaceful election, CCM won the 2010 election with 50.1% of the vote. CUF got 49.1% of the vote. The peace was still maintained, and the GNU was established (see ILPI 2010).

References

Allport, G. (1954/1988). *The nature of prejudice.* Cambridge, MA: Perseus Books.

Bakari, M. A. (2011). Understanding obstacles to political reconciliation in Zanzibar: Actors, interests and strategies. In M. Baregu (Ed.), *Understanding obstacles to peace. Actors, interests, and strategies in Africa's Great Lakes region* (pp. 222–270). Kampala: Fountain.

Braun, V., & Clarke, V. (2006). Using thematic analysis in psychology. *Qualitative Research in Psychology, 3*, 77–101. doi:10.1191/1478088706qp063oa

Bourdieu, P. (1990). *The logic of practice.* Cambridge, UK: Polity Press.

Brubaker, R. (2004). *Ethnicity without groups.* Cambridge, MA: Harvard University Press.

Dovidio, J. F., Gaertner, S. L., & Saguy, T. (2009). Commonality and the complexity of "we": Social attitudes and social change. *Personality and Social Psychology Review, 13*, 3–20. doi:10.1177/1088868308326751

Dovidio, J. F., Gaertner, S. L., Saguy, T., & Halabi, S. (2008). From when to why. Understanding how contact reduces bias. In U. Wagner, L. R., Tropp, G. Finchilescu & C. Tredoux (Eds.), *Improving intergroup relations. Building on the legacy of Thomas F. Pettigrew* (pp. 75–90). Malden: Blackwell Publishing.

Fielding, N. (1982). Observational research on the national front. In M. Bulmer (Ed.), *Social research ethics: An examination of the merits of covert participant observation* (pp. 80–104). London: Macmillan.

Gaertner, S. L., & Dovidio, J. F. (2000). *Reducing intergroup bias: The common ingroup identity model*. Philadelphia, PA: Taylor and Francis.
González, R., & Brown, R. (2003). Generalization of positive attitude as a function of subgroup and superordinate group identifications in intergroup contact. *European Journal of Social Psychology*, *33*(2), 195–214. doi:10.1002/ejsp.140
Hewstone, M. (1996). Contact and categorization: Social psychological interventions to change intergroup relations. In C. N. Macrae, C. Stangor, & M. Hewstone (Eds.), *Stereotypes and stereotyping* (pp. 323–368). New York: Guilford Press.
Hornsey, M. J., & Hogg, M. A. (2000). Subgroup relations: A comparison of mutual intergroup differentiation and common ingroup identity models of prejudice reduction. *Personality and Social Psychology Bulletin, 26*, 242–256. doi:10.1177/0146167200264010
ILPI. (2010). *Elections in Zanzibar. Consolidating peaceful multiparty politics.* Report 43/2010. Oslo: International Law and Policy Institute.
Levine, M., Prosser, A., Evans, D., & Reicher, S. (2005). Identity and emergency intervention: How social group membership and inclusiveness of group boundaries shape helping behavior. *Personality and Social Psychology Bulletin*, *31*(4), 443–453. doi:10.1177/0146167204271651
Moss, S. M. (2014). Beyond conflict and spoilt identities: How Rwandan leaders justify a single recategorisation model for post-conflict reconciliation. *Journal of Social and Political Psychology, 2*, 435–449. doi:10.5964/jspp.v2i1.291
Moss, S. M. (2016). "Country first, politics later." Reasons for dual recategorization in Zanzibari narratives. *Peace and Conflict: Journal of Peace Psychology, 22*(4), 318–328. doi:10.1037/pac0000223
Moss, S. M. & Tronvoll, K. (2015). We are all Zanzibari! Identity formation and political reconciliation in Zanzibar. *Journal of Eastern African Studies, 9*(1), 91–109. doi:10.1080/17531055.2014.985357
Moss, S. M., & Vollhardt, J. R. (2016). You can't give a syringe with unity: Rwandan responses to the government's single recategorization policies. *Analyses of Social Issues and Public Policy, 16*(1), 325–359.
Mullen, B., Brown, R., & Smith, C. (1992). Ingroup bias as a function of salience, relevance, and status: An integration. *European Journal of Social Psychology, 22*, 103–122. doi:10.1002/ejsp.2420220202
Reckwitz, A. (2002). Toward a theory of social practices: A development in culturalist theorizing. *European Journal of Social Theory 5*(2), 243–263. doi:10.1177/13684310222225432
Schatzki, T. (1996). *Social practices. A Wittgensteinian approach to human activity and the social.* Cambridge, UK: CUP.
Sherif, M. (1966). *In common predicament: Social psychology of intergroup conflict and cooperation*. Boston, MA: Houghton-Mifflin.
Tajfel, H. (1982). Social psychology of intergroup relations. *Annual review of psychology*, *33*(1), 1–39. doi:10.1146/annurev.ps.33.020182.000245

Author Biography

Sigrun Marie Moss is associate professor of political psychology at the Department of Psychology, University of Oslo, Norway. Her research focuses on identity processes in conflict, with particular focus on the balance between national identities and group identities. Moss looks at this at both leadership levels and general population levels. Her regional focus is East Africa and the Horn of Africa.

Chapter 9
"She Didn't Know I'm Black, You See". Practices, Body Signs, and Professional Identity

Ellen Andenæs

9.1 Introduction

Within workplace discourse research, professional identity has been studied most frequently from a gender perspective (Marra and Angouri 2011, p.11), and research on diversity most often deals with ethnicity and 'race' as differences between given social categories that are hierarchically ordered. This chapter offers instead an interactionist, practice based approach to professional identity. A professional identity is commonly understood as the image a person has based on the way she performs a job, and as related to particular kinds of knowledge and competencies shared with colleagues (Karlsson and Nikolaidou 2011). However, identity is embodied, and the relationship between competencies and bodies is not as straightforward as it may seem. This chapter is about the bodies of nurses; how they are interpreted by patients, and how such interpretations figure in negotiations of nurses' professional identity.

In this chapter, I will present research in Norwegian nursing homes for the aged with an ethnically diverse staff and an unusually high proportion of male employees. Residents were mainly white ethnic women, some of whom would reject nurses they disliked or distrusted on the basis of the nurses' appearance. Certain skin colours, accents, and markers of gender were 'body signs' (Søndergaard 1996, 2005) that could be construed as grounds for residents to accept particular nurses or to dismiss them as inappropriate, i.e. as not meeting the expected standard. This challenged the nurse's professional identity, and also the work flow on the ward. Challenged identities need to be reconfirmed, and the

E. Andenæs (✉)
Norwegian University of Science and Technology, Trondheim, Norway
e-mail: ellen.andenaes@ntnu.no

S. Bagga-Gupta et al. (eds.), *Identity Revisited and Reimagined*,
DOI 10.1007/978-3-319-58056-2_9

chapter investigates how nurses account for such situations in research interviews, and what kind of identity work their accounts accomplish.

9.2 Gender, 'Race', and Challenged Professional Identities in Healthcare

To meet the demand for health care services, high-income countries increasingly depend on importing health care workers from low-income countries (Marchal and Kegels 2003; Smith 2007). This accelerates a workforce diversity that represents a challenge for institutions as well as for professionals. Hierarchies of race, ethnicity, and social class are sources of conflict in caregiving and working relationships in nursing homes (Ryosho 2011; Seeberg 2012; Gullikstad 2010; Andenaes 2010). Numerous studies reveal tensions related to ethnicity and 'race', and their intersections with gender, and also to language and communication, in the healthcare system (Dreachslin et al. 2004; Allan et al. 2004; Timonen and Doyle 2010; Mapedzahama et al. 2011).

Based on several studies, Likupe (2006) concludes that "most foreign nurses have a negative experience working in the United Kingdom", where they experience deskilling, various forms of harassment and discrimination. Berdes and Eckert (2001, 2007), who researched race relations in eldercare in the US, describe the problem as deserving of urgent attention, and state that much work needs to be done to recognize and intervene in the problem. There are also tensions related to gender (Evans 2002), though there seems to be less research on this issue. A common finding in the interview-based studies is that foreign-born nurses report being subjected to offensive behaviour, ranging from blatant racism to subtly insulting comments. Male nurses, irrespective of colour, may be met with scepticism from colleagues (McMillian 2006) and prospective employers (McGregor 2007) and with resistance from patients (McGregor 2007; Evans 2002; Gullikstad 2010). All of the above are challenges to the nurses' professional identity.

Dodson and Zincavage (2007, p. 921) conclude that racial slurs and abuse are often presented as"a disturbing if inevitable experience for workers of color in nursing homes", and Jönsson (2007, p. 90) points out that this parallels a tendency to view violence from care recipients in nursing homes as a normal part of care work. Such incidents are obvious threats to the 'good encounters' between patients and nurses (Westin 2006; Bergland and Kirkevold 2006), and to the welfare of nurses and patients alike. Nurses must also be able to handle situations where normative expectations are not met—and to do so in a professional manner. That entails having access to professional practices for handling such situations, for instance when professional identity is at stake. There are, however, few studies that deal with micro level analysis of actual discourse and with accounting practices, which is my topic here.

9.3 Theoretical Underpinnings

9.3.1 "Pretty Is as Pretty Does": An Interactionist, Practice Based Approach to Professional Identity

The literature on identity is, in the words of Brubaker and Cooper (2000, p. 6 in Tracy, 2011, p. 176) an "amalgam of constructivist language and essentialism argument". Researchers see identity along a continuum ranging from a psychological mechanism of self-classification that is reflected in people's social behaviour, to something that is constituted through social action and interaction. The present research is grounded in interactionism and belongs in the latter category, together with views of identity as performance or construction that is interpreted by other people. Such constructions take place in discourse[1] and other social and embodied conduct, such as how we move, where we are, what we wear, how we talk and so on (Benwell and Stokoe 2006).

One basic tenet of interactionism is that identities, like other forms of social meaning, cannot be taken for granted, but must be accomplished, or *done*, continuously, in interaction with others (West and Zimmerman 1987; Butler 1990). This orientation is basic to discourse-based studies. Recent research on workplace identity in this vein is lucidly set out in edited volumes like Angouri and Marra (2011), Holmes (2006). Until recently, discourse research has privileged talk (or text), but recent research on embodied communication has investigated the multimodality of language, examining bodily conduct that functions as integrated aspects of talk (e.g. Couper-Kuhlen and Selting 2006; Goodwin 2000; Kita 2003; Streeck et al. 2011). In the research presented here, the focus is somewhat different: not on what bodies *do*, but on what they *are*—or, rather, what they are taken to be; how they are invested with meaning, and the implications of such meaning for interaction.

Discursive approaches focus on the constitutive power of language and discourse in communication to create, maintain or oppose meaning, including impressions of ourselves and each other, and what we experience as the reality of a particular social situation. A central concept in analyses of the relational aspects of interaction is the Goffmanian concept of face, the positive social value a person effectively claims for her- or himself (Goffman 1971, p. 319). As pointed out by Tracy (2011), the notion of identity-work also is rooted in the work of Goffman (1967, 1971). It has been further shaped by the perspective offered by Ochs (1992) on the linguistic constitution of gender identity, and in the positioning theory developed by discursive psychologists (Harré and van Langenhove 1999; Wetherell 1998).

Akin to these approaches, the notion of identity I deploy here can be described through five points. First, identity is the product of situated practices rather than

[1]The term 'discourse' is used here in accordance with established usage in various forms of linguistics, about what conversation analysts often call talk-in-interaction.

their source and therefore is a social and cultural rather than primarily internal psychological phenomenon, and, second, identities are relational and interactional, constructed through the relationships between self and others (Bucholtz and Hall 2005, p. 585). Third, identities are subject to negotiation. In any encounter I can suggest an identity for myself—how I wish to be perceived—but ultimately it is up to other people to validate or reject this proposed identity. Bucholtz (2003, p. 408) uses the term authentication for “the assertion of one’s own or another’s identity as genuine or credible”. In the course of the interviews nurses offered a number of stories about challenged identity or lack of authentication. These stories highlight the situated, relational and interactional nature of identities. They also demonstrate my fourth point: that local negotiations on the micro level are connected to conditions, relations, and processes on the macro level. Our bodies are imbued with cultural meanings—in this case, gender, ethnicity, and ‘race’ are ostensibly relevant dimensions. Cultural identities are brought *into* the encounter, but they are also brought *about* in the encounter (Roberts and Sarangi 2005, p. 634), and there is a dialectic between meaning production on the micro and the macro level. From these four points follows the fifth: that no person has one, single and stable, identity, but several. To have an identity is also to be cast into a social category, and the question is which one is brought to the forefront and made relevant in any given interaction.

Linell (2009, p. 190) defines practices as “socioculturally established ways of carrying out recurrent types of projects and activities”, including ways of organizing social relations. Performing professional practices entails both following procedures and creative application of skill, and is routinely embedded in institutional and organizational rules and procedures (Sarangi and Candlin 2010, p. 3). Such practices define and delineate who and what will be seen as professional. In this study, mandatory practices were ascribed to ‘good’ (i.e. professional) nurses, and prohibited practices attributed to those who lacked the proper background or ‘feeling’ for the work and could be dismissed as unprofessional. Practices are basic to both identities and relations. As persons with a professional identity are licenced to perform professional practices, so very often a person seen performing such practices is taken to have a professional identity. Discourse practices are central to nursing and care work, and talk often accompanies the body-work, or enables it (as in, for instance, “talking the patient into care”).

Ideally, the nurse-patient relation is a harmonious and reciprocal role relationship. As Shattell (2004, p. 16) writes: “In the sick role, a patient is a willing passive recipient of care provided by a knowledgeable health care provider. The patients freely give up their power to professionals [...]”. The normative expectation is that the patient will cooperate and thereby authenticate the nurse’s professional identity. ‘Normal’ practices are geared to these normative expectations: that the nurse will be competent, and that the patient will cooperate. In practice, though, patients may—and some do—resist, refusing to let themselves be cared for at all, or by one or a category of nurses. My focus here is on the latter, specifically on cases where residents are reported to have refused care from nurses they categorize as ‘men’, ‘foreigners’, or ‘dark-skinned’. Gender, ethnicity or race seemed not to influence the institutional organization of work in the facilities. Even so, it was evident that the normal (or proper) nurse's body was recognizable as white, female, and a native speaker of Norwegian, and any body differently marked could be seen as a "body out of place" (Ahmed 2002, 2012). Søndergaard (1996, 2002) introduced the term 'the sign on the body' with reference to gender, and the term has been extended to racialized body signs (Staunæs 2003). It refers to observable marks on the bodily surface that are interpreted as cues for categorizing subjects.

With Benwell and Stokoe (2006), we can understand the term 'identity' here in its broadest sense, in terms of who people are to each other, and how different kinds of identities are produced in interaction. This is analytically useful because it invites us to differentiate the rather vague concept 'work identity' and ask who the nurses are *to whom*, and how this is accomplished. Nurses' professional identity is many-faceted; as professionals nurses manage relations to patients, to their relatives, and to colleagues. While all three relations can be seen as practice based, both the specific practices and the way they are conducted and displayed vary with the setting and interactional partners. Karlsson and Nikolaidou (2011) distinguish between professional, institutional and personal aspects of work identity,[2] which are grounded in types of knowledge and can be connected to what Sarangi and Roberts (1999) call discourse modes. In this chapter, I focus on the professional identity vis-à-vis patients, and on the professional discourse. Generally, to speak like a professional is to speak like an expert. For nurses this means to speak like an expert *on* patients' conditions and care needs and to demonstrate how these are the grounds for work practices, including how nurses speak *to* patients.

9.3.2 Accounts and Accounting

The ethnomethodological concept of accountability refers to a general feature of action—that actors are responsible for their actions and can always be *taken to account*, having to explain or justify them (ten Have 2007, p. 217). I use it here in the narrow sense defined by Scott and Lyman (1968), to refer to linguistic devices that are used after so-called 'failure events' to re-present or re-contextualize the unfortunate event by creating a preferred meaning for it.

Research on accounts and accounting in professional contexts (Mäkitalo 2003; Hall et al. 2006) demonstrate that the competent handling of accounts is an important aspect of work activities, and also that having a repertoire of valid accounts is a necessary resource for constituting professional identity. In the words of Scott and Lyman (1968, p. 59): "*Every account is a manifestation of the underlying negotiation of identities*" (italics in the original). The accounts presented here are typical of those offered by nurses in the interviews, and are analysed as

[2]While professional identity is grounded in a body of knowledge shared with colleagues, institutional identity is derived from position in the institutional hierarchy, and personal identity is built on personal experience.

both professional and authoritative descriptions of the institutional order (Mäkitalo 2003, p. 495–496).

9.4 Data and Research Sites

The study reported here is part of a more comprehensive investigation into gender and ethnicity in Norwegian working life.[3] In search of good practice with respect to handling workforce diversity, we wanted to study workplaces with a diversified workforce, and where the institutional hierarchy was not obviously gendered or racialized. These criteria led us to four wards in medicalised nursing homes for the elderly, all of them municipal (as part of the Nordic welfare state model, Norwegian eldercare has traditionally been provided through public social services, though this is changing). These wards had active and successful diversity recruitment policies with regard to both gender and ethnicity, and they were explicitly committed to promote anti-discriminatory practices and to create equality in the workforce. The selected wards employed an unusually high proportion of men, varying between 15 and 30% and of foreign-born nurses (between 30 and 66%).[4] The main data was generated through qualitative interviews, and interviewees were selected so as to correspond to these patterns for each ward.

While highly medicalized tasks were the exclusive responsibility of registered nurses, both care-workers and nurses conducted care-work, bringing them into close contact with residents. Also, all nursing/care-working staff wore identical uniforms, obscuring the institutional hierarchy to residents and visitors. In this chapter I refer to them all as ‘nurses’, without distinguishing between different categories (registered nurses, auxiliary nurses, trained care-workers, assistants), even if this strongly misrepresents the hierarchical relations between nurses and care-workers (Dahle 2005; Seeberg 2012). Also, I refer to all categories as professionals, regardless of their educational level. The words ‘patient’ and ‘resident’ are used interchangeably, in keeping with the local usage.

Nurses were selected by researchers from employee lists and invited by us to participate. They were advised of their right to decline participation or to withdraw at any time, and that full anonymity was guaranteed. The project and our research interests were described in staff meetings and printed material left in staff rooms.

35 interviews totalling about 50 hours were audiotaped and transcribed in various degrees of detail. All transcripts were anonymized. Through thematic discourse analysis (Roberts and Sarangi 2005) we identified particularly interesting sequences, which were then transcribed according to principles for capturing interactional

---

[3]The project *Gender equality—a boundary between ‘us’ and ‘them’?* was funded by The Norwegian Research Council and was approved by the privacy ombudsman for research in Norway, NSD.

[4]For an analysis of how eldercare is situated in the crossroads of the national gender regime and globalised distribution of care-work, see Seeberg 2012.

qualities of talk-in-interaction (such as speed, stress, prosody, pauses and gaps, overlapping talk, laughter, voice quality, etc.). All extracts quoted here have been analysed on the basis of these finely grained transcripts, repeated listening to the tapes, and researchers' field notes. For the purposes of this chapter I have chosen a simplified rendering in order to facilitate reading. This means editing out quite a lot of information on the interactional aspects of the talk, and I include a few comments on those in the analysis.

9.5 Analysis

9.5.1 Analytic Approach: Interviews as Discourse

> Interviews tell us about the cultural resources people have available for telling their patch of the world. This is particularly so when the corpus of interviews is relatively large, there is a lot of homogeneity, and repetition and clear patterns emerge (Wetherell 2004, p. 13).

Accounts for actions are local, cultural resources for representing and interpreting people, actions, and events and orienting ourselves in the world. They are based on assumptions of shared background knowledge of roles and relationships and on what constitutes proper conduct in particular relations and situations, demonstrating their cultural and moral character. Scott and Lyman narrowed the concept down to refer to devices used after 'failure events', that is, when interactional expectations have not been met, or when obligations have been ignored (Mäkitalo 2003, p. 496). In this sense, accounts are "designed to recast the pejorative significance of action, or one's responsibility for it" (Buttny 1993, p. 1). As mentioned above, this is the sense in which I use the term here, but more as an analytical perspective on the data than as a categorization device. It is distinguished from other explanations and descriptions because it is only the occurrence of improper conduct that necessitates an account, which according to Scott and Lyman (1968) will be either an excuse for or a justification of the improper act, to "bridge the gap between actions and expectations". When patients reject a nurse, they demonstrate a gap between what they expect a nurse to be like on the one hand and the actual nurse on the other. From the point of view of the nurse, there is a gap between their expectation to engage in care-work and being rejected. And obviously, the verbal rejection is an act that deviates from the institutional order and must therefore be accounted for.

As noted by De Fina (2009), in some research traditions interviews are discarded as poor substitutes for 'real data' on what people ordinarily do in social situations. In the discourse analytic approach used here, the point is not to discover what people ordinarily do, but how they talk about what they do. Interviews are seen as situated social interactions and must be analyzed as such. Stories told, incidents reported and accounts offered are produced in the frame of this particular activity type (Sarangi 2004) at specific points in that talk, and do certain kinds of work there. This does not imply that accounts offered in interviews are any more or less true than alternative versions. It is simply a reflection of the fact that in any interactional event, people tell stories to do something: to explain, to alert, to counter an argument or support one, etc. (Schegloff 1997, p. 97). We invited nurses to participate as professionals, and the talk centered on the everyday work routines, and so it came as no surprise that nurses' talk was primarily in a professional mode. As will be demonstrated below, the accounts can be seen as resources for each participant in establishing and maintaining a professional identity vis-à-vis interviewers.

Since our interviews were conducted with the help of a thematic guide rather than by a predetermined sequence of questions, we were free to let each conversation run its individual course, picking up and elaborating on topics we found interesting along the way. While this generated clearly different conversational trajectories and stories, it also let us see striking similarities and patterns across interviews, allowing us to identify a professional discourse. This discourse defined standards for good care work and good care workers, primarily as a set of practices which were either prescribed (as professional) or prohibited (as unprofessional).

9.5.2 Interpreting Marked Bodies

We interpret bodies in our environment so routinely that we are often unaware of doing so. Certain signs or markings indicate what kind of body this is, and what someone like me can anticipate from it: how can it be expected to act, and how will it react to what I do?

In the nursing home, the uniform signifies that the body belongs here in a certain capacity: it has been trained and employed to offer assistance and care. But the uniform appears together with several other signs. The *normal* uniformed body is marked as 'white', as female, and as Norwegian. Because this configuration of signs and appurtenances marks the body as 'normal' in this setting, the body also appears as invisible, and the person can be understood as a 'disembodied mind', able to discipline and control the body and its reactions, pleasures, and inclinations (Moser 2006). Or, put in another way, it can be trusted not to be distracted from conducting itself professionally. The good—that is, professional—nurse is expected not to respond to provocation but to appear unfailingly as kind, patient, and cheerful.

A body that is perceived as dark-skinned, marked as male, or with an accent, becomes visible. Such a body must be interpreted, its implications considered. The darker the hue, the more obvious the maleness, the stronger the accent, the more conspicuously embodied the person appears to be. Not all old women want their bodies to be washed and cared for by a male body, and some residents dislike having a dark skin very close to their own. A few old men misinterpret the female sign, responding to it as an indication of sexual availability. Occasionally, one sign is singled out as so potent as to overshadow the others. Possibly it was the nurses’ uniform, traditionally associated with women, that had misled one patient to conclude that Daniel, her favourite nurse, was a woman. She was appalled to learn the truth: “Are you a man? Bloody hell! I’ve given you two hugs! And you have washed down there!”

9.5.3 Restoring the Moral Order Through Accounts

Goffman (1967) pointed out that normal conduct is moral in nature, and its norms are both acquired and sustained through interaction. When a breach of norms troubles the moral order, one or more interactants will normally take steps to restore it. The examples in this section are chosen to demonstrate how nurses do this in interviews by offering an account for troubling incidents, and how these accounts function as resources for professional identity.

The accounts presented here are retrospective representations of problematic episodes, offering preferred meaning for problematic episodes and distributing blame and responsibility for them. According to Morris et al. (1994), they provide insight into the local moral order by allowing us to see what actually happened as opposed to what should have happened. Or, rather, they let us see the narrator’s *representation* of what happened, in the frame of the interview. In the words of Johnstone 1990, p. 100: “… all tellings, by their nature, are fictions, in the sense that all tellers make choices about what to present and how to give it meaning as they present it”.

As mentioned above, Scott and Lyman (1968) distinguished between two main types of accounts: excuses and justifications. The main finding is that nurses, rather than blaming residents for rejecting nurses, often provided excuses or justifications for them. Both are represented in the data, but excuses are by far the more common.

A justification is an account that asserts that an action (in this case, for a patient to reject a nurse) is generally wrong, but also claims that in this particular case, the action was permissible. In this data, justifications made by ethnic Norwegian nurses often referred to ‘foreign’ nurses as having poor language or communication skills —making it legitimate for the patient to ask for another nurse. Transcript 9.1 below is from the interview with Anders, a qualified nurse’s assistant in a supervisory position. The extract consists of one extended turn, divided into sequences here for practical reasons.

Transcript 9.1: “Go get Anders”

1a.

Patients haven’t got the energy to start explaining to someone they find it difficult to talk to.

```
1b.

They're trying to express that "I have some pain somewhere,
some diffuse place".

1c.

It's difficult to concentrate, difficult to express what they
want, and then someone comes in and says (mimics strong for-
eign accent) "What did you want?"

1d.

Then you get "No, go get Anders".
```

In 1a-1c, Anders offers what comes across as a patient's perspective on the situation. Framed by the statement in 1a, 1b-1c provide further details which give credibility to the description and invites the interviewer to empathize with the vulnerable patient and their need to see the nurse as a competent communication partner. The nurse's accent, mimicked by Anders in "What did you want?", is taken as a mark of low communicative competence, which makes it easier to accept as legitimate the patient's response in the constructed conversation in 1c-1d. Anders does not imply that he personally is a better or more popular nurse; it is simply the accent (or lack of it[5]) that makes him the patients' preferred choice. The account constitutes Anders' identity as a caring and competent professional, knowledgeable about patients, and as a fair colleague. It also implies that an accent-free Norwegian is a prerequisite for being a fully competent nurse.

This account asserts that the patient's act—rejecting a nurse—is generally wrong, and so the account supports the existing moral order. In the frame of a professional nursing discourse, centered on accommodating patients' states and needs, it also claims that the patient was entitled to do so. Going back to Shattell (2004): patients are not obliged to embrace the sick role vis-à-vis a nurse they do not see as having the requisite competence to fill the nurse role. In other words, that nurse is denied a professional identity.

An excuse differs from a justification in that it admits that the action really *was* wrong, but claims that the person was not, or not fully, responsible for it (Scott and Lyman 1968). In this data, excuses were typically offered by nurses on grounds of dementia, mental disorder, fear, or modesty in patients. These examples are prototypical: "She doesn't really mean it, she's ill"; "They're not racist, they're scared"; "they don't know what they are saying", "they're not used to being undressed and washed by a man". These excuses occur frequently in the interviews, and that is in accord with findings in several other studies. (Berdes and Eckert 2001; Jönsson 2007; McGregor 2007). They all imply that no racism or sexism is intended and therefore no offense should be taken.

[5]'Accent' in Norwegian usage never refers to regional dialects, but exclusively to 'foreign' accents.

Transcript 9.2: "She didn't know I'm black, you see"

Whether or not Maria is 'black' is a matter of interpretation. Staunæs (2003) explains racialized body signs as *configurations* of physical features: 'black' and 'white' is not only about skin colour, but about facial features, quality of hair, etc. M'charek (2010) demonstrates how a sign can be interpreted in the light of accompanying appurtenances, a particular social setting, and even proximity to other people. Below, we see that while one resident categorises Maria as black—like she does herself—the other has seen her as white.

Maria's account is extended over a stretch of talk in the interview. It is rendered in full, as it unfolded, but in a simplified transcription. To facilitate reading, I have divided it into numbered sequences, and I provide comments along the way.

The extract starts with Maria's coda to the previous talk, a story about a resident who had called her a 'blackskull', a derogatory term.

2a. Maria

He wasn't used to it, I think. But it's normal, really, because in their day there weren't so many foreigners, none, almost, when they were young, youngsters, right? But it doesn't happen to me often, really.

In this part of the extract, Maria offers an excuse for the resident's behaviour and explicitly normalises it. Even so, she closes the topic with stating that this sort of thing doesn't happen to her often.

In 2b, Maria proceeds to present a narrative about another resident. Her orientation to the interviewer is evident from the embedded comments providing context for the encounter she is about to report (in **bold**).

2b. Maria

But I've heard one here who said…she didn't know (laughs), I don't know … **she didn't know I'm black, you see?** so she said… **there's a man and he is dark, tall…he is darker than me, you know** …

Maria starts her narrative in 2c, again breaking off to provide a contextual comment:

2c. Maria

She said to me, "guess what?", she said…**I was giving her a shower, you see**.
"Yes, what?" I said.
"You should have seen, yesterday!"
"Well, what happened?", I said.
"There was a dark-skinned one who had intended to give me a shower!"

2d. Berit bursts into laughter and Maria joins in.

The resident's "guess what?" and "you should have seen…" are devices that build up a narrative tension, which is emphasized in Maria's animated enactment of the conversation. The tension climaxes with the resident's moral point: it is quite unacceptable for her to be given a shower by a "dark-skinned one" (presumably the "dark, tall" one that Maria referred to in 2b above). That the resident offers this story, in this particular manner, and while she is being showered by Maria, triggers joint laughter from Berit and Maria. This way, the tension that might have ensued from the story is dissolved, and the incident is framed as comical and therefore unthreatening. Maria then proceeds in 2e to enact the subsequent conversation with the resident:

2e. Maria

And I just: "So am I".
"Are you? I'm sorry, but you aren't so dark."
"Well, but I am…" (laughs). **She apologised**.
"You know, we aren't used to it", she said.

Harré and van Langenhove (1999) define positions in talk as "momentary clusters of rights and duties to think, act, and speak in certain ways". Positions may change quickly, as we see in the transition from 2c to 2d. In 2c, the resident had taken it for granted that Maria would agree with her, seeking to forge an alliance between the two of them as white. This created an ambivalent position for Maria. She might have let it go, but in 2e, we see how Maria avails herself of the opportunity to demonstrate to the resident that it *is* quite appropriate to be given a shower by "a dark-skinned one". Negotiating the possible meanings of skin colour in this way, Maria in effect undermines what had been presented as 'obvious' and 'natural' implications of skin colour. And in Maria's story, the old lady accepts this. She apologizes for having made a statement which she now apparently sees as rude and offers an account for it; "we aren't used to it". Thereby, she creates a position for Maria to demonstrate a forgiving and generous attitude, assuring the resident that her previous comment was "quite understandable" and that no offence has been taken, as we see in 2f:

2f. Maria

"Yes, that's quite understandable", I said to her, "no problem".

2g. Maria

That's just the way it is. You know, they aren't racist, but they are scared. She was scared. So it's like… But I don't think it… they're used to it, I feel now.

Maria's coda in 2g sums up the incident with a condensed excuse, stating that residents are scared, not racist. While this may or may not be so, it is a convincingly professional interpretation of residents, and by stating that this is "just the way it is"

Maria implies that it must be accepted. The seeming contradiction between 2a and 2g—that residents aren't used to 'dark-skinned' people, but they are [getting] used to it now—can be seen not as a contradiction, but as a testimony to ongoing change.

Transcript 9.3: "Maybe you are angry with me because of some other thing?"

In contrast to the previous examples, and less frequently in this data, rejection is attributed to actual racist or xenophobic views in the patient: "She doesn't like foreigners"; "He was so angry with foreigners he wouldn't allow me in his room". These typically occur embedded in descriptions of the patient in question, leading up to stories about the nurse's professional strategies for coping with such behaviour. They differ from the other accounts in that they do not excuse or justify patients' behaviour, but instead explain the breach in the institutional, or moral, order and placing the responsibility on patients.

The extract starts just after I (Ellen) have asked whether Yasmin has a favourite resident, to which she responds by stating that it is the work itself—helping people—she likes, not particular residents. This is of course a more professional attitude than holding favourites. In 3a, Yasmin starts to explain how residents sometimes make it difficult for her to demonstrate her professional abilities by "saying things". She offers an example with a lady who "fusses a lot" and "dislikes foreigners", and reports a dialogue between the two of them.[6]

Laughter can have more than one function in dialogue. In this extract, Yasmin speaks partly in a 'laughing voice' in turns 3a-3c (that voice quality is indicated by the symbol @ and angle brackets around the relevant stretches of talk).

3a. Yasmin:

<@And then when she says "go get someone Norwegian. You don't have a high standard"@ > and so on? Then it gets a little…

We see that Yasmin delivers the patient's blunt rejection and her stated reason for it, in a laughing voice. I noted at the time that the laughter never came across as an attempt to frame something as laughable or humorous, and I did not respond to it as an invitation to join in. Instead, I provided a clue for Yasmin to proceed:

3b. Ellen:

What do you *do* then?

3c. Yasmin:

Well, I then just look at her, I smile, she just < *@"no you @@. You don't do what I tell you."@* > I say to her, *"No. I can't do anything if you say—because maybe you are angry with me? Because of some*

[6]Again, while the transcription is simplified, the talk is rendered as it unfolded between us in the interview.

other thing, and then you < @say such things@ >." And then, but after…after a while she gets quiet and so on. Herself. Then it is a little easier.

Again, it is troubling statements from the patient that are produced with a laughing voice quality, and without generating laughter from either of us.

3d. Yasmin:

But… if for example I speak to her at the same time she speaks to me, then it gets even worse. Then she… She is ill. We must… bear with … what she says and such. Because it is, it is okay (little laugh).

[2 lines omitted]

In 3d, Yasmin demonstrates a professional understanding of patients as ill and frail, and therefore not morally accountable for their own behaviour.

3e. Ellen:

But what … what does it do to you? Do you get upset and angry?

3f. Yasmin:

No, not because of … the old ones. If they do something. Because they, they … maybe they don't know what they are saying.

3h resonates with 3d above, and adds an implicit comparison between categories of people, i.e. residents and others. Unpleasant behaviour from "the old ones" should not provoke negative feelings, but be excused. "They don't know what they are saying" alludes to the fact that about eighty percent of residents have some degree of dementia.[7]

There is an ambiguity in this account, too, but different to the one in example 2. When introducing the enacted dialogue, Yasmin described the resident in question as a lady who "doesn't like foreigners", whereas the coda is a general statement about "they" who "don't know what they are saying". Whether or not this applies to the lady is unclear. Anyway, it is made obvious that it is up to the nurse to handle troublesome behaviour from residents. It is clear from elsewhere, in this interview and others, that similar behaviour from residents' relatives or from work colleagues —people who do know what they are saying—is seen as much more offensive. In their interviews with auxiliary nurses, Berdes and Eckert (2007) identified a practice they call "constructive confrontation", where the nurse counteracts racist remarks in an attempt at 'educating the patient', and that may be what Yasmin was attempting in this episode.

[7]This means that, even in milder cases, they are prone to anxiety, fear, and confusion. This group also has reduced tolerance for linguistic ambiguity, and may find it hard to cope with unfamiliar accents.

9.5.4 *Characteristics of the Accounts*

Sarangi and Roberts (1999, p. 15) point out that a given professional account will have identifiable linguistic features "which are not only durable, but also legitimate and authoritative". Certain characteristics make the above extracts representative for the many accounts offered during the interviews. One is the way the narrators recruit patients' voices in their accounts, in reported speech or enacted dialogue. Especially in combination with descriptive details, these voices provide credibility, creating an impression that this was exactly how things happened, these were the exact words uttered – even if the dialogue is constructed (Tannen 2007; Holmes 2006, pp. 173–174). Another characteristic is that each accounting episode contains one or more kernel statements as comment or coda to the core narrative; most frequently along the lines of "they're not racist, but they are scared".

9.6 Professional Identity, Body Signs and Accounts

The concept of body signs invites us to look into the complex processes in which the surfaces of bodies are interpreted as evidence of qualities and dispositions on the inside of those bodies, and sometimes in quite unexpected ways. All bodies are marked, but while some bodies are deemed as appropriate in a particular setting or for a particular role, others are deemed inappropriate. While some interpretations of bodies support a professional identity, others seem to contradict it.

In the nursing homes, some problems related to inappropriate bodies were met by institutionalized solutions, like entering in a residents' journal that they should not be cared for by a male or a black nurse. In most cases, though, it was up to the problematic body itself to take on the extra work required to neutralize or accommodate itself (Ahmed 2007; Star 1990). The extra work was tailored to the way nurses categorized residents. Having first attributed patient resistance to modesty, male nurses would then explain to woman patients that professional nurse training had made the nurses indifferent to the sex of patients' bodies. The point was to stop the old women feeling shy about their own bodies. It is difficult to imagine a black nurse employing a parallel strategy, assuring white patients that they do not need to feel shy about the whiteness of theirs. Hierarchies and asymmetries of gender and race are similar, but not identical, nor are the social meanings attached to gendered and raced bodies parallel.

Challenged identities need to be reconfirmed, and accounts are excellent resources for doing just that. When accounting for encounters that undermine their professional identity nurses take up positions that allow them to repair and authenticate it. Accounting practices are central to any professional discourse. In this case excuses and justifications frame residents as so ill, frail, and vulnerable that they are not accountable for their actions. Such accounts are professional practices where nurses present themselves as knowledgeable, empathizing, and respectful of patient integrity. The accounts also support the 'incorrigible proposition' (Morris et al. 1994) that the patient-nurse relationship is harmoniously reciprocal.

In this manner, an account offered by one nurse would contribute not only to constitute the professional identity of that particular nurse, but also to that of the group. Throughout the interviews we were told about various tasks and of how nurse should conduct themselves when performing them. The core of these explanations was expressed as concern for residents' well-being and sympathetic insight into their mental and physical needs, evidenced in practices like "talking the resident into accepting care" and then washing that patient "with the heart, not just with the sponge". The collective character of professional identity became evident through choice of words: unfailingly, it was "we", not "I" who "must leave our personal problems at the door" or "can never force a patient into accepting care".

As pointed out by, among others, Potter and Wetherell (1987), discursive practices in organizations do not just describe things, they *do* things. Through regular repetition these statements are turned into institutional truths, part of the collective knowledge base and a basis for performing and evaluating practice. This knowledge base is largely concerned with quality care, 'good encounters' and the demands they place on nurses and care workers. As stated by Karlsson and Nikolaidou (2011), the professional identity of nurses is closely related to this shared body of knowledge. But with identities, there are always bodies involved, and always ideas about bodies, representations, categories, and negotiation. Together with accounts, the concept of body signs provide a basis for reflecting on how such interpretations impact on identities, including professional ones.

References

Ahmed, S. (2002). *Strange encounters: Embodied others in post-coloniality*. London: Routledge.

Ahmed, S. (2007). *A phenomenology of whiteness. Feminist Theory, 8*(2), 149–168.

Ahmed, S. (2012). *On being included: Racism and diversity in institutional life*. Durham: Duke University Press.

Allan, H. T., Larsen, J. A., Bryan, K., & Smith, P. A. (2004). The social reproduction of institutional racism: Internationally recruited nurses' experiences of the British health services. *Diversity in Health and Social Care, 1*(2), 117–125.

Andenæs, E. (2010). 'Nok norsk' til å være 'norsk nok'? Språk, arbeidsliv, likestilling. In A.-J. Berg, A. B. Flemmen & B. Gullikstad (Ed.), *Likestilte norskheter. Om kjønn og etnisitet* (pp. 195–224). Trondheim: Tapir Akademisk Forlag.

Angouri, J., & Marra, M. (Eds.). (2011). *Constructing Identities at Work*. New York: Palgrave Macmillan.

Benwell, B., & Stokoe, E. (2006). *Discourse and Identity*. Edinburgh: University Press.

Berdes, C., & Eckert, J. M. (2001). Race relations and caregiving relationships: A qualitative examination of perspectives from residents and nurse's aides in three nursing homes. *Research on Aging, 23*(1), 109–126.

Berdes, C., & Eckert, J. M. (2007). The language of caring: Nurse's aides' use of family metaphors conveys affective care. *The Gerontologist, 47*(3), 340–349.

Bergland, Å., & Kirkevold, M. (2006). Thriving in nursing homes in Norway: contributing aspects described by residents. *International Journal of Nursing Studies, 43*(6), 681–691.
Brubaker, R., & Cooper, F. (2000). Beyond "Identity". *Theory and Society, 29*(1), 1–47.
Bucholtz, M. (2003). Sociolinguistic nostalgia and the authentication of identity. *Journal of Sociolinguistics, 7*(3), 398–416.
Bucholtz, M., & Hall, K. (2005). Identity and interaction: A sociocultural linguistic approach. *Discourse Studies, 7*(4–5), 585–614.
Butler, J. (1990). *Gender trouble. Feminism and the subversion of identity*. New York: Routledge.
Buttny, R. (1993). *Social accountability in communication*. London: Sage.
Couper-Kuhlen, E., & Selting, M. (2006). *Prosody in conversation: Interactional studies*. Cambridge: Cambridge University Press.
Dahle, R. (2005). Dirty work in a Norwegian health context (the case of Norway). In H. M. Dahl & T. R. Eriksen (Eds.), *Dilemmas of Care in the Nordic Welfare State: Continuity and Change* (pp. 101–111). Aldershot: Ashgate.
De Fina, A. (2009). Narratives in interview—The case of accounts: For an interactional approach to narrative genres. *Narrative Inquiry, 19*(2), 233–258.
Dodson, L., & Zincavage, R. M. (2007). "It's like a family": caring labor, exploitation and race in nursing homes. *Gender and Society, 21*(6), 905–928.
Dreachslin, J. L., Hunt, P. L., & Sprainer, E. (2004). Workforce diversity: Implications for the effectiveness of health care delivery teams. *Social Science and Medicine, 50*(10), 1403–1414.
Evans, J. A. (2002). Cautious caregivers: Gender stereotypes and the sexualization of men nurses' touch. *Journal of Advanced Nursing, 40*(4), 441–448.
Goffman, E. (1967). *Interaction ritual. Essays on face-to-face behavior*. New York: Pantheon Books.
Goffman, E. (1971). *Relations in public: Microstudies of the public order*. New York: Basic Books.
Goodwin, C. (2000). Action and embodiment within situated human interaction. *Journal of Pragmatics, 32*(10), 1489–1522.
Gullikstad, B. (2010). Når likestilling blir ulikhet. Interseksjonalitet i arbeidslivet. In A.-J. Berg, A. B. Flemmen & B. Gullikstad (Eds.), *Likestilte norskheter. Om kjønn og etnisitet* (pp. 101–132). Trondheim: Tapir Akademisk Forlag.
Hall, C., Slembrouck, S., & Sarangi, S. (2006). *Language practices in social work: Categorisation and accountability in child welfare*. London/New York: Routledge.
Harré, R., & van Langenhove, L. (Eds.). (1999). *Positioning theory: Moral contexts of intentional action*. Oxford: Blackwell.
Holmes, J. (2006). Workplace narratives, professional identity and relational practice. In A. De Fina, D. Schiffrin, & M. Bamberg, (Eds.), *Discourse and Identity* (pp. 166–187). Cambridge: Cambridge University Press.
Johnstone, B. (1990). *Stories, community, and place: narratives from middle america*. Bloomington: Indiana University Press.
Jönsson, H. (2007). Is It Racism? *Journal of Gerontological Social Work, 49*(4), 79–96.
Karlsson, A.-M., & Nikolaidou, Z. (2011). Writing about caring: Discourses, genres and remediation in elder care. *Journal of Applied Linguistics & Professional Practice, 8*(2), 123–143.
Kita, S. (Ed.). (2003). *Pointing: Where language, culture, and cognition meet*. Mahwah, New Jersey: Lawrence Erlbaum.
Likupe, G. (2006). Experiences of African nurses in the UK National Health Service: A literature review. *Journal of Clinical Nursing, 15*(10), 1213–1220.
Linell, P. (2009). *Rethinking Language, Mind, and World Dialogically. Interactional and contextual theories of human sense-making*. Charlotte, NC: Information Age Publishing.
Mäkitalo, Å. (2003). Accounting practices as situated knowing: Dilemmas and dynamics in institutional categorization. *Discourse Studies, 5*(4), 495–516.

Mapedzahama, V., Rudge, T., West, S., & Perron, A. (2011). Black nurse in white space? Rethinking the in/visibility of race within the Australian nursing workplace. *Nursing Inquiry, 19*(2), 153–164.
Marchal, B., & Kegels, G. (2003). Health workforce imbalances in times of globalization: Brain drain or professional mobility? *The International Journal of Health Planning and Management, 18*(S1), S89–S101.
Marra, M., & Angouri, J. (2011). Investigating the negotiation of identity: A View from the field of workplace discourse. In J. Angouri & M. Marra (Eds.), *Constructing Identities at Work* (pp. 1–14). New York: Palgrave Macmillan.
M'charek, A. (2010). Fragile differences, relational effects: Stories about the materiality of race and sex. *European Journal of Women's Studies, 17*(4), 307–322.
McGregor, J. (2007). 'Joining the BBC (British Bottom Cleaners': Zimbabwean migrants and the UK care industry. *Journal of Ethnic and Migration Studies, 5,* 801–824.
McMillian, J., Morgan, S. A., & Ament, P. (2006). Acceptance of male registered nurses by female registered nurses. *Journal of Nursing Scholarship, 38*(1), 100–106.
Morris, G. H., White, C. H., & Iltis, R. (1994). "Well, ordinarily I would, but": Reexamining the nature of accounts for problematic events. *Research on Language and Social Interaction, 27* (2), 123–144.
Moser, I. (2006). Mulighetsbetingelser for normalitet. In T. H. Eriksen & J.-K. Breivik (Eds.), *normalitet* (pp. 135–166). Oslo: Universitetsforlaget.
Ochs, E. (1992). Indexing gender. In A. Duranti & C. Goodwin (Eds.), *Rethinking context: Language as an interactive phenomenon* (pp. 335–358). Cambridge: Cambridge University Press.
Potter, J., & Wetherell, M. (1987). *Discourse and social psychology*. London: Sage.
Ryosho, N. (2011). Experiences of racism by female minority and immigrant nursing assistants. *Affilia: Journal of Women and Social Work*, *26*(1), 59–71.
Roberts, C., & Sarangi, S. (2005). Theme-oriented discourse analysis of medical encounters. *Medical Education, 39*(6), 632–640.
Sarangi, S. (2004). Institutional, professional, and lifeworld frames in interview talk. In H. van den Berg, M. Wetherell, & H. Houtkoop-Steenstra (Eds.), *Analyzing race talk: Multidisciplinary perspectives on the research interview* (pp. 64–84). New York: Cambridge University Press.
Sarangi, S., & Candlin, C. N. (2010). Editorial: Applied linguistics and professional practice: Mapping a future agenda. *Journal of Applied linguistics and professional practice, 7*(1), 1–9.
Sarangi, S., & Roberts, C. (1999). The dynamics of interactional and institutional orders in work-related settings. In S. Sarangi & C. Roberts (Eds.), *Talk, work and institutional order: Discourse in medical, mediation and management settings* (pp. 1–57). New York: Mouton de Gruyter.
Schegloff, E. (1997). "Narrative analysis" thirty years later. *Journal of Narrative and Life History, 7*(1–4), 97–106.
Scott, M. B., & Lyman, S. M. (1968). Accounts. *American Sociological Review, 33*(1), 46–62.
Seeberg, M. L. (2012). Immigrant care workers and Norwegian gender equality: Institutions, identities, intersections. *European Journal of Women's Studies, 19*(2), 173–185.
Shattell, M. (2004). Nurse–patient interaction: A review of the literature. *Journal of Clinical Nursing, 13*(6), 714–722.
Smith, P. (2007). Editorial: Overseas-trained nurses, diversity and discrimination: perceptions, practice and policy. *Journal of Clinical Nursing, 16*(12), 2185–2186.
Star, S. L. (1990). Power, technology and the phenomenology of conventions: On being allergic to onions. *The Sociological Review, 38*(S1), 26–56.
Staunæs, D. (2003). Where have all the subjects gone? Bringing together the concepts of intersectionality and subjectification. *NORA—Nordic Journal of Feminist and Gender Research, 11*(2), 101–110.
Streeck, J., Goodwin, C., & LeBaron, C. (Eds.). (2011). *Embodied interaction: Language and body in the material world*. Cambridge: Cambridge University Press.

Søndergaard, D. M. (1996). *Tegnet på kroppen: køn: Koder og konstruktioner blandt unge voksne i akademia*. Copenhagen: Museum Tusculanum.
Søndergaard, D. M. (2002). Poststructuralist approaches to empirical analysis. *International Journal of Qualitative Studies in Education, 15*(2), 187–204.
Søndergaard, D. M. (2005). Making sense of gender, age, power and disciplinary Position: Intersecting discourses in the academy. *Feminism & Psychology, 15*(2), 189–208.
Tannen, D. (2007). *Talking Voices. Repetition, Dialogue, and Imagery in Conversational Discourse*. Cambridge: Cambridge University Press.
ten Have, P. (2007). *Doing conversation analysis. A Practical guide*. London: Sage.
Timonen, V., & Doyle, M. (2010). Migrant care workers' relationships with care recipients, Colleagues and employers. *European Journal of Women's Studies, 17*(1), 25–41.
Tracy, K. (2011). Identity-work in appellate oral argument: Ideological identities within a professional one. In J. Angouri & M. Marra (Eds.), *Constructing Identities at Work* (pp. 175–199). Palgrave Macmillan.
West, C., & Zimmerman, D. H. (1987). Doing gender. *Gender & Society, 1*(2), 125–151.
Westin, I. (2006). Nurses' experiences of caring encounters with older people living in Swedish nursing homes. *International Journal of Older People Nursing, 1*(1), 3–10.
Wetherell, M. (1998). Positioning and interpretative repertoires: Conversation analysis and post-structuralism in dialogue. *Discourse & Society, 9*(3), 387–412.
Wetherell, M. (2004). Racism and the analysis of cultural resources in interviews. In H. van den Berg, M. Wetherell, & H. Houtkoop-Steenstra (Eds.), *Analyzing race talk: multidisciplinary perspectives on the research interview* (pp. 10–30). New York: Cambridge University Press.

Author Biography

Ellen Andenæs is associate professor of applied linguistics at NTNU, Norwegian University of Science and Technology (16). An active researcher and educator, she has published in the fields of second language studies, minority education, gender and ethnicity, and professional discourse. Her research is grounded in dialogical and sociocultural perspectives on learning, communication and identity, and her current work focuses on participatory practices in professional talk.

Chapter 10
The Complexities of Deaf Identities

Irene W. Leigh

> I no longer feel ashamed of who I am; instead, those who treat me as less than I am are now the problem, not me.
>
> Elisa Cimento (2013, p. 44)

Elisa Cimento (2013) transitioned from shame to pride as a deaf person after participating in a national conference focusing on listening and spoken language that included a program track for deaf high school peers. She had worked hard to blend in with hearing classmates at her mainstream school and hide the fact that she was deaf until the conference. Realizing she was no longer alone and now had new connections with other deaf teenagers who were up front about how they dealt with their being deaf and using auditory aids, including hearing aids and cochlear implants,[1] this experience provided her with the motivation to "come out" as who she is, a teenager with a solid, positive deaf identity that included significant social and academic accomplishments.

Considering that 96% of deaf children are born to hearing parents (Mitchell and Karchmer 2004), how these deaf children internalize possible deaf identities is not necessarily straightforward and can be a complex process. Their parents are not deaf nor are they part of Deaf culture[2] so cannot transmit this culture to their deaf

---

Portions of the material presented in this chapter have been excerpted from Leigh (2009, 2012).

---

[1]The cochlear implant is a small electronic device that that provides the ability to hear. The internal portion is surgically inserted into the cochlea of the inner ear. The external portion is placed behind the ear. It has the potential to help deaf individuals develop or understand spoken language.
[2]The use of lower case deaf refers to deaf people with severe-to-profound hearing levels, while upper case Deaf denotes those who identify with and affiliate with Deaf culture.

I.W. Leigh (✉)
Department of Psychology, Gallaudet University, Washington, DC, USA
e-mail: Irene.leigh@gallaudet.edu

S. Bagga-Gupta et al. (eds.), *Identity Revisited and Reimagined*,
DOI 10.1007/978-3-319-58056-2_10

child. Most of these parents have never thought about the possibility of a deaf child and have no idea how deaf people manage in life. Much depends on the language and communication choices that parents make for their deaf children, whether spoken or signed. Much depends on what kind of access to deaf people the children may have and how they feel about not having the sense of hearing that the majority of people around them have. Much also depends on the attitudes toward deaf people that hearing persons may reveal, depending on the situation. These attitudes can reveal curiosity, interest, positive support, rejection, or skepticism about the ability of deaf people to manage for themselves. As such, these attitudes have the potential to influence how deaf individuals feel about themselves. This chapter provides information that elucidates the reasons why internalizing deaf identities can be complicated to understand and research.

10.1 Interpretations of "Deaf"

To embrace "difference" when a deaf person is alone in the mainstream rather than in a school for the deaf can be daunting when this "difference" embodies the perception of deafness as defective. No wonder Elisa Cimento originally tried to look as "hearing" as possible, like her hearing peers. This "defectiveness" is typically exemplified by the belief that the deaf person has to endure a way of life that is a never-ending struggle to overcome the inability to hear and access the spoken language of the surrounding hearing society. The word "deaf" denotes a medical problem that "requires" reparative measures, including medical and technology interventions as well as speech and auditory training. The ultimate goal is to create access to an auditory environment that theoretically minimizes society's cultural constructions of deafness as disabled, impotent and isolated (Branson and Miller 2002; Brueggemann 1999; Davis 1995). This cultural construction is often reinforced by a society that does not understand the potential for deaf people to live rich lives and accomplish their maximum, hearing and speaking issues notwithstanding. Many are not aware that there are culturally Deaf lawyers, medical doctors, stockbrokers, entrepreneurs, school administrators, and an infinite plethora of other occupations. As the deaf population is a low-incidence population, the opportunity for hearing society members to see deaf people functioning well in daily life tends to be limited. Consequently, the perception, either conscious or unconscious, of deaf as a stigma continues. Because of this perceived stigma that, for example, can make it difficult for a number of deaf people to obtain employment, individuals may attempt efforts to conceal their hearing difference as much as possible and deny any sense of a deaf-related identity.

However, there are many ways to be deaf and to achieve a firm sense of self as a deaf person, whether through spoken languages, signed languages, in the mainstream, as a person affiliated with Deaf culture, or as biculturally competent in traversing between the mainstream where spoken language predominates and Deaf culture environs where sign language predominates (Leigh 2009). Each component reflects deaf identities that exemplify the uniqueness of each person. This has come about due to an increased focus on "deaf" as a normal state of affairs, or as an expected component of the diversity spectrum (Leigh 2009). Since time immemorial, deaf people have demonstrated resilience and an ability to create productive lives encompassing family, work, and play, thus counteracting the prevalent notion of "deaf" as a tragedy. This perception has been reinforced by the emergence of Deaf culture as a construct that encompasses the uniqueness and strengths of signed languages and Deaf cultural ways of being (Humphries 2008). Deaf culture represents a conscious social group with a Deaf center that has at its core the value of sign languages, visual ways of understanding the world, and shared experiences as Deaf people in Deaf and hearing environments. It is a rich culture that includes a common understanding of Deaf lives as expressed through stories, literature, theater, and visual art (Holcomb 2013; Leigh 2009).

10.2 Issues to Consider

In considering the complexities of deaf identities, we start with the language of separatism. This language demarcates deaf identity groups into various categories such as Deaf (affiliated with Deaf culture), oral deaf or having a hearing identity (preferring spoken language, interactions with people who hear, and interactions with other deaf individuals who prefer to speak), hard of hearing, hearing impaired, and so on (Breivik 2005). This concept of separatism is too simplistic considering deaf people's typical exposure to both hearing (based on hearing family of origin and the surrounding hearing environment) and Deaf cultural collectives (based on Deaf environmental exposure or having culturally Deaf parents). We lack in-depth understanding of how this "double consciousness" (DuBois 1997) of two contrasting deaf-related internalizations, hearing and deaf (Humphries and Humphries 2010), develops and interacts in the direction of biculturalism. What are specific deaf identities? What is the nature of the experiences that facilitates a positive sense of identity versus a defective sense? How do these experiences lead to the evolving internalization and integration of deaf identities? Does a hearing identity, especially with cochlear implants increasingly prominent, imply the desire to disavow the disability/deaf identity and "pass" for hearing? Related to identities based on ethnicity, religion, gender, sexual orientation, additional disabilities, work, and multiple other dimensions, how do multiple consciousnesses or multiple intersectionalities that include the deaf dimension evolve, interact with, and influence identities, particularly when these identities often are fluid, depending on context (Leigh 2012; Parasnis 2012)? In order to tackle these questions, the next section reviews researchers who have attempted to broaden the understanding of deaf identities and how these develop.

10.3 Theories of Deaf Identities and Research Findings

Researchers have used different theoretical models and data collection methods to define and better understand deaf and hearing identities. This section provides a review of theoretical perspectives based on psychological frameworks together with relevant research findings.

Among the earlier theories in the psychological literature was that of a disability framework utilized by Weinberg and Sterritt (1986). They conceptualized hearing identity as able-bodied, deaf identity as disability-related, with dual identity reflecting identification with both deaf and hearing peers. The authors developed the *Evaluation of Self as a Deaf Person Scale* to categorize study participants as having hearing, deaf, or dual identities. Each of the three subscales had four items reflecting each identity category. However, the internal consistency was 0.22, which is unacceptably low. Additionally, many Deaf people affiliated with Deaf culture do not universally accept the notion of deaf as a disability. They tend to view themselves as able-bodied and feel comfortable in their own skin. Interestingly, the study findings supported this perspective, with dual identity being associated with more positive adjustment outcomes, while hearing identity had the least positive outcomes. It is well known that even when affiliation with hearing people is desired, that can be more stressful if communication access is limited due to difficulties in acquiring spoken language skills. Noteworthy is that later studies involving individuals with cochlear implants show that they can demonstrate positive psychological adjustment even as they affirm a hearing identity that has been facilitated by easier communication access (e.g., Leigh et al. 2009; Mance and Edwards 2012).

Stinson and Kluwin (1996) based their conceptualization of deaf identities on social orientation parameters. They created the *Social Activity Scale* in order to assess both deaf student perceptions of their relationships in and out of school and identity formation based on whom one associates with and feels most comfortable with. This measure produced three factor scores: orientation to deaf peers, orientation to hearing peers, and a measure of emotional closeness to peers in general (both deaf and hearing peers). For deaf high school students participating in this large study, perceived signing skill and degree of hearing loss differentiated among these three groups. Those who were hearing oriented had the lowest factor score for signing skills and had the less severe hearing loss, while those who were deaf oriented had the highest factor score for signing skills and more profound hearing losses. The third group, which consisted of those who affiliated with both deaf and hearing peers or neither, fell in between the other two. Based on these results, it is reasonable to conclude that shared ways of communicating facilitate specific social relationships, which contribute to identity formation. Subsequent researchers have endorsed this perspective (e.g., Bat-Chava 2000; Hardy 2010; Mance and Edwards 2012). Essentially, the importance of language and communication, socialization, and social perspectives about what it means to be deaf, however the individual experiences that, rather than the hearing disability itself, are significant contributors to group identification.

In an effort to more fully explore the parameters of deaf identities, Glickman (1996) explored racial and cultural identity stage development theories and developed a parallel model incorporating four different stages of deaf identity development. He labeled the first stage as culturally hearing, meaning that deafness is viewed as a medical condition or disability to be cured or ameliorated, thereby minimizing the need for signed languages or support services. Hearing ways of speaking, understanding, and behaving as hearing people do are seen as ways of assimilating into hearing society. Individuals who fit this category tend to identify themselves as oral deaf, having grown up using spoken language and interacting primarily with hearing persons, or as late deafened, meaning those who have lost their hearing in adolescence or adulthood after language has been established. Deaf children born to hearing parents are immersed in a hearing environment and may start off as feeling culturally hearing, particularly if they have not been exposed to other deaf people.

Stage 2 covers cultural marginality. This is a state of being that incorporates individuals who do not identify with either hearing or deaf peers and are unable to integrate into either society. Deaf children who do not have full access to communication in their hearing home and have no access to deaf peers may fall into this category. While this category appears to be psychologically problematic, Hintermair (2008) states that this category can also reflect individuals who have personal resources aside from connecting with deaf or hearing groups and may do well in life.

Moving on to *Stage 3*, the individual integrates into Deaf culture to get a sense of belonging, identify as Deaf, and behave as culturally Deaf people do. Hearing people are denigrated as ones who cause problems for deaf people, but eventually, as the individual transitions into *Stage 4*, there is a rapprochement with hearing people while holding on to a Deaf culture identity, such that as a bicultural Deaf person the individual can positively relate to both hearing and deaf people.

Glickman (1996) initially saw these four stages as developing linearly. Linear development, however, is not always the case because deaf persons can start off as, for example, culturally Deaf if they are born to culturally Deaf parents. Also, extensive literature on identity evolution confirms the erratic nature of identity status formation (Côté 2006). In any case, these four identity stages have metamorphosed into identity categories that are reflected in various research studies on deaf identities based on Glickman's (1996) *Deaf Identity Development Scale* (e.g., Maxwell-McCaw and Zea 2011; Moradi and Rottenstein 2007; Most et al. 2007).

After seeing limitations in Glickman's (1996) theoretical underpinnings, which focused on internal dimensions of identity, Maxwell-McCaw and Zea (2011) turned to the paradigm of acculturation to explain Glickman's deaf identity categories. Based on the concept that acculturation patterns vary depending on the level of psychological identification and behavioral competencies with the various cultures within which individuals are embedded, Maxwell-McCaw and Zea developed the *Deaf Acculturation Scale* (DAS) as a means of applying the acculturation paradigm to deaf identities. The DAS consists of a Deaf acculturation scale and a hearing acculturation scale, each of which has five relevant subscales covering five domains: cultural identification, cultural involvement, cultural preferences, language competence, and cultural knowledge. Based on scoring parameters, respondents can be placed in each of Glickman's four identity categories. In an earlier version of the DAS, Maxwell-McCaw (2001) demonstrated that psychological well-being was positively associated with Deaf acculturation and biculturalism (hearing and Deaf).

Interestingly, Rudmin (2003) views work such as the research cited above as too limiting, with two cultures allowing for only four types of acculturation, when in actuality two cultures, two attitudes, two identities, or two languages result in 16 possible types of acculturation, not four. In this era of globalization and exposure to additional cultures, including for example religious cultures, cultures related to sexual orientation, and work-related cultures among others, combinations reflecting various types of acculturation will increase depending on situational variables that create fluidity in identities. Hence, research conclusions cannot be hard and fast since identity boundaries are not absolute.

Utilizing a narrative framework that focuses on self-definition, with data derived from interviews, Ohna (2003, 2004) confirms the fluidity of deaf identities. While researchers have worked to define deaf identity categories, ultimately people shape their identities "in their own way" as they integrate life experiences into coherent identities based on how situations, responses, and external perceptions align (Leigh 2009; McIlroy and Storbeck 2011). Their narratives reflect what they verbalize as their identities.

10.3.1 Implications of Research Findings

According to Corker (1996), deaf identity is not necessarily a core identity but rather one that becomes salient depending on the extent to which deafness is prominent in one's daily life. If the individual is consistently exposed to deaf people, particularly those who use signed languages, whether at home, in school, or socially, the perceived positive quality of this exposure is likely to reinforce the chances of identifying as a culturally Deaf person. Those with less exposure to Deaf culture may be more likely to identify as audiologically deaf, hard of hearing, or hearing impaired (Leigh 1999, 2009).

In general, again emphasizing the importance of social situations and communication, research findings confirm that Deaf environments (schools and organizations for culturally Deaf persons) tend to result in respondents espousing a Deaf-related identity while those more in the mainstream and those individuals with cochlear implants gravitate towards "hearing" oriented identities, possibly as a way of getting around the "difference" of being deaf and finding an identity affiliation. Deaf individuals who are exposed to both environments and feel comfortable in either environment may be more likely to manifest a bicultural identity, meaning they are comfortable interacting with culturally Deaf peers and mainstream hearing colleagues. Those who do not feel a part of either environment are labeled as marginal.

The results cited here are partially influenced by languacultures[3] that influence how diverse signed and spoken languages and minority versus majority cultural group perceptions envelope the deaf person (Horejes 2012). Specifically, whether the deaf person is placed within a culture where either spoken language or sign language predominates, particularly within the school system, will influence that person's identity formation and proclivities toward interacting with Deaf or hearing persons. As schools are embedded in cultures, the use of signed or spoken languages in schools for the deaf as well as mainstream schools have the power to shape one's cultural affiliations and identities. The use of spoken language within schools will reflect the values of hearing societies and reinforce hearing-based identities, while the use of signed languages will reflect the values of Deaf culture and reinforce culturally Deaf identities. Interestingly, those who make languagculture choices for school settings are typically hearing administrators, some of whom are very supportive of Deaf culture values. The culturally Deaf community often agitates for culturally Deaf individuals to take supervisory roles in school systems and therefore ensure a culturally affirmative Deaf environment within schools. The issue of power dynamics is beyond the scope of this chapter, but is one that factors into how languaculture decisions are made.

One longitudinal study (Sheridan 2001, 2008) reflects the power of languaculture and environmental experiences in influencing more nuanced identities via interviews with a deaf cohort in childhood and again in adolescence. As these interviewees moved from preadolescence to adolescence, a critical component in their identity formation was that of communication accessibility, which became more important as these individuals eventually encountered more complex social situations and identified preferred social contexts. Languacultures enter the picture here; if the interviewees were able to experience the ease of access to the language as prescribed by the culture, whether spoken or signed, not only within the family, but more so within school systems, this access had the power to influence their identities as more Deaf oriented or as hearing oriented. As a result, the variation in accessibility means that their identities as hearing oriented or culturally Deaf wax and wane over time depending on individual situations and the fit with languaculture environments.

---

[3]Languaculture is defined as "the transmission of culture by means of a language" (Horejes 2012, p. 156).

10.4 Intersectionality[4]

In recent years, due to globalization and immigration, awareness of diverse identities, diverse ethnicities, and diverse cultural beliefs has become far more salient in discourses about identity formation. With the focus on deaf-hearing identities for deaf individuals, it is easy to overlook the possibility that "deaf" is only one component making up the complex picture of individuals who do have other identities and consciousnesses related to, for example, family background, gender, ethnicity, religion, educational status, social class, sexual orientation, and so on, similarly to their hearing counterparts, that intersect with each other in multiple, complex ways. It has long been thought that being deaf trumps all possible differences and brings diverse deaf people together. However, deaf people are not immune to the perspectives of their larger hearing societies. Exclusion or marginalization from the dominant hearing, or even Deaf society, is a real possibility for deaf individuals of minority status, whether based on, for example, ethnicity, sexual orientation, or additional disability status. Current research literature is only beginning to address the experiences of these individuals.

10.4.1 Ethnic Identities

Clearly, ethnic identity has long since been significant. Corker (1996) believes that ethnic identity emerges before deaf identity does, based on exposure to family of origin. Ethnic identity classification typically reinforces separatism, and this has been true for Deaf persons with minority ethnic identities. For example, in the United States, until well after the 1950s, Black Deaf students were sent to schools that were of inferior quality compared to schools for White Deaf students (Berke 2009). Black Deaf adults were excluded from White Deaf-sponsored recreational and sports activities during that time (Burch 2002; Corbett 2010). While exclusion is no longer sanctioned at this time, Black Deaf adults increasingly tend to view themselves as having a culture with its own standard way of relating and its Black American Sign Language that is distinct from the White Deaf and Black hearing cultures and from American Sign Language (Corbett 2010; McCaskill et al. 2011). Deaf Native Americans are often educated in White deaf schools, thereby strengthening their connections with White Deaf culture. Consequently, their

[4]Intersectionality refers to how different aspects of each individual interact, thereby resulting in different life experiences (Crenshaw 1989). Within the contexts of ethnicity/race or other marginalized identities and being deaf, these experiences will have the potential for creating feelings of oppression.

connections with their home Native tribes may be tenuous at best, depending on their access to communication and integration within their tribal family systems. Nonetheless, they may experience a blending of cultural patterns as they acknowledge their Native American/tribal heritage (Eldredge 2010). Deaf Asian Americans have to integrate their Asian ethnicity, Americanness (referring to North America), and deaf experiences into their own individual identities (Wu and Grant 2010), just as Deaf Latinos and Latinas (Hidalgo and Williams 2010) and Deaf Mäoris from New Zealand (Smiler and McKee 2007) have to integrate their deaf identities with their various cultural identities (culture of origin, host country culture, etc.). If this integration process is cohesive, deaf individuals can shift identities and cultural affiliations as needed depending on situation and do not have to choose one identity aspect over another.

This process, however, can be complicated if there is no Deaf home culture entity (e.g., Asian, Latino/a, Mäori, etc.) to identify with. A study in Great Britain involved researching deaf Pakistani Muslims and noting their preference for a Deaf identity to protect themselves from an inaccessible hearing environment (Ahmad et al. 2002). The paradox is that this implied endorsement of a White, Christian-based Deaf identity even while affirming their Pakistani Muslim identity. This can easily lead to cultural stress and internal identity conflict if they perceive this Christian-based Deaf identity as antithetical to their cultural heritage and if their skills at shifting as the situation warrants is insufficient (Atkin et al. 2002).

An added complexity is that Asian, Latino/a, Native American, Arabic, African, and other such comprehensive hegemonic terms in actuality cover many cultural identities depending on country, tribe, or religion of origin that differ from each other, thus adding to the complexity of identity formation. To clarify, "Asian" encompasses numerous countries and cultures in Asia, and the same is true for the other hegemonic terms. Compounding that is the immigration experience for those who emigrate to other countries. This subjects one to the acculturation experience of the new host country, necessitating a shift in self-perceptions and identity when dealing with unfamiliar cultural paradigms while at the same time continuing to identify with the home culture.

Studies of how ethnic identities evolve in tandem with deaf identities are still in their infancy. However, the field is beginning to recognize that the deaf-hearing paradigm by itself is too simplistic considering the reality of intersectionalities. This is exemplified by a factor analysis study of Black Deaf participant responses to the Deaf Acculturation Scale (DAS) that resulted in a sixth factor not accounted for in the original five factor result for a large majority Caucasian sample in the United States (Nelson Schmitt and Leigh 2015). This result suggests that different groups of deaf individuals may experience their deaf identities differently depending on context and additional group/ethnic affiliations in contrast to a stereotypical perception of deaf people as a homogenous group based on the predominance of White Deaf culture frames of reference in the literature.

10.4.2 Sexual Minorities

Lesbian, gay, bisexual, transgendered, and queer (LGBTQ) individuals face significant challenges in societies that allow for heterosexuality as the only permissible norm for couples and families, taking into account the fact that in some countries this norm is changing. When minority ethnic groups and Deaf persons are added to this category, you have multiple minority status issues that compound the ease of identity formation depending on the salience of each identity component (Leigh 2012). The decisions to disclose, to shift identities as situations demand, and to move towards self-acceptance all become critical issues that these individuals have to confront, depending on what is acceptable in each situation. On top of this, other issues such as health, geographic location, socioeconomic structures, historical antecedents, and politics create complexities in determining the meanings of each identity component. Naturally, the pull for synthesis to resolve competing identities is compelling, but can be accomplished under certain conditions, i.e., if there are accepting communities that provide safe havens.

Recent research indicates that Deaf community traditions of cohesiveness, strong interpersonal connections, and LGBTQ visibility may create more positive attitudes toward LGBTQs who are Deaf (Gutman and Zangas 2010). Yet, since the Deaf community is not immune to societal discriminatory attitudes towards those who are "different," the deaf LGBTQ individual will have to contend with these depending on context or situation. Dealing constantly with different contexts, each having different levels of acceptance, can take an emotional toll. For example, deaf LGBTQ individuals, particularly those of ethnic minority status, may have to struggle with identities related to their relevant majority Deaf community group (in the United States, typically White Deaf groups), their hearing ethnic minority group, their Deaf ethnic minority group if one is available, and being LGBTQ. Each of these groups harbors their own unique attributes and potential oppression possibilities. Then we have the question: Do these various identities harmoniously juxtapose with each other, or do these clash? For example, a Black African Deaf lesbian female in an European country may have to face issues with being Black and African in a White majority society, as a lesbian in a Christian community that is not quite accepting of homosexuality, and deal with the lack of a Deaf community that is similar to her in identity composition, plus explore whether she will be accepted in the White Deaf community. How situations transpire will influence which hidden identity component she will allow to emerge.

10.4.3 Additional Disabilities

Deaf persons with additional disabilities such as blindness, cerebral palsy, autism, and intellectual disabilities have largely been ignored in the deaf identity literature (Leigh 2009, 2012). The labeling of disabilities has to influence one's identity formation. Additional disabilities are not additive in terms of identity formation, but rather interact with other constellations to create one's unique identity. Current research indicates that having additional disabilities is associated with less positive psychological adjustment (e.g., Brunnberg et al. 2008; Danermark and Möller 2008). Additional disabilities will have unique bodily and experiential constellations, based on ethnicity, class, sexual orientation, and ideology surrounding the specific disability (Nielson 2006). How the deaf person integrates the additional disability identity with all other relevant identity categories begs for research to address this unique developmental issue.

10.5 Conclusions

This chapter has focused on the complexity of identities when the individual is deaf, but has taken into account only a few of the multiple identity constellations that deaf persons may incorporate into their identities. Historically, the focus has been on deaf identity classification. Current theories and research projects on deaf identities have yet to explore in depth how these deaf identities develop, with the exception of narrative explorations of emerging deaf identities based on life stories, such as the study conducted by Breivik (2005). Most of the deaf identity category research has been conducted with White participants, with too few studies focusing on diverse deaf populations. Missing are in-depth psychological studies of ethnically diverse individuals as well as those who are dealing with sexual orientation issues, differing disability status, and other categories such as religion and social class and how these identity categories develop and interact within the context of deaf identities. Not to be ignored is the role of language in creating a sense of culture and identity within the individual person. For example, does a Deaf gay male require certain language specifics to understand who and what he is?

Researchers would do well to refrain from utilizing only essentialist categories and investigate not only how multiple identities manifest independently, but also interactionally. This is an area ripe for research, considering that intersectionality is an inescapable fact of life that is rarely researched, due in part to its complexity. The importance of this research is highlighted by the possibility of conflict between various identities that can lead to mental health issues. For example, the Black African Deaf lesbian residing in a European country mentioned in the Sexual Minorities section above will often find herself in conflicting situations where she may have to suppress sensitive identities depending on her environment. How can she handle these without overwhelming struggles? A better understanding of how intersectionalities coexist or conflict with each other can lead to the development of appropriate mental health strategies to minimize identity conflicts. It is important to constantly keep in mind the fluid and dynamic nature of identities that are continually influenced by biology, cognition, social/historical contexts, and language choice/languaculture (Cramer and Gilson 1999; Leigh 2009, 2012).

References

Ahmad, W., Atkin, K., & Jones, L. (2002). Being deaf and being other things: Young Asian people negotiating identities. *Social Science and Medicine, 55,* 1757–1769.

Atkin, K., Ahmad, W. I. U., & Jones, L. (2002). Young South Asian deaf people and their families: Negotiating relationships and identities. *Sociology of Health & Illness, 24,* 21–45. doi:10.1111/1467-9566.00002

Bat-Chava, Y. (2000). Diversity of deaf identities. *American Annals of the Deaf, 145,* 420–428.

Berke, J. (2009). *When skin color separated Black and White Deaf kids.* Retrieved from http://deafness.about.com/cs/featurearticles/a/segregated.htm

Branson, J., & Miller, D. (2002). *Damned for their difference: The cultural construction of deaf people as disabled.* Washington, DC: Gallaudet University Press.

Breivik, J.-K. (2005). *Deaf identities in the making*. Washington, DC: Gallaudet University Press.

Brueggemann, B. (1999). *Lend me your ear: Rhetorical constructions of deafness.* Washington, DC: Gallaudet University Press.

Brunnberg, E., Boström, M., & Berglund, M. (2008). Self-rated mental health, school adjustment, and substance use in hard-of-hearing adolescents. *Journal of Deaf Studies and Deaf Education, 13*(3), 324–335.

Burch, S. (2002). *Signs of resistance: American Deaf cultural history, 1900 to 1942.* New York, NY: New York University Press.

Cimento, E. (2013, May/June). LOFT-y connections: Accepting my deafness and getting an internship. *Volta Voices,* 44–45.

Corbett, C. (2010). Mental health issues for African American deaf people. In I. W. Leigh (Ed.), *Psychotherapy with deaf clients from diverse groups* (pp. 161–182). Washington, DC: Gallaudet University Press.

Corker, M. (1996). *Deaf transitions.* London, UK: Jessica Kingsley Publishers.

Côté, J. (2006). Emerging adulthood as an institutionalized moratorium: Risks and benefits to identity formation. In J. J. Arnett & J. L. Tanner (Eds.), *Emerging adults in America* (pp. 85–116). Washington, DC: American Psychological Association.

Cramer, E., & Gilson, S. (1999). Queers and crips: Parallel identity development processes for persons with non-visible disabilities and lesbian, gay, and bisexual persons. *Journal of Gay, Lesbian, and Bisexual Identity, 4*(1), 23–37.

Crenshaw, K. (1989). Demarginalizing the intersection of race and sex: A black feminist critique of antidiscrimination doctrine, feminist theory, and antiracist politics. *University of Chicago Legal Forum, 140,* 139–167.

Danermark, B., & Möller, K. (2008). Deafblindness, ontological security, and social recognition. *International Journal of Audiology, 47*(Suppl. 2), S119–S123.

Davis, L. J. (1995). *Enforcing normality: Deafness, disability, and the body*. London, UK: Verso.

Dubois, W. (1997). *The souls of black folk.* Boston, MA: Bedford Books.

Eldredge, N. (2010). Culturally responsive psychotherapy with deaf American Indians. In I. W. Leigh (Ed.), *Psychotherapy with deaf clients from diverse groups* (pp. 183–209). Washington, DC: Gallaudet University Press.

Glickman, N. (1996). The development of culturally deaf identities. In N. Glickman & M. Harvey (Eds.), *Culturally affirmative psychotherapy with deaf persons* (pp. 115–153). Mahwah, NJ: Lawrence Erlbaum.

Gutman, V., & Zangas, T. (2010). Therapy issues with deaf lesbians, gay men, bisexuals and transgender individuals. In I. W. Leigh (Ed.), *Psychotherapy with deaf clients from diverse groups* (pp. 85–108). Washington, DC: Gallaudet University Press.

Hardy, J. (2010). The development of a sense of identity in deaf adolescents in mainstream schools. *Educational and Child Psychology, 27*(2), 58–67.

Hidalgo, L., & Williams, S. (2010). Latino deaf individuals and their families. In I. W. Leigh (Ed.), *Psychotherapy with deaf clients from diverse groups* (pp. 237–257). Washington, DC: Gallaudet University Press.

Hintermair, M. (2008). Self-esteem and satisfaction with life of deaf and hard-of-hearing people—A resource-oriented approach to identity work. *Journal of Deaf Studies and Deaf Education, 13*(2), 278–300.
Holcomb, T. (2013). *Introduction to American Deaf culture*. New York, NY: Oxford University Press.
Horejes, T. (2012). *Social constructions of deafness: Examining Deaf languacultures in education*. Washington, DC: Gallaudet University Press.
Humphries, T. (2008). Scientific explanation and other performance acts in the reorganization of DEAF. In K. Lindgren, D. DeLuca, & D. J. Napoli (Eds.), *Signs and voices: Deaf culture, identity, language, and arts* (pp. 3–20). Washington, DC: Gallaudet University Press.
Humphries, T., & Humphries, J. (2010). Deaf in the time of the cochlea. *Journal of Deaf Studies and Deaf Education, 16*(2), 153–163.
Leigh, I. W. (1999). Inclusive education and personal development. *Journal of Deaf Studies and Deaf Education, 4,* 236–245.
Leigh, I. W. (2009). *A lens on deaf identities*. New York, NY: Oxford University Press.
Leigh, I. W. (2012). Not just deaf: Multiple intersections. In R. Nettles & R. Balter (Eds.), *Multiple minority identities* (pp. 59–80). New York, NY: Springer.
Leigh, I. W., Maxwell-McCaw, D., Bat-Chava, Y., & Christiansen, J. (2009). Correlates of psychosocial adjustment in deaf adolescents with and without cochlear implants: A preliminary investigation. *Journal of Deaf Studies and Deaf Education, 14*(2), 244–259.
Mance, J., & Edwards, L. (2012). Deafness-related perceptions and psychological well-being in deaf adolescents with cochlear implants. *Cochlear Implants International, 13*(2), 93–104.
Maxwell-McCaw, D. (2001). Acculturation and psychological well-being in deaf and hard-of-hearing people (Doctoral dissertation, The George Washington University, 2001). *Dissertation Abstracts International, 61*(11-B), 6141.
Maxwell-McCaw, D., & Zea, M. C. (2011). The Deaf Acculturation Scale (DAS): Development and validation of a 58-item measure. *Journal of Deaf Studies and Deaf Education, 16*(3), 325–342.
McCaskill, C., Lucas, C., Bailey, R., & Hill, J. (2011). *The hidden treasure of Black ASL*. Washington, DC: Gallaudet University Press.
McIlroy, G., & Storbeck, C. (2011). Development of deaf identity: An ethnographic study. *Journal of Deaf Studies and Deaf Education, 16,* 494–511.
Mitchell, R., & Karchmer, M. (2004). Chasing the mythical ten percent: Parental hearing status of deaf and hard of hearing students. *Sign Language Studies, 5,* 83–96.
Moradi, B., & Rottenstein, A. (2007). Objectification theory and deaf cultural identity attitudes: Roles in deaf women's eating disorder symptomatology. *Journal of Counseling Psychology, 54* (2), 178–188.
Most, T., Wiesel, A., & Blitzer, T. (2007). Identity and attitudes towards cochlear implant among deaf and hard of hearing adolescents. *Deafness and Education International, 9*(2), 68–82.
Nelson Schmitt, S., & Leigh, I. W. (2015). Examining a sample of Black Deaf individuals on the Deaf Acculturation Scale (DAS). *Journal of Deaf Studies and Deaf Education,* 20(3), 283–295.
Nielson, K. (2006). Was Helen Keller deaf? Blindness, deafness, and multiple identities. In B. J. Brueggemann & S. Burch (Eds.), *Women and deafness* (pp. 21–39). Washington, DC: Gallaudet University Press.
Ohna, S. E. (2003). Education of deaf children and the politics of recognition. *Journal of Deaf Studies and Deaf Education, 8*(1), 5–10.
Ohna, S. E. (2004). Deaf in my own way: Identity, learning and narratives. *Deafness and Education International, 6*(1), 20–38.
Parasnis, I. (2012). Diversity and deaf identity. In P. V. Paul & D. F. Moores (Eds.), *Deaf epistemologies: Multiple perspectives on the acquisition of knowledge* (pp. 63–80). Washington, DC: Gallaudet University Press.
Rudmin, F. (2003). Critical history of the acculturation psychology of assimilation, separation, integration, and marginalization. *Review of General Psychology, 7,* 3–37.
Sheridan, M. (2001). *Inner lives of deaf children*. Washington, DC: Gallaudet University Press.

Sheridan, M. (2008). *Deaf adolescents: Inner lives and lifeworld development*. Washington, DC: Gallaudet University Press.
Smiler, K., & McKee, R. (2007). Perceptions of Mäori deaf identity in New Zealand. *Journal of Deaf Studies and Deaf Education, 12*(1), 93–111.
Stinson, M., & Kluwin, T. (1996). Social orientations toward deaf and hearing peers among deaf adolescents in local public high schools. In P. Higgins & J. Nash (Eds.), *Understanding deafness socially* (pp. 113–134). Springfield, IL: Charles C. Thomas.
Weinberg, N., & Sterritt, M. (1986). Disability and identity: A study of identity patterns in adolescents with hearing impairments. *Rehabilitation Psychology, 31,* 95–102.
Wu, C., & Grant, N. (2010). Asian American and Deaf. In I. W. Leigh (Ed.), *Psychotherapy with deaf clients from diverse groups* (pp. 210–236). Washington, DC: Gallaudet University Press.

Author Biography

Irene W. Leigh, Ph.D. is a deaf psychologist and Professor Emerita, having taught in the clinical psychology doctoral program at Gallaudet University in Washington, DC and chaired its Department of Psychology. Her numerous presentations, research and publications focus on deaf people and identity, multiculturalism, parenting, attachment, depression, and cochlear implants. She is an American Psychological Association Fellow and was Associate Editor for the Journal of Deaf Studies and Deaf Education.

Part IV
Identity Work in Institutional and Technology Mediated Environments

The final part of the volume "*Identity Revisited and Reimagined. Empirical and Theoretical Contributions Across Time and Space*" presents four chapters that empirically focus upon the making and shaping of identities in technologically mediated environments at work and in educational contexts.

Chapter 11 by Elisabeth Keating constitutes the first chapter in Part IV of the book. In "They Blame, They Complain but They Don't Understand": Identity Clashes in Cross-Cultural Virtual Collaborations," the point of departure is the taken for grantedness among members of a community with regards to the relationships between identity and culture, even as they expertly manipulate them interactionally. Contexts where the negotiated nature of identity can be challenged, however, illuminate varied and conflicting ideas about identity, and cross-cultural collaborations, where dissimilar ways of talking and different models and interpretations meet. Keating deploys Erwin Goffman's concept "spoiling" of identity and Harold Garfinkel's word on ritual status degradation when she describes identity conflicts in cross-cultural virtual collaborations where professionals from across the world work together. Her main point is that without some attention to how cultural patterns influence identity practices, those working in global teams can inadvertently spoil others' identities or participation in the status degradation of others.

Keating argues that the performance of identity is a fundamental aspect of human society and that identity is "talked into being" in interactions with others. This negotiated nature of identity, however, can be challenging in cross-cultural interactions, where dissimilar ways of talking and different models and interpretations meet. Keating highlights that communication technology has made it routine for members of certain professions to work together from different cultural locations in sparsely furnished virtual spaces where it is not always clear that multiple systems of identity are in play (or at work). The chapter analyzes one such context, engineers working in virtual collaborations. Keating shows how differences in the way cultures organize identities (e.g., along priority axes of self versus social role identity) are influenced by cultural ideas of the person.

In Chap. 12, Johan Hjulstad highlights which of a person's multiple intersecting identity-positions are most prevalent and what they come to mean. These, he argues, constantly shift across various discourse contexts. The chapter "Identity Negotiations in a Visually Oriented Virtual Classroom" explores some of the identity negotiations performed by sign language learning students in a video conferencing classroom. These students come together in a distance education program which has the explicit aim of strengthening student's "deaf" identity. The chapter illustrates how a seemingly simple exercise has a powerful effect on what "deaf" identity means for hearing non-signing friends from the students' local classes: through working with a teaching plan on "friendship," where the signing students plan for and invite hearing friends, to the renegotiation of what "deaf" comes to mean in the inclusive setting of a local school.

The chapter explores identity negotiations by Norwegian Sign Language (NSL) learning students in a video-only mediated environment (VME). Hjulstad asks how mainstreamed deaf students can reach the goal of learning NSL so that it can form the basis of a positive subject formation and identification with positive dimensions of the signing community in the geopolitical spaces of Norway. By investigating a "friendship" teaching plan and the invitation of hearing non-signing classmates to the distance education virtual classroom, Hjulstad illustrates how the embodied interactional organization of participation gets cooperatively crafted and sustained through simultaneous co-occurring influences. He highlights the dynamic, changing, and complex ways in which identity negotiations are accomplished by the participants in the VME, and how the identity of "deaf" is renegotiated in unique ways. The chapter raises a number of implications for issues of identity development, the role of technology, and inclusive education.

In the third chapter in Part IV, "'Janne X Was Here'. Portraying Identities and Negotiating Being and Belonging in Informal Literacy Practices," Annaliina Gynne presents a study where young people's identity work and informal literacy practices are examined in two separate but intertwined settings: in a bilingual school context and at a social network site. The study draws on ethnographic data, and the concepts of language and identity-as-agency are explored from a discourse analytic perspective. In Chap. 13, Gynne argues that portraying identity positions and negotiating being and belonging are possible in and through practices where multiple aspects of communicative repertoires and modalities are employed.

Drawing on sociocultural approaches and (n)ethnographic data, the chapter aims to expand understandings dealing with identity work and heteroglossic languaging, including informal literacy practices, in settings across the offline–online continuum. Through analysis of data sets consisting of video recordings, photographs, and screen grabs, Gynne illustrates the ways in which interactions, agency, and social positionings emerge at the intersection of people, discourses, spaces, practices, and technologies.

The final chapter in Part IV constitutes the final chapter in this book. Here, Elina Tapio focuses on the conflicting discourses in relation to English language learning by deaf Finnish sign language signers. In the chapter titled "A Moment of Self-Revelation as a Turning Point in Understanding Language," Tapio documents how a deaf Finnish sign Language signer, Hanna, suddenly realizes that what she herself has taken for granted—that she has limited resources for language learning—is not true at all. Hanna's revelation is based on her own daily communication practices and opens up for a new understanding of herself and her linguistic resources. The hegemonic discourse in deaf education highlights that deaf sign language learners have limited resources for language learning. Tapio contributes to recent empirical studies of communication practices among signers and challenges this view. Through the case study of Hanna, she illustrates how an individual becomes aware of the conflict between a dominant, authoritative discourse—the perspective she has adopted from others—and the contrasting practices with English in her everyday life. This moment of revelation, a rupture of taken for grantedness during an interview, leads to new self-positionings. Tapio argues that such moments of self-revelation offer possibilities for reverse discourses where new identity spaces can emerge.

Chapter 11
"They Blame, They Complain but They Don't Understand": Identity Clashes in Cross-Cultural Virtual Collaborations

Elizabeth Keating

11.1 Introduction

The performance of social identity is a fundamental aspect of human society. Yet it is a process that is unstable and highly contingent, influenced by sociocultural knowledge, both tacit and formalized, and by individuals' unique perceptions and representations (Bucholtz and Hall 2005; Benwell and Stokoe 2006). Identity depends on the ratification of others (Goffman 1963) and others' attributions of identity affect those they classify (Hacking 1986). With the increasing mobility and diversity of groups, intercultural negotiations of identity are growing in frequency (Gumperz and Cook-Gumperz 2007). The use of communication technologies, for example, makes it possible for people who inhabit diverse settings geographically and culturally to work together, which means negotiating identities across sense-making systems. When technology facilitates arenas for intercultural collaboration, exciting potentials emerge. Often, however, these technologically-mediated spaces are rather devoid of cultural content other than language. The technological interface appears uniform, a technical ground within which identity practices figure, but missing important contextual background material: the unique sights, sounds, stories, and artifacts of particular cultures. In this paper, I describe some implications of these context-poor, technologically-mediated spaces in the case of identity negotiation, an important part of working together–important enough to influence the success or failure of a project.

The case I examine is one where engineers suddenly (due to decisions from upper management) find themselves working with engineers from another culture, that is, they are technologically joined to engineers living and working in different

E. Keating (✉)
University of Texas, Austin, USA
e-mail: elizabeth.keating@austin.utexas.edu

S. Bagga-Gupta et al. (eds.), *Identity Revisited and Reimagined*,
DOI 10.1007/978-3-319-58056-2_11

parts of the world. They are tasked to work on a complex project, one that proves to be complex both in terms of engineering and in terms of culture. In spite of the engineers attesting that in terms of identity "an engineer is an engineer," I found that due to unshared cultural expectations, identity was a source of conflict among the engineers. And when identity issues emerged, they were attributed not to differences in cultural ways of expressing and ratifying identity, but to impoliteness and incivility. I argue that if the engineers (and others engaged in technologically mediated, cross cultural work) could focus particularly on one aspect of culture, identity, especially how it hinges on ratification and yet how its expression varies cross culturally, then some recurrent sources of conflict could be addressed, and the role of identity in conflict attributed. Communication technology has made it routine for members of certain professions to work together from different cultural locations in the sparse furnishings of virtual space, a text and voice-dominant space with very little extra-situational cultural or social context available, including information about each other's habits and values. Social science has much to contribute to better understanding these settings.

In discussing identity, I find two concepts useful for gaining insights into identity problems the engineers reported while working together in technologically-mediated office interactions: The "spoiling" of identity (Goffman 1963) and the concept of ritual status degradation (Garfinkel 1956). These are discussed further below, with examples from the anthropological literature and examples from the engineers.

11.1.1 Study Background

This paper describes research conducted among several teams of engineers (Keating and Jarvenpaa 2011; Jarvenpaa and Keating 2011; Keating and Jarvenpaa 2016). The data consists of conference calls, interviews and participant observation during periods of weeks or months over a three year span of time, in a case where technology linked Romanian, Indian, Brazilian and American engineers. The engineers were prepared to adapt to different engineering contexts and design aesthetics, and were all speaking English. They were collaborating on designing advanced processing plants for fossil fuels.

It is well recognized that identity is "talked into being" (Heritage 1984), and is a creative performance (Butler 2002; Rampton 1999; Blommaert et al. 2005; Hasnain et al. 2013), a process that maps shared symbolic resources, or at least assumes them, and a process that is richly dialogic. With this in mind, interviews and extracts from intercultural conference calls are examined here for what they show about talk and identity, particularly to illustrate how the engineers talked with each other and how they explained instances of affront to their identities, as well as their strategies to make sense of each other and to account for unanticipated, unfamiliar contingencies.

11.1.2 Identity and Technological Mediation

A good deal of the work on the relationships between language and identity has focused on speakers’ specific linguistic features and styles, how people express class, ethnic and gender identities, and identities based on sexuality, and to a lesser extent age, and (dis)ability. Work on language and identity has focused on how social categories are staged in terms of dominant and subordinate categories and entitlements, as well as understanding the particular linguistic resources people use in establishing and maintaining identities and linking them to context.

Global work flows make plural identity systems apparent (Ong 1999), and although there is no longer the same confidence in linking linguistic features to a certain locality (Auer 2007; Cutler 2003), there are still many features of identity (as expressed in language and other semiotic modalities) that vary from group to group. With digital technologies, new types of identities are being displayed (Androutsopoulos and Georgakopoulou 2008) to new audiences.

A well-known example of technological mediation of identity is the call center industry where workers located in one country, e.g. India, work with often unhappy customers calling from another culture, e.g. the US. The call center workers, unlike the engineers discussed here, have undergone training to understand the culture of their clients, and have accepted as part of their work practice the adoption of certain identity markers familiar to and understandable by their clients. They take Anglicized names for their workday, and are trained in the American practice of “smiling down the phone” (Taylor and Bain 1999). The call center workers adapt to different cultural expectations for the expression of identities of entitled supplicant and soothing company representative, and how people are expected to perform in a culture of service providers foreign to them (notably, the clients undergo no orientation to their new providers, on the contrary, they are often led to believe they are interacting with local providers). In virtual engineering, the focus of this chapter, however, taking a phone call in India or Brazil or the U.S. or Romania from another engineer doesn’t include being required (at least consciously, or in terms of company manuals) to adapt to another country’s identity practices and expectations of reciprocal relationships. In fact, the issue of behavioral expectations and identity attributions is rarely explicitly addressed (as it is in the case of call center operators) if at all, even when problems develop. Rather, expressions of identity are interpreted within an engineer’s local meaning system. As one engineer said: “There are a lot of people who have not been out of Texas, outside Houston; so they blame, they complain but they don’t understand.” As Garfinkel showed in his famous breeching experiments, we shouldn’t be surprised that when interactional expectations fail to be met, there is not only initial confusion, but hostility in the reactions of interactants.

The engineers this paper discusses were experts at interpreting engineering symbols and trained problem solvers. They daily exchanged shared symbols representing aspects of design, for example, on engineering documents as they created complex piping diagrams of a processing plant together. They enthusiastically described the technology and the ease of sharing engineering documents across the globe:

> …And it is just a click of a second… I [here in India] can give control to my counterpart in Houston and they can give to me the control, they can open up their document on their server I can open mine from our server, they can take control on our document, we can take control on their document, it's amazing, and it's real-time. There is no time difference in between.

The fact that they were all speaking English (though in the case of Romania and Brazil most were not native speakers), that they shared engineering training, and the agile way that both technology (as described above) and features of language such as pronouns provide an easy switch of perspective (for example, people easily switch between the first person "I" and third person "you"), however, ill prepared them for the complexities in understanding the other's cultural context, such as what identities the term "you" or "I" might actually refer to, and the historical and social contexts in which I and you live and make sense.

Though it was easy to send documents to each other and to share the same technologically mediated work space, there was a notable absence of means for the transmission of cultural information or extra-situational information. There was, for example, no virtual spot which could function like the proverbial water cooler, an informal space for sharing and socialization to novel aspects of 'I' or 'you' cultural identities or to observe environments and structures in action. For the engineers, there was little opportunity for observing each other's identity performances outside of technical or planning emails, comments on drawings, and conference call status meetings. The engineers felt this loss and were nostalgic about face-to-face contexts for engineering work and the importance of informal learning and multimodal communication. As a Romanian engineer said:

> It is better to see each other face-to-face, to know the equivalent and to understand each other in the future…I consider that it's necessary, not mandatory, but it's necessary that the Romanian and the [Houston, Texas] people meet each other to know each other and to have a little accommodation.

Face-to-face interaction to learn to accommodate to each other's different ways of expression and expectations was rarely possible for them, though, since the whole idea of the virtual collaboration was to find cost effective ways of working globally. The virtual engineering collaborations had little if any travel budget for the engineers to visit each other and learn about different cultural environments. Instead, nostalgia was countered by attitudes about technology, a ruthless attitude of conform or be left behind, as illustrated by one engineer:

> Oh, yes. We have one old guy [an older engineer] and he didn't like what I was doing, he was complaining about it, and I just told the CAD [computer aided design] coordinator, "This is the way it's going to be. Either he comes up to speed or we'll leave him behind. Make your choice."

Here, "old guy" (resisting technology) is an identity not worthy of inclusion, but rather of outdatedness or obsolescence. Technology influences how identities are ratified in an office setting, and technology is often unrecognized for its potential as a site of identity spoiling and status degradation. Below I discuss relationships between identity and culture more broadly, to highlight the importance of focusing on identity and the importance of cultural as well as technical virtuosity. Relations between culture and identity are typically taken for granted among members of the same culture, even as they expertly manipulate them interactionally. Certain contexts, however, illuminate varied and conflicting ideas about identity, such as diasporic contexts, efforts to shape national identity, and, the context focused on here, cross cultural collaborations.

11.2 Identity, the Person, and Context

Identity conflicts in diasporic or immigration contexts have been much discussed by scholars looking at representation and identities (e.g. Bhabha 1994; Said 1979), and are relevant to global work contexts. In such settings, attributes that were once positive identity assets (such as language) are suddenly liabilities. Cases have been studied from the Indian diaspora or Latin American diaspora where first generation immigrants are not recognized for their capabilities because their language abilities in the new locale are stigmatized. A few words can play a pivotal role in identity boundary positioning in immigrant and other cross cultural situations (Cornips and de Rooij 2013). In global English office encounters, like the engineers were managing, speakers with "foreign" accents are, like in other contexts, often given a less favorable identity in status level (Sebastian and Ryan 1985). From uttering a few sounds, people are judged as having an identity that is scored lower in trustworthiness, friendliness, kindness and benevolence.

In such encounters, identity anticipations and normative expectations are influenced by different and sometimes opposing cultural beliefs and categories. People remain perpetual strangers in certain ways. Their strangeness to each other is influenced by differences in boundaries of the self and how a moral person should act, since individual performances of identity are related to beliefs about the person (Shweder and Bourne 1984). When American and European social workers went to Romania after the collapse of the political system in 1989, Romanians described the western workers as generous, but at the same time disempowering and demeaning the Romanians. The western workers were described as lacking the ability to lay aside their "individual" views and values (Dümling 2004). Anticipations and normative expectations clash in such cases, including the proper expression of relationality of self to others, public versus private territories of identities,[1] historical

[1]The public/private dichotomy has been widely critiqued, but I am using it here as a way to talk about the creation of social relationships in the sense of intimate/distant.

influences on identity categories, to what extent identity is an assertion of free will or the acceptance of an assigned role, or to what extent identity is considered to be personally achieved or to be mostly beyond a person's control, or how a combination of the two is expressed.

Several examples show just how diverse expectations about personhood and identity can be. For the Piraha, of Brazil, new spirits regularly invade the body and fundamentally change who they are; the Piraha in turn try to resist being taken over by the spirits' identity by frequently changing their names. In another example, western young people make sense of identity instabilities, too, when they have an "identity crisis," but this is explained differently; not that the person is possessed, but rather has not yet reached maturity. In many cultures, identity is something aggregated over multiple lifetimes, whether in the case of the last names passed down by powerful families, or beliefs about the persistence of karmic consequences of individual actions over generations. In some societies, the boundary of individual identity even more specifically includes the ancestors (Rasmussen 2008). In scholarly attempts to illustrate different views of the person, Indian personhood and identity and American personhood and identity have been compared to the difference between porous and buffered selves (Taylor 2007). The porous self is expected to change as a person moves through places and relationships. The buffered self is expected to maintain identity through constancy. While western ideas of the person tend to separate behavior and person (as parents are coached to criticize the child's behavior and not the person), in other places actions and codes of conduct are not considered separable from the person (Marriott 1976). I cite these examples both to illustrate the range of differences as well as to show ways scholars have attempted to translate them across meaning systems.

Some anthropologists have used the word "dividual" (Marriott and Inden 1977) to heighten awareness of the extent of cross cultural differences in personhood or stimulate discussion on culturally-based ideas of the person. In this scheme, the dividual is divisible, made up of heterogeneous material influences, the accumulated effects of the mixing and separation of others and one's own essences in interaction (not just dialogically), so that each person contains mixed and separated essences with something of the nature of the persons they interacted with (Marriott 1976), a product of "what comes and goes" (Lamb 2000; Majumdar and Madan 1956). In western terms, the South Asian idea of the constantly changing person, though, has been described as such a radically different account of personhood as to be a "sign of a rather severe psychopathology" (Spiro 1993). This negative description is an example of the challenges of translating across systems and of how identity spoiling and status degradation can take place based on the common practice of interpreting one cultural framework in terms of another.

The following is an example of the challenges of interpretation expressed by one engineer in making sense of the identities displayed by others:

> I cannot understand the philosophy in this area [Houston]. You are a parent, teach your children to [age] 12, and at sixteen years you put your children in the car. Why? There is no communication here between the people. They come to work, they go home, that's it. They

> communicate only with the car. They don't talk unless they don't have [something]. I can't understand so well this philosophy but that's it. To stay only in the car.

This comment reflects how each person's identity is at risk in interactions because the social value that a person claims has to be verified by others (Goffman 1967). People in a cross cultural collaboration are especially vulnerable to the possibility that the social value that they claim (their public identity) is not verifiable by others. Since people have a profound concern about identity ratification and a concern to be included within the bounds of normative moral behavior (rather than someone "tainted" or "discounted"), it is not surprising that identity conflicts can have serious effects on team work. As Goffman states:

> When a stranger comes into our presence, then, first appearances are likely to enable us to anticipate his category and attributes, his "social identity"… We lean on these anticipations that we have, transforming them into normative expectations, into righteously presented demands …While a stranger is present before us, evidence can arise of his possessing an attribute that makes him different from others in the category of persons available for him to be, and of a less desirable kind–in the extreme, a person who is quite thoroughly bad, or dangerous, or weak. He is thus reduced in our minds from a whole and usual person to a tainted, discounted one (Goffman 1963: 2–3).

In the case of the Americans and their car-centered life, characterized above, their identities as a "fast forward family" (Ochs and Kremer-Sadlik 2013) struggling to maintain upper middle class status is discounted, as strange or even pathological (e.g. anti-family). Identities are not only indexed through labels, implicatures, stances, styles, or linguistic systems but through miscommunications (see Gumperz et al. 1979).

Without much visibility on each other's distinctive cultures and cultural ideas of the person, or visibility on normative interactional entitlements in terms of recognition and ratification (e.g. what is the proper form of address), and without any formal preparation for the multiple systems of meaning that might be in play, the engineers (as Goffman described for others) relied on interpretations based on their local value systems. In the following example, Indians are communicating to me their interpretation of another aspect of the American engineers' identity, that they are complacent, lack dedication and don't share responsibility for the team compared to the Indian engineers.

> In the U.S. they watch the clock more than India, they only work to 5 [o'clock]. Hire and fire at will. In India it's more family-like… In the U.S. life is easier. In India it's a struggle to get to and from the office.

The individual versus family priority axes of self and society are differently expressed and interpreted in the US and India in the workplace. A characterization of "only working until 5" is presented, not as evidence that Houston engineers are indeed "family-like" (like Indians), by going home to fulfill their family role obligations. Rather the Americans are seen as a lacking the will or desire to work until the job is done (past 5, if necessary) and relying on their Indian counterparts.

The issue is, from the Indian point of view, that they are not being family-like towards their colleagues. Watching the clock signifies a person whose identity is not even professional grade. The Indian speaker described American life as easier compared to India, even though that contradicted somewhat the hire and fire at will brutality also mentioned as a negative aspect of the American worker's life. Several Brazilian engineers interpreted their American colleagues' behavior as not demonstrating caring for other people because they didn't take time to informally get to know their virtual colleagues; they were always in a hurry. For their part, the American engineers stereotyped Romania as a country where the rules were changing all the time (and vice versa!). This comment especially shows that expectations were difficult to calibrate.

In the following comment about how behaviors are interpreted variously, an engineer relates how he experienced the same ways to treat a person in one place (the way of directing a subordinate) turn into a violation in another:

> There is no doubt [in countries such as those in South America] that boss is boss. When I came to this country [the US], and my boss called me, I used to say 'Yes Sir.' My boss used to say "you get back to me by tomorrow" and I would get back…But I was formed in that way too [in South American country X]. In this country [the U.S.] they don't have that. That is a cultural difference there is no doubt about it…here [the U.S.] I need to be very careful when I speak to a guy. He will just call the Human Resources. You don't see that [in other countries]. They won't call the Human Resources. They say 'Yes Sir.' I don't know it's good or bad. But it's their culture…I am an old fashioned one. Here we are too democratic.

Attempts to make sense of the unexpected too often took the shape of negatively charged generalizations about identity ('Americans,' 'Romanians,' 'Brazilians,' 'Indians'), even though the engineers' comments showed that they recognized that these stereotypes could be dismantled in face-to-face settings with opportunities for experiencing a more varied range of activities together. I argue (employing insights from Goffman and Garfinkel) here that generalizing about identity in a different way, by orienting to a shared human vulnerability (that at any moment identity is susceptible to spoiling and degradation) can provide an approach for engineers and others like them to orient to sociological principles of identity ratification, rather than highlighting stereotypical differences, in collaborative environments where plural identity expectations are in play.

11.3 Identity Spoiling

A rejection of particular identities such as "only working till 5" (as mentioned above) can be seen as part of a suite of practices included in identity construction and maintenance that includes the practice of finding negative mirror images in the behavior of others, so that values that are opposed are "found" in the other group (cf. Auer and Dirim 2003; Bucholtz 1999; Cutler 2009; Rampton 1999). This kind of identity spoiling of the other group is frequently used in building distinctive national culture identities, for example, how "repudiation of the west" was used to create a distinctive Romanian identity under Ceaușescu (Iordachi and Trencsényi 2003). A western identity was the spoiling one, a threat to the traditional values of the Romanian village, the mythical receptacle of the Romanian soul (Daskalov 1997). Among the engineers, the global collaboration at first was considered threatening and suffered from a kind of identity spoiling. An engineering manager told us:

> At first the engineers thought Bengal [engineers] would "take our jobs" and "we shouldn't share our intellectual property with them." For the first 6 months they wouldn't send any work to India. Then they were told they have to; [they were told] we have the same legal agreement with them; that economic issues [survival of the company] are critical.

In similar examples of spoiling identities, the identity of young, westernized Indian women has been a target of criticism in India (Lukose 2008). In the Netherlands, Surinamese men's identities and Moroccan men's identities have been viewed negatively in media discourses as threatening Dutch social order (Geschiere 2009; Cornips and de Rooij 2013). Some children of immigrants in the U.S. view their family's ethnic identity as spoiled and create oppositional lifestyles and identities or "oppositional youth culture" (Ogbu 1978; see also Shankar 2008). In colonial situations, people are forced to re-experience their culture, expertise, language, identity and history negatively viewed through the categories of another culture (see e.g. Spivak 1985). Gender is an example of an identity that is either categorically spoiled (even leading to rationalizations of female infanticide) or constantly at risk of being spoiled, and elaborate rules are established to manage gender identity. The idea that a woman's identity can be permanently spoiled sexually, for example, makes traveling through public space risky, and the woman's identity in public arenas being made into a de-stabilizing and volatile presence (Lukose 2008). The subtle ways identity spoiling can proceed in the workplace is illustrated by the following example from an American female computer science graduate student:

> I was working at a fairly small company whose communal coffee was awful. A group of 6 of us (4 men, 2 women) bought our own coffee maker and had decent coffee which we paid a few cents for to defray the costs of coffee and cream. Anyway, I usually bought the coffee and my male coworker usually bought the cream. A new member to the group (male) approached me and told me we were out of cream. I told him that M2 usually bought the cream. Later that same day, M1 again comes up and tells me we are out of cream. I once again tell him that M2 gets the cream. To this he says, 'But how can I bother M2 with something as insignificant as buying cream?' Needless to say, I told this fellow exactly what I thought about that (Spertus).

These examples of identity spoiling show a type of identity work and identity negotiation that is deeply influenced by cultural categories. The examples show the vulnerability of each individual's identity to others. A type of identity spoiling among the engineers similarly took the form of assertions of what was 'right' to do, or normative versus what was deviant. In one discussion, for example, an American engineer concluded that his own (culturally based) engineering idea "will look RIGHT" in contrast to the design the Romanian team had spent time preparing. A Romanian engineer defended the design, though, as normative to other professional engineers.

Romanian engineer:	I uh I just came from a visit from uh [describes similar design used by another engineering project] and they used more or less this uh solution. Okay! But I will agree and we will move, we'll act at your request. ((conversation between US engineers on US side))
US engineer:	yeah well you could put [description of his own solution] and it's not gonna hurt that at all. And it will look RIGHT.

The Romanian design was influenced by a unique history of material shortages chronic in Romania in the period before 1989, where designs were oriented toward using a minimum of raw materials.

When claims about one's identity (such as "competent engineer with important global skills, including engineering and multilingualism") are unratified, according to Goffman, a person feels "righteously indignant" (Goffman 1963). Romanians expressed indignant feelings when their identity as innovators in the face of difficult engineering problems was not ratified. In an attempt to explicitly get his identity ratified, one engineer said during a conference call to his counterparts across the world: "The information is not reaching you, I have leadership qualities, have had a management position, like to take initiative." In global office settings, the co-existence of multiple systems of meanings, when it comes to identity ratification, presents workers with new challenges to being alert to signs that another's identity claims have been rejected.

It is common to hear that a sense of humor is a valued resource, and a sense of humor can create a space for metacommentary on culture. A sense of humor usually entails being able to, in a way, spoil one's own identity through self-mocking. A manager in Romania told us, jokingly: "our folk stories are pretty pathetic, about melancholy shepherds." This type of joking can be an opportunity to negotiate identities and stances, encourage informal learning and play. But humor in cross cultural settings is hard to make work, because it builds, like identity performances, on shared background, just the sort of cultural background missing when what is shared is a standardized computer interface of buttons and choices, which are primarily focused on ways of establishing or leveraging electronic relationships. Awareness of the role identity plays in shaping the judgements of those who are inputting selections on a screen would be a step in bringing sociological theory to the challenges of the workplace, such as the potential for identity spoiling and status degradation in cross cultural teams with different ideas about the nature of a person and how a moral person interacts with others.

11.4 Degradation Rituals: Status Degradation

The concept of status degradation, as developed by Garfinkel (1956) concerns public rituals of degradation. An example might be the two-day pulling down of the statue of Lenin in Bucharest in 1990, where the "degradation ceremony" reclassified the former leader as no longer entitled to veneration. Another example is the case of imprisonment, such when under Ceaușescu, people, including one engineer's father and brother, "were put in prison, and were more or less killed." Although the technologically-mediated global engineering settings are not sites of formalized transformations of identity such as Garfinkel described or Romanians experienced under Ceaușescu, the concept of status degradation is useful for understanding the surprising number of comments engineers made about feeling disrespected. The notion highlights a person's vulnerability to humiliation through a process of identity transformation in the act of cross cultural interpretation.

The sociolinguistic literature is filled with examples of the unique habits of sociopragmatic conduct across cultures and languages. Politeness has been extensively studied, for example, the daily ceremonial ways that people recognize the appearance of others in their midst. Cross culturally, politeness has been analyzed as derived from efforts to ensure a person's identity is recognized and acknowledged (a range of acts from flattery to merely greeting someone) (Brown and Levinson 1987) as well as a way to demonstrate something about one's own identity (Matsumoto 1988; Ide 1989). People are typically only expert in the idioms of politeness recognition in their own societies. Jacquemet has discussed "metapragmatic attacks" (Jacquemet 1994) where different metapragmatic awareness (Silverstein 1993) across members of different cultural groups results in one person rejecting another's language use and implicitly their identity.

Bailey's study of Korean storekeepers and African American customers in Los Angeles (Bailey 1997) is a good example of how different expressions of personhood can contribute to feelings of status degradation. Bailey showed how Korean storekeepers' way of interacting with their African American customers was perceived by the African American customers as too distant, which in terms of their expectations was interpreted as a sign that they were not considered worthy human beings by the storekeepers. The friendly self-disclosure the customers valued, and the way they shared their lives during the sales transaction, was perceived by Korean shop owners, on the other hand, as embarrassing and disrespectful, because it was too intimate by their own norms (there is also racism to account for the hostile feelings between the two groups, but racism itself is maintained through processes of status degradation). Different cultural beliefs about the person resulted in each side interpreting that they were excluded from the identity category of respected human being. As Bailey's example shows, for some groups in the U.S., self-disclosure is seen as a way to establish equality (there is also evidence of this on personal social media pages), and lack of self-disclosure can be viewed as refusing to engage as equals (Hastings 2000). In other groups, too much individual identification with a position is seen as an aggressive action.

Some engineers experienced a similar status depreciation through feeling unratified participants, forgotten or "disappeared." Their partners in the technological mediation forgot to address them as full-status participants:

> Sometimes it seems like [the U.S. location] can forget that…you know, there's [India] in the room, you know…maybe because there was no visual, they would start talking among themselves sometimes.

Status degradation resulted from applying the term "normal" from one's own local engineering practice and rejecting other people's practices as odd or "an oddity," as previously described and as shown below:

> That's the normal scheme. That's just what's normally done industry wide. No matter which industry you're talking about, power industry, this industry, that industry…what we've got here is somewhat of an oddity, will it work? Sure…but the other concern I have [he explains].

The constant process of exchanging documents electronically, without face-to-face personal mediation resulted in a situation where status depreciation was an all too common experience. The example below shows how receiving a document that's been unexpectedly corrected or changed by a counterpart, with no accompanying communication or account, is treated with incredulity and experienced as humiliating.

> We're told not to change [the specifications] and they [the Americans] go ahead and change it. They never called me and asked "what was your thinking." They just change it. It's embarrassing…They don't follow their own established rules. Half of the job is done and they are changing the rules.

Status degradation was partly an effect of the geographical "nowhere" of virtual space. A Romanian engineer commented on Americans' lack of interest in anything about his real location, his national identity or history: "Americans don't know where Romania is." He interpreted this lack of knowledge as evidence of Romania being relegated to insignificant status. He worked to elevate the status of his national identity not only through inferring that Americans were less knowledgeable than Romanians, but through normalizing knowledge about Romania, and assertions such as: "Romania, the civilization is okay, the life conditions are okay… Romania is a very nice country."

The engineers made references to status degradation when they described being treated with a lack of humanity. The Brazilian engineers felt dehumanized by the American engineers' style of getting "straight to the point" in emails, what the Brazilians called "leaving out the human." They said: "the human factor matters more outside the U.S. [than to Americans]." Similarly the Indian engineers pointed to the lack of a salutation such as "Dear Rajesh" or lack of signature such as "Regards, Bill," as status depreciation: "I feel his arrogance." The importance of greetings in avoiding status degradation was not communicated effectively or not able to be heard. This was shown by a comment by an American engineer working with the Brazilians, who said the Brazilians complained "over even simple things" like "the [American] manager didn't say good morning" to them.

The common type of IT platform through which the engineers interacted brought them into contact with a diverse range of expectations but didn't provide a means to reshape their expectations. Unresolved differences in how to explicitly maintain human to human dignity and respect in some cases destroyed the credibility professionals had worked long hours to achieve. As one engineer said, joint projects are not possible without clear recognition of the others' identity:

> Without [engineer's name] there I think it [the collaboration] would not have taken the shape it's taken today because he's familiar with our names, our culture, he knows all of us. He has developed a kind of liking for us, supporting us, so without all those I think it's impossible.

He lists several familiar features of identity–recognition, aspects of cultural background, affirmation, appreciation, and ratification.

11.5 Conclusion

Technology has enhanced the mobility and diversity of people working together, meaning that intercultural negotiations of identity are more and more part of a work day. In technologically-mediated settings, however, there is little cultural or social context available to facilitate learning about identity practices or how to accommodate to diverse cultural notions of personhood influencing identity construction in these settings. Identity work varies with cultural beliefs about the person, and how each person shows a culturally-informed relatedness to others. Unfortunately, without some attention to how cultural patterns influence identity practices, those working in global teams can inadvertently spoil others' identities or participate in the status degradation of others. In the settings described here, people are alert to processes of identity negotiation and meanings within their own culture, but overgeneralize their own local practices.

Technology is making it routine for members of certain professions to work together from different cultural locations, and social science has a role to play in bringing a discussion of language, culture, and identity to these spaces. In this paper I have argued that attention to two sociological concepts, identity spoiling and status degradation, can help prioritize attention to ensuring regular and consistent identity ratification in cross cultural virtual professional collaborations.

Acknowledgements My sincere thanks to the many engineers who gave generously of their time and ideas. This work was supported by the National Science Foundation under Grant 0729253 (any opinions, findings, conclusions or recommendations expressed in this material are those of the author and do not necessarily reflect the views of the National Science Foundation). Many thanks to the organizers of the REID conference 2013, and all the participants of that conference, and to the reviewers of this article whose thoughtful contributions enhanced this chapter.

References

Androutsopoulos, J., & Georgakopoulou, A. (2008). Youth, discourse, and interpersonal management. In G. Antos & E. Ventola (Eds.), *Handbook of interpersonal communication* (pp. 457–480). New York: Mouton de Gruyter.

Auer, P. (Ed.). (2007). *Style and social identities*. Berlin/New York: Mouton de Gruyter.

Auer, P., & Dirim, I. (2003). Sociocultural orientation, urban youth styles and the spontaneous acquisition of Turkish by non-Turkish adolescents in Germany. In J. Androutsopoulos & A. Georgakopoulou (Eds.), *Discourse constructions of youth identities* (pp. 223–246). Amsterdam: John Benjamins.

Bailey, B. (1997). Communication of respect in interethnic service encounters. *Language in Society, 26*(3), 327–356.

Benwell, B., & Stokoe, E. (2006). *Discourse and identity*. Edinburgh: Edinburgh University Press.

Bhabha, H. (1994). *The location of culture*. New York: Routledge.

Blommaert, J., Collins, J., & Slembrouck, S. (2005). Polycentricity and interactional regimes in 'global neighborhoods'. *Ethnography, 6*(2), 205–235.

Brown, P., & Levinson, S. (1987). *Politeness: Some universals in language usage*. Cambridge: Cambridge University Press.

Bucholtz, M. (1999). "Why be normal?": Language and identity practices in a community of nerd girls. *Language in Society, 28*(02), 203–223.

Bucholtz, M., & Hall, K. (2005). Identity and interaction: A sociocultural linguistic approach. *Discourse Studies, 7*(4–5), 585–614.

Butler, J. (2002). *Gender trouble*. New York: Routledge.

Cornips, L., & de Rooij, V. (2013). Selfing and othering through categories of race, place, and language among minority youths in Rotterdam, The Netherlands. In P. Siemund, I. Goglin, M. Schulz, & J. Davydova (Eds.), *Multilingualism and language diversity in urban areas: Acquisition, identities, space, education* (pp. 129–164). Amsterdam: John Benjamins Publishing Company.

Cutler, C. (2003). "Keepin' it real": White hip-hoppers' discourses of language, race, and authenticity. *Journal of Linguistic Anthropology, 13*(2), 211–233.

Cutler, C. (2009). "You shouldn't be rappin", you should be skateboardin' the X-games: The coconstruction of whiteness in an MC battle. In H. Alim, A. Ibrahim, & A. Pennycook (Eds.), *Global linguistic flows: Hip hop cultures, youth identities, and the politics of language* (pp. 79–94). New York: Routledge.

Daskalov, R. (1997). Ideas about, and reactions to modernization in the Balkans. *Eastern European Quarterly, 31*(2), 141–180.

Dümling, B. (2004). Country notes: the impact of western social workers in Romania—A fine line between empowerment and disempowerment. *Social Work and Society, 2*(2), 270–278 (University of Duisburg-Essen, Center for Social Work and Social Policy).

Garfinkel, H. (1956). Conditions of successful degradation ceremonies. *American Journal of Sociology, 61,* 420–424.

Geschiere, P. (2009). *Perils of belonging: Autochthony, citizenship, and exclusion in Africa and Europe*. Chicago: University of Chicago Press.

Goffman, E. (1963). *Stigma: Notes on the management of spoiled identity*. New Jersey: Prentice-Hall.

Goffman, E. (1967). *Interaction ritual: Essays on face-to-face behavior*. New York: Anchor Books.

Gumperz, J., & Cook-Gumperz, J. (2007). Discourse, cultural diversity and communication: A linguistic anthropological perspective. *Handbook of Intercultural Communication, 7,* 13–29.

Gumperz, J., Cyprian, T., & Roberts, C. (1979). *Crosstalk: A study of cross-cultural communication*. Southall: National Centre for Industrial Language Training.

Hacking, I. (1986). Making up people. In T. Heller, M. Sosna, & D. Wellbery (Eds.), *Reconstructing individualism: Autonomy, individuality, and the self in Western thought* (pp. 222–236). Stanford: Stanford University Press.

Hasnain, I., Bagga-Gupta, S., & Mohan, S. (Eds.). (2013). *Alternative voices: (Re)searching language, culture, identity*. Newcastle upon Tyne: Cambridge Scholars Publishing.

Hastings, S. (2000). Self-disclosure and identity management by bereaved parents. *Communication Studies, 51,* 352–371.

Heritage, J. (1984). *Garfinkel and ethnomethodology*. Cambridge: Polity Press.

Ide, S. (1989). Formal forms and discernment: Two neglected aspects of universals of linguistic politeness. *Multilingua, 8*(2/3), 223–248.

Iordachi, C., & Trencsényi, B. (2003). In search of a usable past: The question of national identity in Romanian studies, 1990–2000. *East European Politics and Societies, 17*(3), 415–435.

Jacquemet, M. (1994). T-offenses and metapragmatic attacks: Strategies of interactional dominance. *Discourse and Society, 5*(3), 297–319.

Jarvenpaa, S., & Keating, E. (2011). Hallowed grounds: the role of cultural values, practices, and institutions in TMS in an offshored complex engineering services project. *IEEE Transactions in Engineering Management, 99,* 1–13.

Keating, E., & Jarvenpaa, S. (2011). Interspatial subjectivities: Engineering in virtual environments. *Social Semiotics, 21*(2), 219–237.

Keating, E., & Jarvenpaa, S. (2016). *Words matter: Communicating effectively in the new global office*. Berkeley: University of California Press.

Lamb, S. (2000). *White saris and sweet mangoes: Aging, gender and body in north India*. Berkeley: University of California Press.

Lukose, R. (2008). Empty citizenship: Protesting politics in the era of globalization. *Cultural Anthropology, 20,* 506–533.

Majumdar, D., & Madan, T. (1956). *An introduction to social anthropology*. Bombay: Asia Publishing House.

Marriott, M. (1976). Hindu transactions: Diversity without dualism. In B. Kapferer (Ed.), *Transaction and meaning: Directions in the anthropology of exchange and behavior* (pp. 109–142). Philadelphia: Institute for the Study of Human Issues.

Marriott, M., & Inden, R. (1977). Toward an ethnosociology of South Asian caste systems. In K. David (Ed.), *The new wind: Changing identities in South Asia* (pp. 227–238). The Hague: Walter de Gruyter.

Matsumoto, Y. (1988). Reexamination of the universality of face: Politeness phenomena in Japanese. *Journal of Pragmatics, 12,* 403–426.

Ochs, E., & Kremer-Sadlik, T. (2013). *Fast-forward family*. Berkeley: University of California Press.

Ogbu, J. (1978). *Minority education and caste: The American system in cross-cultural perspective*. San Diego: Academic Press.

Ong, A. (1999). *Flexible citizenship: The cultural logics of transnationality*. Durham: Duke University Press.

Rampton, B. (1999). Styling the other: Introduction. *Journal of Sociolinguistics, 3*(4), 421–427.

Rasmussen, S. (2008). Personhood, self, difference, and dialogue. *International Journal of Dialogical Science, 3*(1), 31–54.

Said, E. (1979). *Orientalism*. New York: Vintage.

Sebastian, R., & Ryan, E. (1985). Speech cues and social evaluation: Markers of ethnicity, social class, and age. In H. Giles & R. St. Clair (Eds.), *Recent advances in language communication and social psychology* (pp. 112–143). London: Lawrence Erlbaum.

Shankar, S. (2008). Speaking like a model minority: "FOB" styles, gender, and racial meanings among desi teens in Silicon valley. *Journal of Linguistic Anthropology, 18*(2), 268–289.

Shweder, R., & Bourne, E. (1984). Does the concept of person vary cross-culturally? In R. Shweder & R. LeVine (Eds.), *Culture theory: Essays on mind, self, and emotion* (pp. 158–199). Cambridge: Cambridge University Press.

Silverstein, M. (1993). Metapragmatic discourse and metapragmatic discourse. In J. Lucy (Ed.), *Reflexive language: Reported speech and metapragmatics* (pp. 33–57). New York: Cambridge University Press.

Spertus, E. http://people.mills.edu/spertus/Gender/pap/node7.html, Accessed December 15, 2014.

Spiro, M. (1993). Is the western conception of the self "peculiar" within the context of the world cultures? *Ethos, 21,* 107–153.

Spivak, G. (1985). The Rani of Sirmur: An essay in reading the archives. *History and Theory, 24*(3), 247–272.

Taylor, C. (2007). *In a secular age*. Boston: Harvard University Press.

Taylor, P., & Bain, P. (1999). 'An assembly line in the head': Work and employee relations in the call centre. *Industrial Relations Journal, 30*(2), 101–117.

Author Biography

Elizabeth Keating is Professor of Anthropology at the University of Texas at Austin, USA. Her research interests include linguistic anthropology, human-computer interaction, virtual collaborative work, language and power, language and social inequality, multimodality, and cross-cultural communication. She has published widely and has served as an editor of the *Journal of Linguistic Anthropology* as well as Director of the Science, Technology and Society Program at the University of Texas at Austin.

Chapter 12
Identity Negotiations in a Visually Oriented Virtual Classroom

Johan Hjulstad

All I really want to do
Is, baby, be friends with you.
Bob Dylan—*Another Side of Bob Dylan* (1964)

12.1 Introduction

This chapter explores some of the identity negotiations performed by signed language learning students in a videoconference classroom—that is, in a video-only mediated environment (VME). Seeking to better our understanding of the subject formation processes by which people come to identify and ascribe membership to

J. Hjulstad (✉)
Department of Language and Literature, Norwegian University of Science and Technology, Trondheim, Norway
e-mail: johan.hjulstad@statped.no

S. Bagga-Gupta et al. (eds.), *Identity Revisited and Reimagined*,
DOI 10.1007/978-3-319-58056-2_12

the deaf[1] community, the focus in this chapter is not on being deaf, but on becoming deaf (culturally). Identities are inevitable, but the most prevalent of a person's multiple intersecting identities, and what these come to mean, constantly shift across various discourse contexts. Bringing signing students (i.e., students who are deaf), enrolled in local municipality schools, together in a distance education program can strengthen their deaf identities. However, this chapter investigates how a simple exercise had a powerful effect on what deaf identity meant, also vis-à-vis deaf students' (hearing) non-signing friends in their local classes. Through working on a "friendship" teaching plan, which involved the signing students inviting their hearing non-signing friends from their local classes to the VME, the students re-negotiated what "deaf" came to mean, also at their local school. In the investigated data, the students and their teachers describe the invitation to the lesson and its consequences as particularly successful, as consequential for identity development, and as a contribution to bridging the gap between deaf and hearing students in mainstream settings. The investigation demonstrates the intertwined and significant role played by technology in the balancing act of stabilizing a positive outcome while negotiating multiple intersecting identities of "deaf" and "friend" across what can be seen as "primary modality orientation." The findings have a number of implications for how we might think about identity development, the role of technology, and inclusive education. While there is an extensive literature on

[1]I use the term "deaf" in this chapter to refer to persons with any degree or kind of hearing loss consequential for participation in "audiologically oriented" (Bagga-Gupta and Holmström 2015) learning activities. While I am sympathetic to the deaf/Deaf distinction used by many researchers, is not commonly reflected in Norwegian or Norwegian Sign Language usage (the languages of the data). Rather, I use "deaf" both when referring to individuals or groups of people with "hearing loss" or "hearing impairment" *and* when referring to people who are members of the deaf community, belonging to a (signing) linguistic and cultural minority (which implies some "deaf" who are fully hearing). I also avoid using the audiological categories (mild, moderate, severe, and profound). Neither do I use the more widely accepted "deaf and hard of hearing." Exceptions are made in cases when I cite or otherwise refer to other researchers who apply any of the terms noted above. I choose this practice because my interest is not in being deaf, but in becoming deaf (culturally), and the aim of the study is to explore the participants' own identity negotiations. Thus, it is important to avoid assigning them unsolicited membership categories. However, because the study investigates a school setting, the most relevant category is "student"; this means that "deaf" often comes with "student." I am well aware of the "non-handicapping language" convention of always putting the impairment after the noun. However, since the topic of this chapter is active encouragement of the positive aspects of developing a deaf identity, such a practice can actually reinforce the idea that the "differently abled" category is always undesirable. Therefore, I often write "deaf students," stressing that this does not imply that deaf is a more (or less) important category than "student" (or "boy," "son," "ice hockey player," and so on), but that this is always situational. However, since the VME is muted, it is for the studied virtual classroom interaction simply not relevant if and how much the students hear. Thus, I refer to the participating students as "signed language learners," because this refers to the purpose of their participation in the distance education. While all students in the dataset were deaf, kodas (kids of deaf adults) who are fully hearing also participate in the distance education program. I would also like to add that not all deaf students use signed language or are particularly skilled in visually oriented ways of communicating.

identity, few studies have examined how technology affects identity in deaf communities or in deaf education (for recent work, see, e.g., Holmström et al. 2015; Bagga-Gupta and Holmström 2015).

12.1.1 *Ethnographic Background*

The issue of deaf identity has, throughout the last decades, attracted a lot of academic and public interest. No less than "a profound revolution in our understanding of human language and culture" is said to have taken place when signed languages were validated as fully linguistic, and a subsequent rewriting from "deaf" to "Deaf" could be made in the sense that Deaf now signifies a cultural identity of a linguistic minority (Bauman 2008, p. 1). The changes that have occurred since the 1960s have provided a new vocabulary for the way in which Deaf individuals can emancipate and empower themselves, and it has been strongly argued that identification with Deaf culture and Deaf community represents a "gain" (e.g., Bauman and Murray 2010).

The unique ways of socializing in deaf communities have long since challenged language socialization theory (Erting and Kuntze 2008). Because only a small percentage of deaf children are born into deaf culture (i.e., to deaf parents), the path to identification for most deaf children with hearing parents is not straightforward. This means that the primary sites of socialization for most deaf people are deaf schools, deaf clubs, and deaf congregations. In previous times, most deaf children attended government run residential schools for the deaf; thus, the schools played an important role as the arena wherein deaf children would meet culturally deaf peers and deaf adults, who served as significant role models. The role of deaf education in the identification processes of deaf students is widely acknowledged. In Norway, development of a positive deaf identity through identification with signed language users and deaf communities has, throughout the last decades, been an important goal of deaf education. The national curriculum for the school subject Norwegian Sign Language (NSL) explicitly states that "Norwegian Sign Language is a key subject with regard to cultural understanding, communication, enlightenment and developing an identity. One key objective of the tuition given in Norwegian Sign Language throughout primary and secondary education is to generate linguistic self-confidence and confidence in one's own culture as a basis for developing an identity, respect for others, and lifelong learning" (Norwegian Sign Language Curriculum 2013).

12.1.1.1 Deaf Identity in New Educational Settings

Over the last decades, a range of significant changes have been made regarding deaf education in Norway, as well as deaf children and their families. The number of students attending residential schools for the deaf on a full-time basis is decreasing.

Instead, students are increasingly enrolling in their local municipality schools. Aside from a general trend towards the principle of inclusion of all special needs students (e.g., as seen in the Salamanca Statement (UNESCO 1994)), the decreased full-time enrollment in schools for deaf students can in general be related to higher expectations of these children's development of intelligible speech, literacy skills, and goal attainment (Simonsen et al. 2009). Early screening of newborn babies' hearing has led to earlier discovery and earlier diagnosis of deafness. Parents receive counseling and measures are taken to start and progress their children's language development (either signed and/or spoken) at an early stage. Further, between 90 and 95% of all children with congenital or pre-lingual profound hearing loss in Norway are now fitted with cochlear implants (i.e., advanced hearing aids) (Kirkehei et al. 2011). However, the trend of parents enrolling their children in local schools must, paradoxically, also be seen in light of the mentioned breakthrough and consequences of the view that deaf children should have the right to signed language tuition and bilingual education. In 1998, the Education Act was amended to include a section (§2.6) giving deaf students "the right to tuition in the use of sign language and through the medium of sign language" (Ohna 2005, p. 168, original in English). This made bilingual education for deaf students "normal" education and not tied to schools for deaf students. The responsibility of these students' education was placed on the local schools, which were expected to provide a teacher or teaching assistant with competence in NSL at the minimum level of 30 ECTS-Credits (European Credit Transfer and Accumulation System) (Ohna 2005). Local schools were also expected to cooperate with deaf schools (which, in 2000, were organized as units within a network of resource centers called "Statped"); this usually meant that the students were offered "part-time education" (i.e., receiving parts of their education—usually a few weeks a year—at schools for the deaf), while their teachers were offered courses at the resource center. National curricula in four school subjects were developed, and a substantial amount of teaching material was made to support teaching in and about NSL. From 1996, parents have been offered participation in an extensive (40-week) signed language training program until their children reach the age of 16, with the aim of improving communication at home. Such factors have made it easier for parents to justify having their child attend a local school, even though the child may be the only (deaf) student learning signed language at that school.

The new situation means that there are great variations in the amount of exposure to signed language and contact with deaf peers and adults these students actually receive. Adding further to the diversity is that many of these students (including their parents and teachers) enter the various programs for signed language training and part-time education at various ages, with some entering at a late stage. It is common for professionals and parents to have a "wait and see" approach, and only when they see that their child's development is not optimal do they decide to "fall back" on signed language training as a "last resort" (cf. Galåen 2008).

In response to the decreasing number of full-time students in schools for deaf students, the Norwegian government recently changed its policy. In 2014, they closed down three out of four state schools for the deaf and turned the part-time education program into a new model for deaf education. In the new model, one of the main tasks of the former deaf schools is to support local municipality schools in providing deaf students bilingual education. Thus, the focus has shifted to providing part-time education within rich signed language environments as a supportive measure for mainstreamed sign-bilingual students.

Concerning the focus of this chapter, as part of the new model, a distance education program was established to provide mainstreamed students an additional arena for learning signed language (i.e. NSL) together with other signing students also in the periods in-between the part-time education. In this program, advanced videoconferencing technologies are used to create a multi-party virtual classroom in which up to five differently located students connect to a teacher at the school for the deaf. The findings from the first six months of the program highlight some of the implications and results of this dramatic change in the education of deaf students in Norway.

12.1.1.2 Deaf Students Struggle in Mainstream Settings

The fact that deaf students often struggle in mainstream settings is not new. It has been well documented that they easily become communicatively isolated in mainstream settings, where they are often the only deaf student among a majority of hearing peers and teachers (Keating and Mirus 2003; Holmström et al. 2015). A recent Norwegian study (Kermit et al. 2014) confirms this international trend for the Norwegian setting, as well. The findings suggest that adolescents with sensory impairments report significantly lower self-esteem and greater loneliness than their peers. Almost one out of four report that they experience solitude. An overall finding in the interview study is that all students with sensory impairments express the wish "to be like everyone else," but their effort to self-present as similar to their peers is a project that none fully succeed with (possible exceptions, according to the study, are signing students attending a part-time education). The study found that many adolescents are well included in many settings. However, this inclusion is first and foremost the result of the adolescent's own effort, and the "informants tell the story of how they themselves, to different degrees, have to strive to adapt to other students or peers in school or during leisure activities" (Kermit et al. 2014, p. xv).

The limited signed language environment at the local school does not typically provide satisfactory conditions for the development of signing skills or a process of subject formation allowing for a positive deaf identity. Therefore, the justification for implementing a distance education program was partly based on reports from students' and teachers' experiences with part-time education stays. It was said that many of the students experienced a sense of having to "start all over again" when returning to a part-time education stay, due to the long time apart and the lack of continuation between stays at the school for the deaf. Thus, the distance education program studied in this chapter was set up as a supplement to the part-time education program, to provide a more continual offer to mainstreamed students.

The background described above makes it relevant to ask how such a goal—to learn signed language to a level at which it can form the basis of a positive subject formation and identification with the positive aspect of the signing community—can be reached, given the present situation.

12.1.2 Theoretical Background: Researching Identity in New Settings

The theoretical approach to identity in this chapter aligns broadly to a sociocultural linguistic framework (Bucholtz and Hall 2005), wherein five principles are proposed as the basis of an analysis of identity: (1) the emergence principle, (2) the positionality principle, (3) the indexicality principle, (4) the relationality principle, and (5) the partialness principle. Following these principles implies seeing identities as emergent, rather than pre-existing, products. This means that identity is something that is situationally accomplished in moment-to-moment interactions with others and the world, and thus a fundamental social and cultural phenomenon. The aim of this chapter is to explore the students' own identity negotiations, seeking to avoid assigning unsolicited membership categories and rather to understand how they negotiate their subject positions. While identities encompass macro-level demographic categories and local ethnographic cultural positions, the analysis for this chapter is mainly concerned with the temporary and interactional stances and participant roles taken by the students. Identity relations emerge in interaction, through several indexical processes (Bucholtz and Hall 2005) spanning mention of identity categories and labeling to use of implicatures and presuppositions, evaluative and epistemic orientations, interactional footings and participant roles, and linguistic structures and systems associated with specific persons and groups—all of which were taken to be important ingredients of students' identity negotiations in the studied VME. Identities are relational and intersubjectively constructed through overlapping complementary relations, including similarity and difference. Further, any given construction of identity may, in part, be deliberate and intentional, and may also, in part, be habitual and hence less than fully conscious. Identities are thus partly an outcome of negotiation and contestation, partly an outcome of others' perceptions and representations, and partly an effect of ideological processes and material structures relevant for the interaction. Thus, identities are inevitable, but they shift as interaction unfolds and across various discourse contexts (Bucholtz and Hall 2005).

My argument is partly based on research that emphasizes the importance of interactive spaces for identity development. In particular, I draw on work done by: the feminist geographer Valentine (2007); the related "Deaf geographies" initiative (Gulliver and Kitzel 2015); similar arguments in linguistic anthropology (Keating 2008); and a "spatial turn" in recent studies in linguistic pragmatics, discourse studies, and sequential analysis of interaction (McIlvenny et al. 2009; Streeck et al. 2011). Seeking to advance the theorization of intersectionality and the relationships between multiple identity categories and subject positions (i.e., "disability," gender, race, sexuality, etc.), Valentine (2007) argues for an appreciation of the significance of space in processes of subject formation. She sees identities as "situated accomplishments" and builds on Judith Butler's theory (1999) that identity categories are performative. She also finds resonance with actor-network theory's (Latour 2005) notion that "things" do not have fixed or stable properties, but properties that emerge in practice (Valentine 2007, p. 14). Valentine argues:

> [t]he identity of particular spaces—the home, the school, the workplace, or a community space such as a Deaf club—are in turn produced and stabilized through the repetition of the intersectional identities of the dominant groups that occupy them. [...] When individual identities are "done" differently in particular temporal moments they rub up against, and so expose, these dominant spatial orderings that define who is in place/out of place, who belongs and who does not. (Valentine 2007, p. 19)

Thus, stabilization and de-stabilization of intersecting identities are often seen to be connected to various spaces through the interactional work that shapes these spaces. However, while it is assumed that space matters for subject formations and the way in which people identify and dis-identify—there is common agreement that this is done at a situated interactional level—little is known and few empirical studies exist on the way in which such spaces are constituted.

In line with this theorizing, and given that different places stabilize different identities, one can easily conclude that deaf "segregated" school settings stabilize a positive deaf identity and affiliation with a community of deaf people, while mainstream school settings de-stabilize a positive deaf identity and stabilize identities of "*dis*-ability" and *loss* of hearing. Such a conception is, however, too simple, and must be nuanced. Based on investigations of a VME that blurs the traditional spaces of segregation and mainstreaming, this chapter argues that we must instead investigate how stabilization is actually accomplished. The chapter entertains the simple idea that the things we do in various places (i.e., home, school, the workplace, etc.), are performed in typical ways. Through recurrent embodied interactional organization and joint coordination of talk and participation, our ways of doing things becomes conventionalized. This, I argue, contributes to the stabilization of these spaces as certain places. As I further argue—implied in the title of the chapter—the participants turn this VME into a "visually oriented space." The concept "visual-orientation" I have borrowed from Bagga-Gupta (2004). I also build on Goodwin and Goodwin (2004), who revisited and expanded the notion of participation (Goffman 1981) within an embodied interaction perspective, which links works in linguistic anthropology with works on participation in other fields, such as education. Focusing on the practices that actors use to collectively participate in the endogenous courses of action in their lifeworlds, powerful tools are provided for analyzing and linking details of moment-by-moment language use to embodiment, culture, social organization, and material structure in the environment (Goodwin and Goodwin 2004). The "embodied interaction in the material world" perspective (Streeck et al. 2011) holds that all interaction is intrinsically multimodal. Thus, the visual orientation of signed language does not imply that the language interaction is any less multimodal, nor that only one modality is employed. However, in order for people to properly understand each other, it is fundamental that they take into account each others' publicly displayed embodied signs of where they are and what they are attending to Goffman (1964). Such embodied displays—that participants are mutually oriented towards each other, particular places, objects, and events in the surrounding environment—creates what Goffman calls "an ecological huddle," or what the Goodwins (2004) call "embodied participation frameworks." The sociolinguistic practices for establishing and sustaining such frameworks are often not shared between deaf and hearing people, because signed and oral communication differs in primary modality orientation. I further suggest that participation is typically co-organized in frameworks that enable and constrain "who" the participants are allowed to be in that particular setting. However, as will be demonstrated in the analysis, the students' agency is demonstrated through their negotiation and cooperative organization of participation. In addition, it is suggested that there is a relation between well known participation frameworks—allowing for "experienc[ing] the sense of sameness and belonging that comes from the ability to communicate freely with others like ourselves" (Valentine 2007, p. 17)—and the feeling of being "at home with" or belonging to a particular place.

Compared to studies of peer communication between deaf-and-deaf persons and hearing-and-hearing persons, studies investigating deaf-and-hearing peer communication in natural settings are scarce. It is a paradox that while a substantial amount of research has reported that deaf students in mainstream settings struggle in social relations with their hearing peers (cf. Xie et al. 2014), very few studies have actually studied the emerging interaction, which becomes critical with mainstreaming. Only a few observational studies of classroom practices with deaf or hard of hearing students within mainstream education have been conducted (e.g., Holmström 2013, focusing on students with cochlear implants), and some studies have focused primarily on teaching practices (e.g., Ohna 2005). How deaf and hearing peers interact inside classrooms has attracted very little attention. Keating and Mirus (2003) investigated peer interactions during recess and lunchtime in the school cafeteria, and found that "unshared sociolinguistic practices and hearing-oriented participation frameworks are crucial aspects of communicative failure between hearing and deaf children in mainstream elementary school settings" (Keating and Mirus 2003, p. 131).

The study in this chapter was initially set up to study the classroom interactions in a new VME with exclusively signing participants (peers). However, a unique opportunity presented itself when—on the initiative of students in one group—hearing, non-signing friends from the students' home classrooms were invited to a lesson. This provided interesting data that demonstrated not only that the technology brought these students together—providing an opportunity for establishing a "we" and the collective work of negotiating and interpreting what it is like to be deaf—but also that the (use of) technology could be appropriated to strengthen the students' sense of positive identity, also vis-à-vis their hearing classmates. Consequentially, the usual roles were reversed, with deaf students no longer at a disadvantage in the classroom. Rather, the hearing students needed special intervention in order to participate in a framework that favored skills and abilities they did not possess. However, as the data demonstrates, this situation still seemed to work out fine; that is, it worked fine *as a result of* the careful planning and preparation for the invitation of the hearing classmates.

The "friendship" teaching plan and the invitation of classmates to the distance education lesson was described as a success. This led me to pursue whether it would be possible to unravel what had most likely made it a success. In particular, I discovered that what most likely constituted the success could be revealed by scrutinizing the preparation process leading up to the successful lesson. This process, I argue, has a number of further implications for how we should think about identity development, the role of technology, and inclusive education.

12.2 Methodology and Data

Inspired by methods of micro-ethnography (Streeck and Mehus 2005), the data for this study was gathered from a range of sources, spanning documents relevant to this project and deaf education to observations of teachers' lesson planning meetings and interviews with teachers and students. However, the most important data were video recordings of the coordinated activities inside the distance education "virtual" classroom. The setup of the VME made it technically easy to record the same live images (video) the participants used to interact with in the VME (see Fig. 12.1). This recording was carried out by the program's technician by a streamer that recorded the lessons and saved them into video files. The project involved 20 students—in 6th to 10th grade (approximately 11–15 years old)—and five teachers, who were organized in five groups. All groups had one lesson of approximately 45 min a week, and additional homework in relation to those

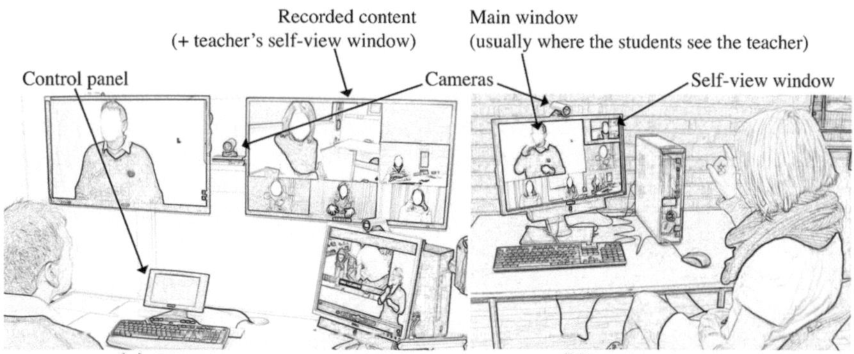

Fig. 12.1 Virtual classroom environment: **a** The studio at the school for the deaf, **b** Set-up at a student's local school

lessons. The period of data collection lasted six months and 67 lessons were recorded. The focus was primarily on 15 consecutive lessons in one group of five regularly participating students (Oscar, Ruth, Wilma, Gail, and Tina—all fictive names). The 15 lessons were logged in order to produce a general overview of the material and to deal with the theme of "friendship" covered in this chapter. A total of 57 min was transcribed in detail.

ELAN, a tool for interaction analysis, was used to transcribe the signed language interactions, combining adapted transcription conventions from conversation analysis (CA) with conventions from signed language linguistic research for glossing manual signs. Analysis of signed language discourse poses several methodological and conceptual challenges. In the process of adapting and preparing recorded material containing signed interactions for analysis and presentation, the analyst is bound to confront issues connected to how the data is transformed into a more permanent form—usually text, but often images and other graphical representations (cf. Heath et al. 2010). Detailed annotation of the interaction seriously challenges the readability of the transcripts—a concern shared by researchers who work to incorporate multimodal and embodied aspects of interaction. Therefore, in the presentation of the findings, a combination of sketched frame grabs, glossing symbols, and translations into full sentences are used.

12.3 Findings

In this section, observations and findings are presented in four parts. First, I present observations of the participants reporting the "friendship" teaching plan as a success (Sect. 12.3.1). In preparation for analyzing the identity negotiations, I found it useful to first deal with observations concerning the particular VME the teaching took place in—its designs, templates, and teaching formats, and how its ecology constrained but also enabled the exploitation of new participatory possibilities (Sect. 12.3.2). The findings in the third part (Sect. 12.3.3) show that success was related to the fact that the students cooperatively planned for it to be successful, revealing what they were working to accomplish in the successful lesson (being friends across different systems for primary modality orientation). Finally, I return to the successful lesson (Sect. 12.3.4). In retrospect, seeing the lesson in relief against the background of the planning, some of what made this lesson successful stands out.

12.3.1 A Story of Success

I start my presentation with participants' reports about the success of the lesson, which I find, in important ways, to actualize questions of subject formation and identity. The following section covers what the success refers to, what aspect the success concerns, and why it should be considered consequential for the process of subject formation. The success is pointed to on various occasions throughout my data, calling attention to something that was done differently—and better—than before.

12.3.1.1 Extract from Evaluation

The following extract is taken from the evaluation in the lesson *after* the successful lesson, where about five minutes are reserved for evaluating previous lessons. All of the students say that they think the lesson was great, and that even the visiting friends had been enthusiastic about it. In the following sequence, Ruth reveals some of the lesson's consequences (Fig. 12.2).

Ruth speaks about the effect of the invitation on her situation and identity in her local school, citing an apparent change in her classmates' interest in learning signs and signed language, and thus a greater attraction to her. The style in which Ruth speaks about this should be noticed: smiling, with a distinct "sensational news" style (i.e., eyes wide open, torso moved back, chin pulled in), attesting to the positive value this has for her. The teacher also responds to this through a matching of style in line 16. Ruth's facial expression, including the manner in which she performs the signs (i.e., drawing on prosodic features), clearly indicates her stance with respect to what she is saying, making it very clear that even if she chooses to use the sign NAG (nagging), this is to be interpreted as a positive. Because only one of her friends from class is allowed to join at a time, there is competition over who will be invited next. Thus, both the one-at-a-time organization and the fact that she and her deaf friends are now perceived as being in an exclusive group account for the success. The situation is one in which her friends want to sign to her, and she must teach them signs "all of the time."

By speaking about this effect, Ruth indicates that her popularity has increased and that she has become someone whom the others initiate contact with. The reason for their initiatives is that she has attractive knowledge that they want her to share with them. They now have a means of initiating contact and a topic: "learning signs." In light of what these initiatives from her hearing non-signing friends do to her situation and identity, there is a change in the (typical) organization of participation between her and her friends, suggesting a close connection between who she is (or who she can be) for others and the way in which participation is organized.

12.3.1.2 Extracts from Teachers' Interviews

The local teachers also bring attention to the "effect" of the new distance teaching setting and how this "effect" relates to the process of subject formation. In an interview conducted with the students' local teachers at the end of the project period, Gail's local teacher points to "another side" of language learning brought about by the distance education teaching:

1	Teacher:	THEN, THINK TRY EVALUATE LAST TEACHING BEFORE CHRISTMAS, YOU TAKE WITH FRIEND, REMEMBER YOU?:: ***Then, I was thinking we should do an evaluation of the last lessons before Christmas, the one where you brought a friend, do you remember?***
2	Students:	(nods)
3	Teacher:	THINK YOU (.) TEACHING LESSON:, YOU TAKE WITH FRIEND, FUNCTION GOOD, WHAT? ***What do you think (.) of the teaching lesson, when you brought the friend, did it work well, or what?***

(Twelve lines (49 sec.) taken out)

15	Ruth:	VERY FUN, FRIEND THINK FUN, AND- (.) FUN- THEY NAG ALLOW WITH, AND FOR SIGNS IN LESSONS MUCH LIKE:: (.) ***It was very fun, the friends thought it was fun, and- (.) fun- they kept nagging about being allowed to come along, and about signs during the lessons, and stuff.***
16	Teacher:	(sits back - surprised look)
17	Teacher:	THEY FRIENDS LEAR- WANT_TO LEARN SIGN? ***So, these friends lear- want to learn more signs?***
18	Ruth:	YES:: (smiles) ***Ye:ss!***
19	Teacher:	GOOD. PT CONTINUE TEACH SIGNS THEM. ***That's good. You have to continue teach them signs.***
20	Ruth:	YES, SO::- (.) ALL FRIENDS MINE WANT TALK SIGN ALL_THE_TIME. ***Yes, so:- (.) now, all my friends want to use signs all of the time.***
21	Teacher:	MUST. ***you should.***
22	Teacher:	GOOD. CONTAGION EFFECT, SIGN SPREAD. GOOD. ***That's good. It has a contageous effect, it spreads the use of signs. That's good.***

Fig. 12.2 Extract from evaluation

> I think that—that—that language—the language has improved, plus there is another side to this, and that has to do with being proud of the language and of what you have knowledge of, it can be—yes, that ehm, I think that this has contributed in a way to raise the status of the language, this thing, right? This [unintelligible] distance education and all this—like for the self-esteem, that this is something that is important. (Translated from spoken Norwegian)

The teacher highlights being proud of the language and having this knowledge, the raised status, and the self-esteem that derives from the importance of this teaching. Further into the interview, Gail's teacher is even more specific, mentioning:

> [...] they brought on one occasion one friend, right? And it could be—what I wish is, that they would be allowed to bring more—bring more—a few students, on more occasions, just in order for them to see what is going on, a good idea.

Gail's teacher indicates that she would like to have more lessons like the one they had when the students invited a friend from their local class. Further on, she follows up and makes a connection between the invitation of a friend and what this new setting can bring about for the signing students:

> [...] it has something to do with raising the status of these students, very many of these students may, struggle some with—with in a way, of making themselves known [Norwegian: by på seg selv], right? And this is a very fine way to—because this is kind of ex- exclusive and special, so it is something in building status and the interest, to put it that way, this is what I would wish for.

Interestingly, Gail's teacher frames it as common knowledge that these students often struggle with "making themselves known [*by på seg selv*]" in mainstream classrooms settings. Thus, she indicates that identity is a process that takes place over time and that may involve very subtle types of communication, and that a lack of fully shared communication practices can challenge a full display of a person and who they "really" are. This is apparently not only something she has discovered about her own student, but something she understands as a known fact (as displayed in the tag question: "right?"). In addition to being widely documented in research, this topic is often discussed among the local teachers at the regular local teachers' courses that Statped arranges simultaneously with the part-time education periods.

However, while she is pointing this out, she does not give an account of what, more specifically, this situation provides, other than concluding that it is "a fine way" for the students to deal with their difficulties. The rationale for scrutinizing the teaching plan that is claimed to have been successful is precisely that its "effect" built self-esteem and grounds for a positive identity. I suggest that it is not satisfactory to think success happens "out of nothing," or to ascribe it to the "exclusivity" of the technology.

12.3.2 Stabilizing Designs, Templates, and Teaching Formats

Preparing for the analysis of identity negotiations, I will first present a range of observations concerning the particular environment, all which seem significant for the lesson having been a success, all—in different ways—relevant to the way in which participation was organized in the lessons, and all related to the affordances (Gibson 1979) of the environment. The various designs, templates, and teaching formats used in this setting can all be said to contain "inscribed" visions of, predictions of, or scripts (i.e., distributed responsibilities and anticipated actions) for imagined users (Akrich 1992).

When Statped decided to establish a distance education program, the project management had to acquire video conferencing technology for use in the program. The process of selecting equipment and adapting the technology to accommodate visual oriented use revealed interesting information concerning expectations of potential users and how they would typically participate in this new interactional space.

First, it became obvious that even though this particular participation technology was made to enable participants to see each other, it was *not* initially made for video-*only*-mediated communication. Connecting participants at different locations challenges the designers of such technologies to decide how the different windows displaying each of the participants are made visible to the participants. Thus, how the participants in the multi-party setting see each other is "hard-coded" in templates that are chosen to be controlled by sound. Any sound (e.g., speaking) at an endpoint rearranges the order of windows so the location making sound (or speech) is displayed in a bigger "main window" of everyone's screens (see Fig. 12.1). This makes perfectly sense in communication that is primarily spoken, but, in signed language interactions, which are usually produced without sound and where visual orientation is a prerequisite, any accidental sound in one of the connected rooms can cause a sudden shift in the arrangement of windows and thus necessitate shifts in gaze direction. Clearly, we can see that the designers envisioned that the main mediating channel for communication through this technology would be sound, and they scripted this so the video image would follow and be subordinate to sound. This points to the fact that all technologies are designed for an imagined typical user, thus it can be said to be inscribed in the technology's design (cf. Haualand 2012).

The second point is that the choices made by Statped concerning the way in which the technology would be adapted and used attests to their vision of their (imagined) users. In the technology's templates, there is no option to deselect the sound control of the window arrangement. Therefore, the only way to avoid visual disturbance and go around the script is to make all participants mute their microphones. This has the convenient effect of stabilizing the mutual *visible* ways of participation as the only viable ways of organizing embodied participation, and thus enabling a focus on learning and practicing signed language skills. Simultaneously, it de-stabilizes the space as an environment for oral communication skills and makes such skills irrelevant for establishing and sustaining joint attention across the virtual space. It also makes participants' ability to hear (or lack thereof) irrelevant for joint attention and the coordination of activities across the virtual space. This has a curious parallel to signed language interactions in co-present settings where participants typically mute their voices—reportedly to enable signed language grammar. But perhaps more importantly, it puts all seeing participants on an equal footing, regardless of their degree of hearing loss. Here we see a re-distribution of the responsibility for stabilizing the environment as a visually oriented space (or a Deaf space; cf. Gulliver and Kitzel 2015; Valentine 2007), shifting it from a responsibility dealt with through the working consensus of the encounter to something that is accomplished through the way in which the technology is employed.

The studied VME is also stabilized as a school space (i.e., a classroom) through the configuration and physical location of the equipment. Also, the teaching formats, which the teachers prepare and enact, stabilize certain patterns for the typical organization of participation. The tasks given by the teachers are typical activities for the class to accomplish, which are both locally and historically shaped (Mondada and Doehler 2004). The investigated data shows that the tasks are very often explicitly specified in terms of how participation should be organized in the joint collaborative accomplishing of the task. The teachers choose and adjust the teaching format to fit the affordances of the VME and the purpose of the distance education program. The VME can, for instance, be seen not to favor lecturing or students working on an individual task. Instead, tasks that can increase student interaction are typically chosen (e.g., discussions, sharing presentations, and tasks that invite students to comment on each other's contributions)—tasks that facilitate peer interaction and peer learning. This is significant, because peer interaction and peer learning are precisely what seem vulnerable for mainstreamed deaf students, due to their uneven access to communication and partially unshared communicative practices.

When students learn how to communicate and take part in the repeated activities within these designs, templates, and teaching formats, the participation frameworks of the VME become conventionalized, and thus stabilized. But this simultaneously de-stabilizes the possibilities for participation by (hearing) students who have not developed the necessary skills to participate in the setting. However, as is made apparent in the next section, the students who become skilled at communicating in this environment also learn and become able to perceive other possibilities for designing and adjusting the participation frameworks. That is, to grow familiar with the VME allows them to create frameworks for the non-conflictual intersecting identity position of "friend," regardless of ability and skills relating to participating in and through systems based on different primary modality orientation (as in signed vs. spoken language interaction).

12.3.3 Doing Identity Negotiations

This section demonstrates some of the ways in which identity was negotiated in the "friendship" teaching plan. As discussed above, the participants pointed to the invitation lesson, itself, as successful. However, investigating this particular lesson, I did *not* find many examples of identity negotiations, as such; thus, it was somewhat hard to render the ways in which the talk and activities in this lesson were relevant for the students' subject formations. What I found instead was that the invitation lesson was planned to be this way, and it turned out as planned. I also discovered that the previous lesson, in which the students prepared for the successful lesson, was particularly rich with identity negotiations. In this section, I present some of the identity negotiations done by the students while they cooperatively accomplished the task given by the teacher. The task was to plan the activities in the upcoming lesson when their friends were to visit.

12.3.3.1 Designing Participation Frameworks

In the preparation lesson, the teacher gives a task that the students are supposed to prepare as homework. They are to discuss what to do in the following week's lesson, when their invited friend from class will join them. The teacher fulfills multiple purposes through her arrangement of this task. She does not just ask for the students' suggestions of what to do in the next lesson, but makes a task out of it. Nor does she pick a random topic to discuss, but she allows the students to influence the content, as well as the procedure, of the upcoming lesson. Ruth is given the role of "teacher," or moderator, in the discussion. In the following extract (Fig. 12.3), Ruth presents her idea for what to do in the next lesson.

In the above extract, Ruth creates a category, "us," with the characteristics "who know a lot of sign language." She creates this in contrast to "the other friends"—a category she positions with "who know a little less." Thus, Ruth establishes two groups, each with a different level of skill, and uses her background knowledge of her classmates to make this categorization. In other words, she sees herself and her signing friends as "experts," compared to her other friends, in communicating in this environment. Further on in the lesson, these two categories re-occur several times. Ruth could just as well have used hearing status as the difference between the groups. However, I suggest that she does *not* use this construction because the critical difference between them (in this particular membership category) is not whether they are hearing or deaf, but their ability to participate in her suggested quiz in the VME. Notice also how she does not create a category of "the others" as friends, but, with the construction "the other friends," she indexes those "who know a little less" as friends, while at the same time implying that those present are also friends. This implication establishes an encompassing "friends" category.

Further, we learn from what Ruth is saying that "games" (modified with the QUOTATIONS sign) can include quizzes and quiz-like games. While games do not need to include talk, quizzes (games of questions) always involve either spoken or written language. What is important here is that games or quizzes create expectations about the procedure of the activity—that is, how participation will proceed—much as the teaching formats mentioned above do. Quizzes can be seen as

1	Ruth:	YES, I ((lag)) THINK HAVE LIKE (gaze up) GAME QUOTATIONS LIKE (gaze side) QUIZ LIKE (moves head), BOTH TOGETHER^WORK, BUT LIKE ONE- TWO DIFFERENT LEVELS, ONE TO THREE_OF_US KNOW MUCH SIGN LANGUAGE, BUT ONE OTHER LEVEL TO THEY OTHER FRIENDS KNOW LITTLE LESS OR_SOMETHING? MEANS LIKE SOME TASKS TOGETHER^WORK OR_SOMETHING? ***Yes, I think we should have a like "game", like a Quiz kind of, so that both get to cooperate, but the way that it has two different levels, one for us who knows a lot sign language, but another level for the other friends who know a little less, right? So it means on some tasks we have to cooperate, or something.***

Fig. 12.3 Idea for activity in upcoming lesson

pre-formatted templates or scripts for cooperatively organizing participation. A quiz is a particular discourse type that sets strong sequential organization: question—working out an answer; then answering—scoring (i.e., before or after more rounds of questions). Thus, it includes known procedural guidelines on the organization of participation. In relation to this participatory organization, Ruth foregrounds her feeling that expectations should be different for each of the two categories of participants, and that the phase of "working out an answer" should be arranged in such a way "so that both get to cooperate" (i.e., as friends do). In other words, she connects this to the way in which this cooperation should be done—in two levels, each related to the skills categories she creates.

12.3.3.2 Managing Possible de-Stabilization of Participation

In the next step, the other students comment on Ruth's proposal (as specified by the teacher when giving the task). Gail comments first. After a little hesitation, she continues:

Gail (in Fig. 12.4, line 14) points to a possible conflict between Ruth's suggested activity and the guests' ability to participate. I find it interesting that in all of my data related to this visit up until this point, it is never questioned that an invitation of non-signing friends to this environment will in fact "work," and that they will be able participate in this setting at all. Gail anticipates, or rather envisions, how it will be for the friends to participate in this setting, and positions them as insufficiently skilled for taking part in their interactions. At the same time, she positions herself as someone who is concerned on their behalf (as a friend would be). To participate in the quiz, the friends must understand its content; otherwise interactional trouble might de-stabilize and exclude the friends from participation. In this light, her objection appears reasonable. As seen in line 17 (Fig. 12.4), Tina does not agree. However, the issue of exactly how the non-signing friends will be able to follow what the signing students will say remains, for the moment, unresolved.

14	Gail:	I VIEW- THINK DIFFICULT OTHERS UNDERSTAND WHAT THREE_OF_US TALK ABOUT. ***My opinion- I think it will be difficult for the others to understand what we're talking about.***

(two lines 9,5 seconds omitted)

17	Tina:	I THINK GOOD AND F- FUN FOR FRIENDS, FRIENDS THINK CERTAIN FUN TAKE QUIZ: I THINK: GOOD. ***I think it's good, and that it would be f- fun for the friends, the friends will probably think it is fun to do a quiz, that's what I think, I think it's good.***

Fig. 12.4 Comments to activity proposal

12.3.3.3 Securing Balanced Participation for Each Category of Participants

The teacher then takes the floor and asks more precisely what kind of quiz the student has in mind, and if she can give an example of a question. This can be seen as an attempt to work out the above issue. By responding to the teacher through giving a suggestion, Ruth starts by referring not to the quiz content, but to the way in which it should be answered:

Here (Fig. 12.5), Ruth elaborates on the sort of participation a quiz question should imply: (1) some (i.e., "us" who are "regulars here" and "can explain more") should have to explain more and elaborate, (2) the question should be easier for the friends to answer, and (3) there should be cooperation, implying that there should be teams answering the quiz. Next, the teacher suggests a procedure for enacting

1	Ruth:	[(strong nod) OK. ONE TO THREE_OF_US KNOW SIGN LANGUAGE: (gaze up) WELL: EXPLAIN IN SIGN LANGUAGE WHAT (gaze side):- BOTH- BOTH NOW, (gaze side) EXPLAIN WHAT- WHAT HAPPEN- (gaze side) WHAT SPECIAL WITH CHRISTMAS? ***Ok. Here is one for us who knows sign language, umh, well, explain in sign language what- umh, or for both- both now, uhm, explain what- what happens- uhm, what is special with christmas.***
2	Teacher:	(wave) EXAMPLE WELL (gaze up) WHY CELEBRATE CHRIST[MAS? EXAMPLE ONE QUESTION?:: ***Umh, for example, well uhm, why do we celebrate christm[as? Could that be an example of a question?***
3	Ruth:	[YES, BUT, SOME EXPLAIN MORE, MEANS THEY CAN EXPLAIN MUCH, THREE_OF_US REGULARS HERE, BUT LITTLE EASIER TO FRIENDS, AND TOGETHER^WORK TOO. ***Yes, but, some have to explain more, it means those who can explain a lot, that would be us who are here regularly, but it should be a little easier to the friends, and we should also be able to collaborate.***
4	Teacher:	YES, YOU CAN FOR_INSTANCE- IF I MAKE QUIZ I: QUESTIONS, FOR_IN STANCE RUTH PLUS YOUR FRIEND DISCUSS SPEAK+(oral) FIRST DISCUSS SPEAK+(oral), AFTER RUTH ANSWER+(back) WITH [SIGNS, AFTER:? OK. POSSIBLE. ***Yes, you can, for instance if I make the quiz, I'll do it, with th[e questions, and for instance Ruth and your friend have a discussion and speak orally with each other, first discuss, speaking orally, and then Ruth returns the answer by signing, afterwards:? Ok, that's possible.***
5	Ruth:	[YES. ***Yes.***

Fig. 12.5 Securing balanced participation

the quiz. The teacher should be responsible for making the quiz and asking the questions—in the "virtual space" (Keating 2008). Further, the two students at each end—in "real space" (Keating 2008)—exemplified here by Ruth and her friend, should discuss among themselves, using primarily audiologically oriented practices (i.e. spoken language). When they have arrived at an answer, the signing student (Ruth) should respond, using primarily visually oriented practices (i.e. signed language).

The teacher not only distributes the responsibilities of who should answer, but also distributes each of the systems for primary modality orientation (i.e., spoken and signed language) onto the specific sequential parts of the quiz. This also secures balanced participation for each category of student, as both have a "home" space in which to fully master the means and skills of participation (and ability to participate). However, one is embedded within the other as the "game" master (teacher) is only available through the visually oriented virtual space. Thus, a solution is offered to Gail's contestation in Sect. 12.3.3.2.

12.3.3.4 Introducing Friends in Visually Oriented Virtual Space

When it is time for Tina to give her prepared suggestion of what to do when the friends are invited, she proposes that the friends present themselves using signs (Fig. 12.6).

Tina suggests that the friends do something that is easy to perform and learn—for example, fingerspelling and/or learning their name-signs or the sign for the place they come from, and telling their age. This proposal gives the invited friends a chance to present themselves using signs and specifies how they should participate, taking turns presenting themselves in the visually oriented virtual space—or, if you like, the virtual Deaf space (cf. Gulliver and Kitzel 2015). The teacher also indicates that this will be done at the beginning of the lesson (before the quiz); thereby, she is planning the organization of the whole lesson.

1	Tina:	OK, I PROPOSE THAT CAN TELL NAME IS, AND BORN WHERE, AND HOW OLD LIKE, WITH SIGNS. ***Ok, I propose that they can tell their names, and where they're born, and how old they are, using signs***	
2	Teacher:	(wave) THEY TRY SIGN TELL LITTLE, IN BEGINNING ⌐YOU+pl GET_TO_KNOW THEM, OK, GOOD PROPOSAL ***So, they will try to use signs and to tell a little, in the beginning, so you can get to know them, ok, that was a good proposal***	
3	Tina:	YES. ***yes***	└YES. ***yes***

Fig. 12.6 Proposing how to introduce friends

12.3.3.5 Telling a Shared Narrative

After all of the students have given their prepared proposals for what to do when the friends from class join them, the teacher asks what else the friends should (be able to) speak about. In the following extract, Ruth expands on this.

Ruth explicitly brings forward a focus on the friendship category (i.e., the joint category comprising them all) and thereby highlights not their difference, but their sameness. As friends, they have a shared history and a potential shared narrative. Telling this narrative can stabilize their friendship and also legitimize the invitation and their presence in the visually oriented virtual space. It also focuses on the interactional work needed to fill and stabilize the creation of a category we might call “friend of deaf.” Here, it is seemingly foremost the identities of the friends that are addressed; indirectly, this also reflects on the students’ own identities, because a story of how they got to know their friend is also a story about each of them.

12.3.3.6 Technology-Positioned Relation

In the previous extract (Fig. 12.7), Ruth takes the technological configuration into account when forming her utterance, in a way that involves both the material possibilities and the actions afforded. Embedded through I BRING FRIEND NEXT TIME, by a point (PT, translated “she”), Ruth assigns a particular location to her friend. This is a common practice for talking about non-present referents in signed language talk; however, through the very specific way in which Ruth performs this point, she places her friend beside herself within the frame shaped by the technology (i.e., showing where her friend will be seated when she speaks about how she knows Ruth and how they met). In this way, Ruth anticipates or imagines how they will be physically seated in relation to both the technology and each other.

1 Ruth TELL WHAT LIKE DO, WHAT::- HOW THEY GET-TO-KNOW FRIEND LIKE,
I BRING FRIEND NEXT TIME, PT TELL WHY PT GET-TO-KNOW ME LIKE,
HOW TWO MEET LIKE WHAT.
They should tell about what they like to do, wha:t(.)- how they came to know their friend and such, I’m going to bring a friend next time, and she will then tell about why she got to know me and such, how the two of us met and such.

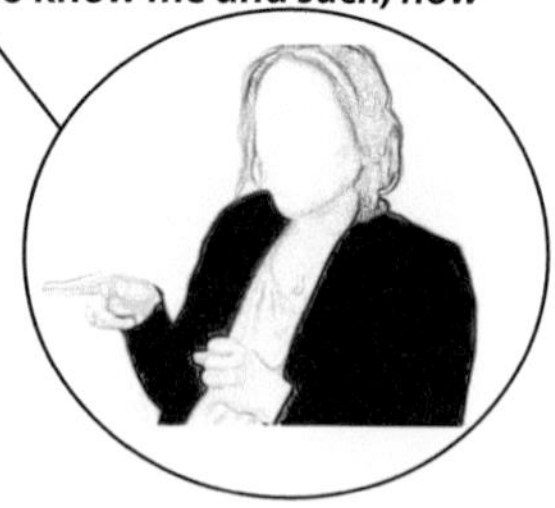

Fig. 12.7 Telling a shared narrative

Moving on, Ruth questions the extent to which their friends know signed language. None of the others' friends know many signs, and, consequentially, Ruth suggests that they give the visiting friend an assignment—to learn some basic signs in preparation for the visit. The teacher adds that she thinks this is a good idea, and that they should practice together and tutor their friend in order to prepare for the visit. They agree that this will make the following lesson more fun. However, in retrospect, this probably also put the signing students in a new position vis-à-vis their friends, compared to what they were used to in the mainstreamed setting. By giving their non-signing friends homework and tutoring them, the students allowed for new patterns of participation (positioning themselves as skilled tutors) that increased the shared repertoire of resources for interacting and sustaining their friendship.

12.3.3.7 What Will They Learn?

In the final extract of this section (Fig. 12.8), Ruth asks what the others think the invited friends will learn from the lesson (the removal of 48 s was due to technical difficulties that left Ruth out of the rest of this sequence).

Gail's answer is expressed with a smiling face, which is further supported by the sign choice CRAM and the manner in which it is performed, indicating that this is a desired result and perhaps even a longed-for situation—their friends will *have to* learn and use signs. The teacher clearly responds to Gail's enthusiasm in line 3. Gail's answer also indicates that after working out this preparation for the invitation, she seems able to envision that this might actually work (compare with Fig. 12.4 in Sect. 12.3.3.2). Tina, in line 6, suggests that this will bring about a situation that will allow the hearing friend to meet and identify with others who are similar to them. Further, in line 7, Tina highlights that this will give the friends the opportunity to meet deaf students as a collective—which perhaps the friends from class will have never experienced. This is an important point for identity building, as it allows the deaf students to present aspects of themselves that their friends have never seen. In this way, the friends get to learn (some) of what it is like to be deaf. The term "deaf," as used by Tina and the teacher, is not about loss of hearing; rather, it confirms "deaf" as a cultural identity category.

12.3.4 The Successful Lesson

The suggested participation frameworks that were collaboratively worked out proceed just as the students and teacher foresaw in their planning, implying that they managed to organize and coordinate the activities in order to create the desired effect and maintain the focus of the activity. Thus, the lack of shared resources for participation does not disturb the main focus of the activity—having fun with friends across primary modality orientation.

1 Ruth: WHAT THINK TWO-OF-YOU, FRIEND TWO-OF-YOU LEARN FROM LESSON?
What do you think, your friends will learn from the lesson?

((approx. 48 sec. taken out))

2 Gail: THEY MUST CRAM SIGN LANGUAGE.
That they have to cram sign language.

3 Teacher: YES, THEY LEARN SI[GN LANGUAGE YES, TOPS[:
Yes, they learn sign language, yes, great.

4 Gail: [TOPS. [(nod)(smile)

5 Teacher: TINA, PT
Tina?

6 Tina: LEARN- *TEACH* SEE- LEARN SEE SIGN LANGUAGE AND (.) MEET FRIEND- KNOW MORE ABOUT FRIENDSHIP, [MEET EACH_OTHER (so) KNOW WHO THEIR FRIEND, SUCH.
They learn- *learn* from see- learn from seeing sign language and (.) get to meet friend- so they know more about friendship, get to meet each other, so they know who their friends are, and such.

((approx. 14 sec. taken out))

7 Tina: AND MEET (collective) MORE [DEAF: DEAF.
And they meet as a collective, more deaf, deaf.

8 Teacher: LEARN HOW DEAF, [THINK YOU?
They get to learn what it's like to be deaf, you mean?

9 Tina: [(nods)

10 Teacher: YES, GOOD.
Yes, good.

Fig. 12.8 What the friends will learn

When the students log on at various times, they sit side-by-side within the frame created by the camera angle (see Fig. 12.9). Initially, there is some waving across the VME or the "virtual space," but most of the interaction in the beginning is conducted in "real space" (Keating 2008) at each end. The students can be seen to talk (primarily orally) about what they observe on-screen, visible at the other ends through the mouth movements and the quick and continuous gazing back and forth between each other and the screen. The students also use occasional gestures and sometimes copy other students at the other end of the VME. The guest students are seen to practice fingerspelling their names and to repeat signs they have learned beforehand, while being guided by the signing-skilled students. This primarily dyadic interaction seems to work fine, representing a communication (participation) framework that deaf students typically manage better than multi-party (oral) settings. The fact that the technology does not transmit sound makes the local setting

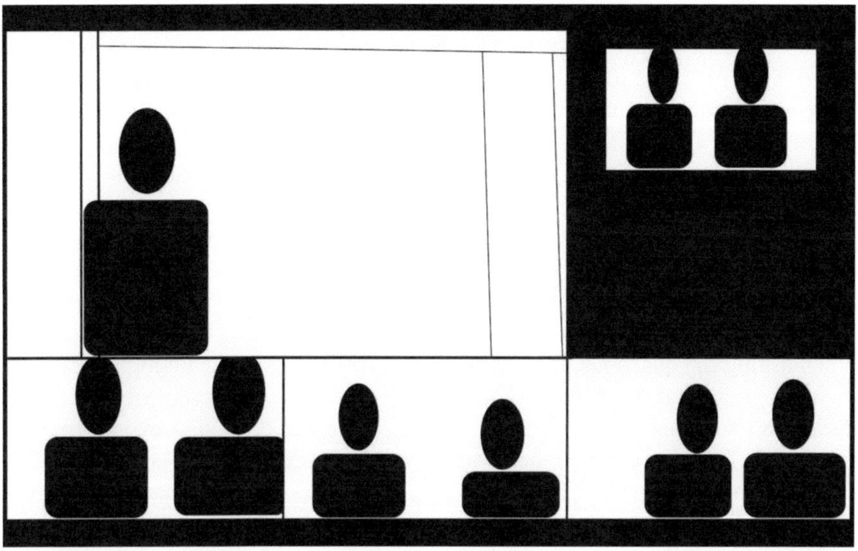

Fig. 12.9 Students' seating in virtual space

much more controllable and easy to cope with in the "real space" at each end, preventing it to develop into spoken multi-party interaction (cf. Keating and Mirus 2003, p. 123). In the "real space" at each local school, the orientation to the visual activity on-screen is embedded within a primarily audiologically oriented participation framework. This dyadic interaction is, on the other hand, embedded within the larger coordinated activity within the visually oriented participation of the virtual space—which is, in large part, mediated and coordinated by the student with signing skills.

The lesson is divided into well defined phases that are framed and enacted by the teacher. The teacher only initiates the start of the actual "lesson" after approximately 10 min. The teacher starts by reminding everyone of the importance of keeping focus on the joint activity on the screen. The lesson begins with a presentation round. Each of the signing students interprets the teacher's instructions (i.e., framings of the upcoming activity) to the visiting friend. The task is for the friend to say in signed language what his or her name is—first in sign, then by fingerspelling the name. Then the teacher writes the name on the whiteboard. This is an example of "local chaining"—a way of linking through presenting the same content in various modalities, sequentially (e.g. fingerspelling, signing, and writing)—a much documented practice in deaf education (e.g., Bagga-Gupta 2002). Occasionally, the signing student turns and helps the friend and tutors her (or him). While one student is presenting, other students simultaneously talk and comment on what is going on online. Since the sound is turned off (and the activity is so well defined), this does not disturb the presenting student. In this phase of the lesson, the teacher is the only one engaged in the main activity at all times.

After approximately 10 min, the teacher frames a new task. The task is for the signing students to take turns telling why and how they became friends with their non-signing friend. In this phase, the signing students add voice to the signing. (At one end, a local teacher/interpreter seems to help by interpreting what the signing students say). The teacher asks follow-up questions.

After another 10 min they start the prepared quiz. The teacher has set up the questions in a pre-made quiz template—a feature of the Whiteboard software. The teacher has prepared the questions in writing, and these are visible on the whiteboard so they can be read by the contestants.

All of the questions have four multiple choice answers in writing presented beneath them. Each choice is also marked with a letter: a, b, c, or d (see Fig. 12.10). When asking the questions, the teacher repeats the question, including the different answers, in signed language. The students have separate responsibilities when answering, and they must decide on an answer together (through mainly oral discussion) before raising their hand to signal they are ready to answer. Usually the guest answers, upon being called (i.e., addressed) with their name-sign by the teacher. The called guest answers by showing the handshape corresponding to the letter in front of the right answer. The participation framework and the firm procedures for anticipated actions likely give the visiting guests a sense of being part of complicated visual interaction across the virtual space.

The quiz takes approximately 15 min to finish. After congratulating the winners, the teacher invites the friends to return on a later occasion, on the condition that they learn more signs and practice more. During the lesson, the students are seen to smile a lot, make jokes, and obviously have a good time—just being friends having fun in class.

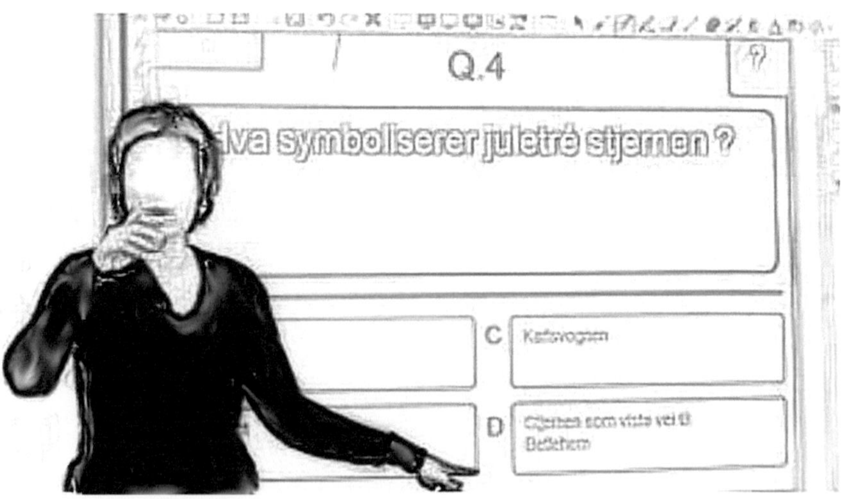

Fig. 12.10 The teacher coordinating the students' answers

12.4 Summary

Summarizing the findings, I first found that the data contained various reports that told a story of the "friendship" teaching plan as a success.

- The "friendship" teaching plan had an effect on the students in their local school. This effect reportedly changed the typical ways in which the students participated in activities with their peers, suggesting a close connection between who they were (or could be) for others and the organization of participation.
- Inviting friends to the VME improved the deaf students' opportunities for making themselves known (*by på seg selv*).

Observations show that the technological configuration was significant for the way in which participation was typically organized in the VME—an ecology that constrains but also enables new participatory possibilities—influencing the interactionally accomplished identity negotiations.

- The videoconferencing technology, through its design, was not initially made for video-*only*-mediated communication.
- With muted microphones, the technology was re-configured as a stabile visually oriented space, re-distributing the responsibility for putting all seeing participants on an equal footing, making participants' hearing abilities irrelevant for joint attention and the coordination of activities, and instead highlighting participation skills in this environment.
- The teachers chose and adjusted teaching formats to fit the affordances and purpose of the VME. Tasks were chosen that favored peer interaction and peer learning, which are vulnerable areas for many mainstreamed deaf students.
- Familiarity with the designs, templates, and teaching formats stabilized participation. However, learning how to participate in this environment implied becoming able to perceive the affordances and actively employ these to cooperatively design and adjust participation frameworks. This allowed for the non-conflictual intersecting identity position of "friend" across different systems for primary modality orientation.

Summarizing some of the identity negotiations accomplished by the students while they were cooperatively accomplishing the task given by the teacher, it was shown that:

- Being allowed to influence the content as well as the procedure of the upcoming lesson, the students suggested participation frameworks (a quiz, a shared narrative, presentation rounds) of relatively known formats and simultaneously established categories based on participation ability (skills level), rather than *dis*-ability.
- The proposals were contested, negotiated, and sorted out (based on the students' own experiences and imaginings of what their friends would enjoy), which drove the arrangement of participation details further. Thereby, they managed a possible de-stabilization of the chosen activity design.

- Stabile participation was secured through cooperatively working out a procedure that dealt with who would do what and in what order in the various planned tasks—for instance through assigning and distributing the various actions (steps in the procedure) of different primary modality orientation to sequences.
- The technological configuration was taken into account when the students formed their utterances and imagined how their friends would act/participate within the VME.
- Giving the visiting friends an assignment (homework) in connection to the visit (to learn some basic signs in preparation) put the signing students in a new position vis-à-vis their friends that allowed for new patterns of participation in the mainstreamed setting outside the VME (e.g., via a tutor role). This increased the shared repertoire of resources for interacting and sustaining the friendship.
- The hearing friends got to experience what it was like to have to learn signed language in order to participate (while having fun doing it). Further, they found themselves in a similar situation as the other hearing friends of the other signing students (also new to the setting). Finally, they got to meet their deaf friend as a member of a collective, allowing the deaf friend to self-present in ways that were new to the hearing friend.
- Seeing the cooperatively crafted (successful) lesson in light of the preparation allows us to see a lesson in which the participants filled their part by coping with the actions that were expected of them, while the mediating technology evaporated into the background (as a stabilized environment). The students and friends were apparently having a good time, just being friends having fun in class.

12.5 Conclusion

Based on the findings, several implications for identity development, the role of technology, and inclusive education emerge.

Identity is accomplished in mundane everyday situated interactions. This chapter has entertained the idea that situated interactions in various environments stabilize certain identities and de-stabilize others. Participation in part-time education and a distance education program with other signing students can foster the development of a positive identity. However, when one is the only signing deaf student in a non-signing mainstream classroom, the meaning of deaf is not easily communicated, negotiated, or even allowed space, and this makes it difficult for deaf students to fully make themselves known. Meeting deaf students as a collective in a VME, on the other hand, provides non-signing friends the opportunity to glimpse who their signing friends are in the company of other signing friends. In the friendship exercise, the identity of "deaf" was re-negotiated (e.g., with the identities of "expert," "leader," and "skillful") in quite extraordinary ways. This was a reversal of the role of "disadvantaged"—instead of "hearing loss" (in the case of the deaf students), there was "visual understanding loss" (in the case of the hearing students). A deaf world was created for the hearing students to enter and experience, and they loved it.

For this to happen, the findings imply that it is a prerequisite for these students to be able to develop signing skills and positive identities in a "segregated" environment in the company of other signed language learning students. In this chapter, it has been shown that a quiz friendship game contributed to bridging the gap between deaf and hearing students. The deaf students were very active in bridging this divide, and the teacher created an environment that was supportive to both deaf and hearing students. Application of the term "inclusive" to mainstream classrooms is supposed to mean that the activities and classroom practices are adapted in such a way that all students can participate on their own premises. This chapter questions whether full participation on equal footing in joint activities in a mainstream classroom is possible in cases where there is only one deaf student and largely unshared sociolinguistic practices and participation frameworks that do not favor visually oriented ways of communicating. However, this chapter has demonstrated that if great care is taken in crafting activities and tasks and their participation frameworks—that is, in ways that work against the identity of "disability"—participants might successfully foster positive identities as students and future members of Norwegian society *and* the signing deaf community.

Through the cooperative crafting of the successful organization of participation, the significant role played by the technology for identity (or who the participants were allowed to be for each other) became foregrounded. Demonstrating how the specific organization of participation is sustained by simultaneous co-occurring influences—such as the design of the mediating technology, the choice of templates for displaying participants, and the setup of teaching formats—reveals the dynamic, changing, and complex ways in which identity negotiations were accomplished by the participants in this VME. It was not the technology, but the ways in which the technology was exploited that made this lesson a success.

References

Akrich, M. (1992). The de-scription of technical objects. In W. E. Bijker & J. Law (Eds.), *Shaping technology/building society: Studies in sociotechnical change* (pp. 205–224). Cambridge, MA: MIT Press.

Bagga-Gupta, S. (2002). Explorations in bilingual instructional interaction: A sociocultural perspective on literacy. *Learning and Instruction, 12*(5), 557–587. doi:10.1016/S0959-4752(01)00032-9

Bagga-Gupta, S. (2004). Visually oriented language use: Discursive and technological resources in Swedish deaf pedagogical arenas. In M. Van Herreweghe & M. Vermeerbergen (Eds.), *To the Lexicon and Beyond: Sociolinguistics in European deaf communities* (pp. 171–207). Washington D.C.: Gallaudet University Press.

Bagga-Gupta, S., & Holmström, I. (2015). Language, identity and technologies in classrooms for the differently-abled. *Journal of Communication Disorders, Deaf Studies & Hearing Aids, 3* (4). doi:10.4172/2375-4427.1000145

Bauman, H.-D. L. (2008). *Open your eyes: Deaf studies talking*. Minneapolis: University of Minnesota Press.

Bauman, H.-D. L., & Murray, J. J. (2010). Deaf studies in the 21st century: "Deaf-gain" and the future of human diversity. In M. Marschark & P. E. Spencer (Eds.), *The Oxford handbook of deaf studies, language, and education* (Vol. 2, pp 210–225). Oxford University Press.

Bucholtz, M., & Hall, K. (2005). Identity and interaction: A sociocultural linguistic approach. *Discourse Studies, 7*(4–5), 585–614. doi:10.1177/1461445605054407

Butler, J. (1999). *Gender trouble: Feminism and the subversion of identity*. New York: Routledge.

Erting, C. J., & Kuntze, M. (2008). Language socialization in deaf communities. In N. H. Hornberger (Ed.), *Encyclopedia of language and education* (pp. 2845–2858). New York: Springer.

Galåen, S. (2008). *"Hvem er det som eier en sannhet?": Rådgiveres vektlegging i arbeid med foreldre til barn med cochleaimplantat ["Who owns a truth?": Counsellors' emphasize when working with parents of children with cochlear implants*]. (M.A. thesis). Oslo: University of Oslo.

Gibson, J. J. (1979). The theory of affordances. In J. J. Gibson (Ed.), *The ecological approach to visual perception* (pp. 127–143). Boston: Houghton Mifflin.

Goffman, E. (1964). The neglected situation. *American Anthropologist, 66*(6), 133–136. doi:10.2307/668167

Goffman, E. (1981). Footing. In E. Goffman (Ed.), *Forms of talk* (pp. 124–159). Philadelphia: University of Pennsylvania Press.

Goodwin, C., & Goodwin, M. H. (2004). Participation. In A. Duranti (Ed.), *A companion to linguistic anthropology* (pp. 222–244). Malden, MA: Blackwell Publishing.

Gulliver, M., & Kitzel, M. B. (2015). Deaf geographies. In G. Gertz & P. Boudreault (Eds.), *The SAGE Deaf Studies Encyclopedia*. Sage Publications.

Haualand, H. M. (2012). *Interpreting ideals and relaying rights: A comparative study of video interpreting services in Norway, Sweden and the United States* (Vol. 2012:51). Oslo: Fafo.

Heath, C., Hindmarsh, J., & Luff, P. (2010). *Video in qualitative research: Analysing social interaction in everyday life*. London: Sage.

Holmström, I. (2013). *Learning by hearing?: Technological framings for participation* (Vol. 42). Örebro: Örebro Universitet.

Holmström, I., Bagga-Gupta, S., & Jonsson, R. (2015). Communicating and hand(ling) technologies. Everyday life in educational settings where pupils with cochlear implants are mainstreamed. *Journal of Linguistic Anthropology, 25*(3), 256–284. doi:10.1111/jola.12097

Keating, E. (2008). *Space shifting: New technologies, new opportunities*. Paper presented at the Texas Linguistic Forum, Austin.

Keating, E., & Mirus, G. (2003). Examining interactions across language modalities: Deaf children and hearing peers at school. *Anthropology & Education Quarterly, 34*(2), 115–135. doi:10.1525/aeq.2003.34.2.115

Kermit, P., Tharaldsteen, A. M., Haugen, G. M. D., & Wendelborg, C. (2014). En av flokken?: Inkludering og ungdom med sansetap—muligheter og begrensninger [One among many?: Inclusion and youth with sensory impairment—possibilites and limitations]. http://www.bufdir.no/global/nbbf/Funksjonsnedsettelse/En_av_flokken.pdf. Accessed May 22, 2016.

Kirkehei, I., Myrhaug, H. T., Garm, N., Simonsen, E., & Wie, O. B. (2011). Kommunikasjonsformer for barn med cochleaimplantat [Forms of communication for children with cochlear implants]. http://hdl.handle.net/10143/193108. Accessed May 22, 2016.

Latour, B. (2005). *Reassembling the social: An introduction to actor-network-theory*. Oxford: Oxford University Press.

McIlvenny, P., Broth, M., & Haddington, P. (2009). Communicating place, space and mobility. *Journal of Pragmatics, 41*(10), 1879–1886. doi:10.1016/j.pragma.2008.09.014

Mondada, L., & Doehler, S. P. (2004). Second language acquisition as situated practice: Task accomplishment in the French second language classroom. *The Modern Language Journal, 88* (4), 501–518. doi:10.2307/3588582

Norwegian Sign Language Curriculum. (2013). http://www.udir.no/globalassets/filer/lareplan/in-english/nor4-04_en_pr.doc. Accessed May 22, 2016.

Ohna, S. E. (2005). Researching classroom processes of inclusion and exclusion. *European Journal of Special Needs Education, 20*(2), 167–178. doi:10.1080/08856250500055651

Simonsen, E., Kristoffersen, A.-E., Hyde, M. B., & Hjulstad, O. (2009). Great expectations: Perspectives on cochlear implantation of deaf children in Norway. *American Annals of the Deaf, 154*(3), 263–273. doi:10.1353/aad.0.0103

Streeck, J., Goodwin, C., & LeBaron, C. D. (2011). *Embodied interaction: Language and body in the material world.* Cambridge: Cambridge University Press.

Streeck, J., & Mehus, S. (2005). Microethnography: The study of practices. In K. L. Fitch & R. E. Sanders (Eds.), *Handbook of language and social interaction* (pp. 381–404). Mahwah, NJ: Lawrence Erlbaum Associates.

UNESCO. (1994). Salamanca statement and framework for action on special needs education. http://www.inclusive-education.org/publications/salamanca-statement-and-framework-action-special-needs-education. Accessed May 22, 2016.

Valentine, G. (2007). Theorizing and researching intersectionality: A challenge for feminist geography. *The Professional Geographer, 59*(1), 10–21. doi:10.1111/j.1467-9272.2007.00587.x

Xie, Y.-H., Potměšil, M., & Peters, B. (2014). Children who are deaf or hard of hearing in inclusive educational settings: A literature review on interactions with peers. *Journal of Deaf Studies and Deaf Education, 19*(4), 423–437. doi:10.1093/deafed/enu017

Author Biography

Johan Hjulstad holds a Ph.D. in applied linguistics from the Norwegian University of Science and Technology, Trondheim, Norway. He currently works as Senior Adviser at Statped (the Norwegian national service for special needs education). His M.A. and Ph.D. research projects have focused on the use of communication technologies and signed language.

Chapter 13
"Janne X Was Here". Portraying Identities and Negotiating Being and Belonging in Informal Literacy Practices

Annaliina Gynne

13.1 Introduction

In contemporary societies of the global North, both physical and virtual settings offer participants, adolescents and others, different kinds of opportunities for what has often been called for *identity work*. Previous scholars have described this core "task" of human beings as *performing identities* (Butler 1990), *negotiating identities* (Pavlenko and Blackledge 2004), *portraying or staging linguistic identities* (Cekaite and Evaldsson 2008) or *writing oneself to being* (Boyd 2008) through participation in various activities. In the core of these activities where individual and group identifications are constantly crafted and portrayed, are *heteroglossic* practices of *languaging*. While heteroglossia here refers to the Bakhtinian notion highlighting the essential variability of all human communication, languaging refocuses scholarly interests towards social actions surrounding and originating from language rather than 'languages' as formal and stable constructions per se (cf. Bagga-Gupta 2014; Bakhtin 1981; Blommaert and Rampton 2011; García 2009).

In the study presented in this chapter, it is proposed that the investigation of people's ways-of-being-with-words—and in particular different representations of literacies—as everyday behaviours, offers a chance to discover human beings' identity work as well as their potentials in participating in social practices and altering them. A central site of investigation are various *writing spaces*, which can be defined as spaces in which a textually mediated world is formed and reformed through human (inter)action (cf. Barton and Lee 2013). In Northern late modern societies, these spaces can be found everywhere; in schools, homes, hospitals, social media and so on. Writing spaces may consist of paper or electronic forms, study books, mobile phones, signs, whiteboards or virtual platforms. Though diverse in their affordances and constraints, most of these spaces carry common

A. Gynne (✉)
School of Education, Culture and Communication, Mälardalen University, Västerås, Sweden
e-mail: annaliina.gynne@mdh.se

S. Bagga-Gupta et al. (eds.), *Identity Revisited and Reimagined*,
DOI 10.1007/978-3-319-58056-2_13

features that invite participants to engage in languaging, including literacies, through drawing on different linguistic and semiotic resources (languages, varieties, styles, genres, images, colours, to name a few).

In this study I analyse and discuss the ways in which aspects of communicative repertoires and modalities are related to portraying and negotiating identities (of both oneself and others) in literacy practices. The main aim of the study is thus to contribute to and expand understandings dealing with identity work in informal literacy practices taking place in so-called multilingual settings across the online-offline continuum. The central research questions are formulated as follows: First, the chapter explores *how "multilingual" young people engage in informal literacy practices in different writing spaces across the online-offline continuum.* Second, the chapter asks *in what ways are the young people's individual and group identifications performed, portrayed and negotiated in and through informal literacy practices.* Third and subsequently I want to discuss *in what ways does the identity work examined contribute to creating a sense of dis-/engagement and belonging among the young people.*

The present study is part of a larger project, DIMuL,[1] Doing Identity in and through Multilingual Literacy Practices, which explores young people's *"multilingual" literacy practices* as well as *social positioning* in everyday life. The project and its substudies operate at different scales: micro-interactional, meso activity levels as well as macro societal discourse levels (Gynne 2016; Gynne and Bagga-Gupta 2013, 2015; Gynne et al. 2016). Broadly, the project and the present study draw on sociocultural perspectives (cf. Säljö 2000; Vygotsky 1986; Wertsch 1991) on communication, identity and learning as theoretical and ethnographic perspectives (cf. Agar 1981; Wolcott 2008), including videotaping, photography and virtual ethnography as methodological points of departure.[2] Furthermore, commonalities between seemingly different kinds of writing spaces and human beings' engagements in and with them form the point of departure for the study presented in this chapter. Thus, the present chapter is anchored in theories that (i) highlight the social construction of reality, (ii) take a critical explorative stance towards essentialist accounts of human communication and formal glossed concepts such as bi- and multilingualism (thus refocusing on heteroglossia), and (iii) underline human beings' active participation in (re)shaping their lives through languaging (Bagga-Gupta 2014; Linell 2009; Säljö 2000).

Earlier scholarly critique (see e.g. Barton 2007; Bruce and Bishop 2008; Lankshear and Knobel 2006; Lotherington and Ronda 2011) has highlighted the fact that formal learning today at times provides limited opportunities for participants. Learning of skills and concepts occurs often isolated from everyday life,

---

[1]DIMuL is a part of the Swedish National Research School *LIMCUL*, Young People's Literacies, Multilingualism and Cultural Practice in Everyday Society. The research school is supported by the Swedish Research Council.

[2]More detailed aspects of both the theoretical framework and ethnographic fieldwork are accounted for in previous and forthcoming writings (Gynne 2016; Bagga-Gupta, Messina Dahlberg and Gynne, forthcoming).

avoiding the aesthetic, moral, ethical, political, or even pleasurable dimensions of participating in the world through the medium of literacy. When considering literacies as a subset of languaging and as such as an intrinsic part of living and acting in the world, rather than skills only to be acquired in the classroom, the present study conjoins this critical vein of studies. It is an attempt to focus attention to how individuals' locally and temporarily emerging identities in literacy practices in different spaces can be explored. From this analytical point of departure, it is argued that examining young people's ways-of-being-with-words and identity work across time and space (Bagga-Gupta 2014; Gynne and Bagga-Gupta 2015) has the potential to deepen our understanding of the connections between school-related practices and communities and social life outside school contexts.

Empirically, the present study is located in two different but interconnected settings; formal education and informal virtual contexts. Both settings offer their participants and users many opportunities for partaking in social action in meaningful ways—and more importantly, function as spaces where identity work through individuals' agency, constantly crafted and negotiated, (Bakhtin 1981; Wertsch et al. 1993) can be considered as a matter of interest. Through presenting analyses of the ways in which the subjects express themselves, communicate and interact with available (linguistic and multimodal) resources and with other participants, this chapter seeks to focus attention to individuals' identity work as it emerges through their agency both locally and temporarily in different writing spaces.

The chapter is organised as follows: Sect. 13.2 sets out the conceptual and theoretical framework used, with a focus on the sociocultural approach to living and learning in the world, and the concepts of languaging, identity and space. In the following section, the outline of the study, its setting, participants and data as well as methods are presented. Section 13.4 presents the empirical findings and analyses with a focus on identity work in different kinds of writing spaces both in and out-of-school settings. The final section discusses the central findings arising from the analyses, including conclusive reflections.

13.2 Theorising Languaging, Identity-as-Agency and Space

The central interest of this chapter is human beings' active involvement in (re) shaping their reality through the means of languaging while they participate in literacy practices. This involvement can also be described as *agency*, through which people can resist, negotiate and put forth different facets of their identities. Simultaneously, even if individuals are accorded agency for their actions, it is here proposed that there remains a social and mediated quality to all higher psychological processes, such as writing and reading (Vygotsky 1978). In this sense, and pertaining to the sociocultural approach, languaging, including literacies, is seen as a socially embedded activity, and identities are considered as locally meaningful within the specific contexts in which they emerge and are crafted. Conjointly, the investigation of sociocultural perspectives on communication, literacies and identities entails taking a stance in which interaction and collaboration between individuals, practices and artefacts/technologies—that is, physical and cognitive resources—are seen as core aspects of human development and learning (Säljö 2000).

In line with the sociocultural approach, the present study draws on a view of language that considers how it functions in the construction of meaning in different social and cultural contexts. The focus here is on *languaging* rather than language (cf. Møller and Jørgensen 2009). This epistemological and conceptual shift leads us towards focusing on the agency of individuals engaged in using, creating and interpreting signs and resources in situated actions, making the social aspects of languaging and people as *languagers* central. Furthermore, literacies are seen as central elements of languaging as well as practices in their own right (cf. Gynne and Bagga-Gupta 2015). Specifically, I take a view of literacies "as situated practices embedded in relations of culture and power in specific contexts" (Prinsloo and Baynham 2008: 2). Moreover, literacy practices entail common patterns of using reading and writing in particular situations where people bring their cultural knowledge to an activity of some kind (Barton and Lee 2013: 12). Consequently, these practices are about the interaction of the written and the spoken, where texts, and talk about texts, make out central mediational means that individuals operate with in different spaces. Furthermore, texts are not viewed as neutral artefacts but as elements that construct and reproduce particular views of the world and influence social interaction (Creese et al. 2008).

This chapter draws on a perspective that refocuses the concept of communication around the multiplicity and interconnectedness of different linguistic and semiotic resources in human interaction. Empirically, literacy practices in different writing spaces are scrutinised. These practices can be considered informal, unofficial (see Maybin 2007), extra-curricular, or self-chosen (see e.g. Björkvall and Engblom 2010). A few of them can be described as non-institutional activities in institutional settings, while others are non-institutional and informal. What is common for them is that they arise from the needs, interests and agendas of the participants themselves. There is a well-grounded body of recent studies that have focused on literacy practices and identity in either classroom settings (Chang 2013; Lytra 2011) or in virtual media sites (Barton and Lee 2013; Livingstone 2008). Moreover, the learning potential of informal literacy activities in formal educational settings has been previously explored by e.g. Björkvall and Engblom (2010) and Maybin (2007). These authors illustrate the importance of self-chosen and unofficial literacy activities for learning in institutional milieu in a way that resembles some of the empirical examples highlighted in the present study. Among contemporary studies investigating spatial perspectives on digital literacy practices in schools, Burnett (2014) can be noted. There exists, however, a relative dearth of knowledge regarding young people's languaging and identity work in practices that stretch across the offline–online continuum. An exception here is Lee (2011), who has empirically illustrated the interplay of "conventional" and "new" literacies in her work.

Within sociocultural studies, *agency* is seen from a perspective that highlights the "extension beyond the skins of individuals" (Wertsch et al. 1993: 343) and it is considered not simply an individual character trait or an activity, but a contextually enacted way of being in the world and doing identity work (van Lier 2008). According to this line of thought, agency is seen as (1) attributable to both individuals and groups, (2) an attribute of individual(s)-operating-with-mediational-means such as language, symbols and artifacts. Agency is thus socially distributed or shared, as well as socioculturally situated because the mediational means employed are "provided and constrained by cultural, historical and institutional contexts" (Wertsch et al. 1993: 352). In the present study, I concur to this view as it highlights continuous, situated and relational aspects of human actions and identity positionings. Moreover, I understand agency, identities and social structures as mutually constitutive, ever evolving and shaping. The reciprocal relationship between identity work and agency is further emphasised through the fact that identity positionings, in turn, can be considered kinds of social action that agency can accomplish (Bucholtz and Hall 2005).

As pointed out by Wertsch et al. (1993: 345), mediational means, such as signs and tools, have fundamental involvement in shaping human agency, as well as creating and maintaining spaces and contexts culturally, historically and institutionally. van Lier (2008) highlights the challenges of empirically locating and analysing agency and suggests relocating the concept of agency as behavior—something that people "do"—rather than a property one owns. This is also in line with focusing on language as "languaging" and taking an explorative, critical stance towards glossed concepts such as "bi/multilingualism". The frameworks of *identity-as-agency* and languaging can be anchored together with the help of the notion of *space*. Spaces, diverging from the geographically constituted and defined places, are socially constructed and reconstructed, products of human activity, a deeply social phenomenon, that in addition are anchored in and by temporal aspects, sometimes named TimeSpace (Lefebvre 1974). Their boundaries are thus seldom clearly marked—rather, most spaces are in a constant state of flux as human beings as creators and co-creators move in and out of them. The concept of space can be examined from a number of different viewpoints, of which a literacy perspective is particularly relevant here. As noted in the introduction of this chapter, Barton and Lee (2013) suggest that literacy practices and people act within "a *textually mediated social world* utilising the *writing spaces* available (2013: 23, italics in original). In a related line of thought, Kress (2003: 34) points out that the logics of spaces affect the logics and meanings of writing (and reading). From this perspective I note that the potentials of these logics are what shape the forms and meanings of literacy practices that people actively contribute to. Both school classrooms and virtual worlds facilitated by the Internet can give rise to writing spaces that can be considered both communicative and discursive, allowing for different types of practices in those particular settings.

In the present chapter, both IRL and virtual writing spaces and human beings' interaction in and with them are deemed particularly interesting in terms of identity work and languaging for participants with access to *multiple linguistic and semiotic resources*. The kinds of cultural tools available in the 21st century classrooms and social media are varied, but what is most often common for them in is that they are permeated with texts, icons and images. It has sometimes been claimed that social networking systems provided by digital communication are ideal for promoting both individuals' identity work and "multilingualism". For instance, previous studies of people's ways-with-words suggest that participation in so-called Web 2.0[3] offers users greater opportunities for interaction and exchange in ways where multiple semiotic resources are employed, both within single communicative discourses and across them (cf. Ivkovic and Lotherington 2009; Livingstone 2008).

13.3 The Study

13.3.1 The Setting and the Participants

The participants of the study presented in this chapter consist of five young people, both boys and girls, between 11 and 13 years of age, who live in the geopolitical space of Sweden and come from so-called multilingual and multicultural backgrounds in terms of their heritage. At least one of each of the participants' parents is of Finnish origin and most of them come from predominantly multilingual (often Swedish-Finnish, Swedish-Finnish-Spanish/Greek/Persian and so on) home settings. During the time of the fieldwork in project DIMuL, the participants belonged to a group of 18 students, "Class 5/6 C", in a school that has an official "bilingual-bicultural" Swedish–Finnish profile. This meant that the school provided bilingual instruction across the curriculum in grades 1–9 and catered to the educational needs of Sweden's largest linguistic minority, Sweden Finns. In formal policy of the school as well as classroom practice, Swedish and Finnish were the dominant linguistic varieties, expected to be used by the participants. Apart from being students in this formally bilingual-bicultural educational setting, many of the young people were also active users of a popular social networking site, Facebook. Facebook was originally founded in 2004 and makes out today (2017) the world's largest social network site with more than 1 billion monthly active users (www.facebook.com). It is structured around user profiles and exhibits a sample of online spaces where people can post status updates, share photos and videos, play online games, send messages and comment on these, building intertextual links between texts and resources available online—and offline (Barton and Lee 2013).

[3]Web 2.0 is a term which describes web-based applications that emphasize user-generated content, social networking and interactivity through the written word and other multimodal content.

The study included two phases. The first part was conducted in the institutional educational setting, focusing on informal literacy practices, and the second part in a social media setting provided by Facebook. Despite their formal separateness, the research sites investigated were interconnected as events, people and practices present on Facebook were present and discussed in the school and vice versa (cf. Gynne, forthcoming). What followed from the participants' engagement in these two settings is that they are here represented as language and literacy users, "languagers" in both environments.

13.3.2 Research Design, Data Sets and Analytic Methods

The present study is based on ethnographic fieldwork, conducted during a 20-month period in 2010–2011. In the study, young people's engagements in languaging and identity work in informal literacy practices are investigated through the analysis of various kinds of data, created in two empirical settings as described above. The combination of different materials and methods—data and methodological triangulation—was employed in order to better map out and discuss the richness and complexity of languaging and identity work in literacy practices that the young people engage in. Through employing (n)ethnographic methods I had the possibility of building an understanding of the participants' uses of different kinds of resources for meaning-making and identity work in their embedded contexts.

The first data set, created during the academic year of 2010–2011, consists of photos and video recordings of the participants' activities in writing spaces related to the school setting. The scrutiny here focuses on young people's informal literacy activities during the school day, within the school setting—but outside the institutional educational agenda. In the selection of these data, the focus was on events and practices where the interplay of different linguistic varieties and modalities comes to life in informal literacy practices within the formal educational setting and where issues of identification were portrayed and negotiated. From a video/photo and field note corpus of approximately 50 instances where these kinds of practices could be observed, two data extracts have been chosen for analysis.

The second data set consists of a data corpus created on the social network site Facebook during a period of (n)ethnographic fieldwork in 2010–2011. This corpus as a whole focuses on posted status updates, both text and images, on the social networking site. From a wider database created through the method of screen grabbing, a data set of 25 photo updates, related to what can be defined as "multilingual-multimodal" identity work, was deemed as particularly interesting for the present study. From this data set, one empirical example and an extract from the discussion thread following it has been chosen for analysis.

In the analysis of both sets of data, a discourse analytical approach has been adopted in order to represent and discuss the different aspects of communicative repertoires and modalities related in doing identity work across time and space in the studied literacy practices. In this analysis, two different analytical extensions have been employed in the process of analysing the data. They comprise a visual analysis, a mapping of linguistic and semiotic resources in each particular data set, followed by a discourse analytical procedure that considers the elements of (inter) action, and the interplay of actors, resources and actions represented in data sets and the practices relating to them. Furthermore, all data sets have been re-examined through taking account of the wider social context in which the actions were taking place. In the latter, ethnographic data originating from participant observations in and around classroom and social networking media environments has been particularly useful in fulfilling the analytical task.

13.4 Doing Being in Different Writing Spaces

In this section, young people's engagement in identity work and literacy practices in writing spaces within a "bilingual" school classroom and a "multilingual" social media site are taken into scrutiny. Differing somewhat from each other in terms of their affordances and functions for users, these spaces provide an ample area for study of the kind of identity work and languaging where the interplay of different communicative repertoires and modalities becomes central. As will be illustrated by the analyses, it is in these spaces that the participants employ different kinds of semiotic resources in order to portray and negotiate individual and collective identity positionings (cf. Creese et al. 2008).

13.4.1 Identity Work and Informal Literacy Practices in Institutional Writing Spaces

The first empirical example illustrates identity work and literacy-related languaging taking place in classroom environment during a recess. The writing space focused here is the whiteboard, which is habitually seen as a tool assigned to the pedagogical staff.

Figure 13.1 illustrates a screen grab from a video recording of an activity occurring at the whiteboard, situated at the front of the class[4] and filled with both hand-written and printed texts. Typically, this is a space and a tool that the teachers claim ownership of, as it is physically located in the space that they commonly use. Consequently, most of the texts appearing in this space are provided by the teachers, conveying institutional information that the students are commonly seen as recipients of. The coloured areas in Fig. 13.1; blue for Finnish, yellow for Swedish and black for English, illustrate different linguistic varieties emerging in the space and underscore the formal bilingualism as well as the presence of the

[4]See Appendix for an illustration of the classroom space.

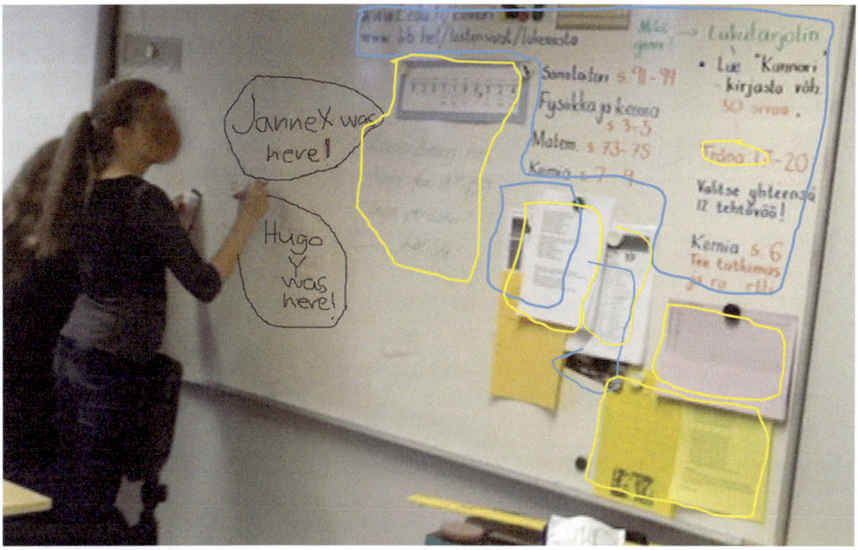

Fig. 13.1 Whiteboard as a space for identity work and languaging

teachers in the classroom despite the absence of their physical bodies. These include (Finnish) hand-written names of subject matters, combined with page numbers in study books, indicating the current matter to study. A number of the many printed documents attached to the whiteboard entail institutional "official" information which is provided in Swedish. Apart from these, two hand-written Internet addresses, referring to Finnish-language educational sites are at the top middle part of the whiteboard.

In this instance, recorded at the beginning of a lesson prior to teacher arriving at the room, two of the students in the class, Iris and Sofia,[5] have taken over the whiteboard and use it for their own purposes, an initiative that entails a sense of autonomy and agency in relation to this writing space. Both girls draw and write silently on the whiteboard, keeping an eye on the classroom door. It is here that Sofia scribbles her fellow (male) students' names on the whiteboard: "Janne X was here!" and "Hugo Y was here!", performing a "speaking personality" (Bakhtin 1981) and employing a voice that speaks with and to an audience of others—her classmates in the classroom as well as the other texts on the whiteboard. When doing so, Sofia's agentive actions also contribute to making the classroom a *heteroglossic* space—which goes beyond the formal Swedish-Finnish bilingualism adopted by the school as an institution. More importantly, the activity represented in Fig. 13.1 can also be examined from the identity work point of view, as it appears that Sofia's agentive actions entail taking on her class mates' identities when claiming that they "were" at the whiteboard.

[5]All names appearing in this paper are pseudonyms.

Creating texts on this writing space can be interpreted as an identity act that entails a kind of *insurgent agency*—a form of revolt which is encoded in at least four ways: First, the sheer act of taking over the institutional space habitually attributed to the teaching staff entails taking on an identity position that could be interpreted as both playful and confrontational as Sofia writes a form of "graffiti" on an institutional wall. This act challenges the particular cultural features related to the writing space and the specific roles or social positionings that the whiteboard as a mediational means and a cultural tool carries in a classroom setting. Second, the rebelliousness of these actions is underlined by both Sofia and Iris keeping an eye on the classroom door, anticipating the teacher coming into the room, which also indicates that the identity act they engage in is at least somewhat in the "forbidden" or extra-curricular zone both temporally and spatially. The literacy activity at hand is possible to conduct only during the in-betweens within formal educational practices (for further elaboration on this, see next example as well as Sect. 13.5). Third, Sofia brings in a linguistic variety, English, that is formally not a part of the school's official bilingual profile, into the linguistic landscape of the classroom (English is, however, recognised in the curriculum and has a central position in the surrounding society). Finally, and fourth, writing the emblematic "somebody was here!" can also be considered similar to "tagging" other individuals in writing spaces provided by virtual media (see below) as well as an element of entextualisation (Kress and van Leeuwen 1996), when a textual element originating from graffiti art in American popular culture[6] ("Kilroy was here") is re-used and resemiotised (cf. Iedema 2003) and its meaning is rearticulated across a new group of individuals. Similar phenomena and elements also apply in the next episode of literacy practices observed in the classroom setting.

Figure 13.2a, b, c illustrates three examples of "speed drawings" created on the classroom computer, situated at the back of the class, by two Class 5/6 C boys, August and Jonas. These literacy practices, like the one represented above in Fig. 13.1, occur typically in time-spaces that can best be described as "in betweens"—most commonly during recesses and lunch breaks or prior to and after the formal school day. What is common for all of these instances is the absence of adults in the physical space of the classroom, which then allows for the students' agentive actions to occur in connection to "institutional" writing spaces in the classroom setting. During some periods of the fieldwork, August and Jonas were observed as engaged in this self-entertaining activity, which entailed particular kind of positioning of oneself and other community members, almost on a weekly basis. Figure 13.2a, b, c illustrates three speed drawings portraying members of Class 5/6 C; a classmate "Hans" (Fig. 13.2a), the author of this paper (Fig. 13.2b) and one of the class teachers (Fig. 13.2c).

---

[6]The origins of the phrase "Kilroy was here" are debated, but the phrase and a distinctive accompanying doodle of a bald male figure peeking from behind a wall became associated with American soldiers in the 1940s.

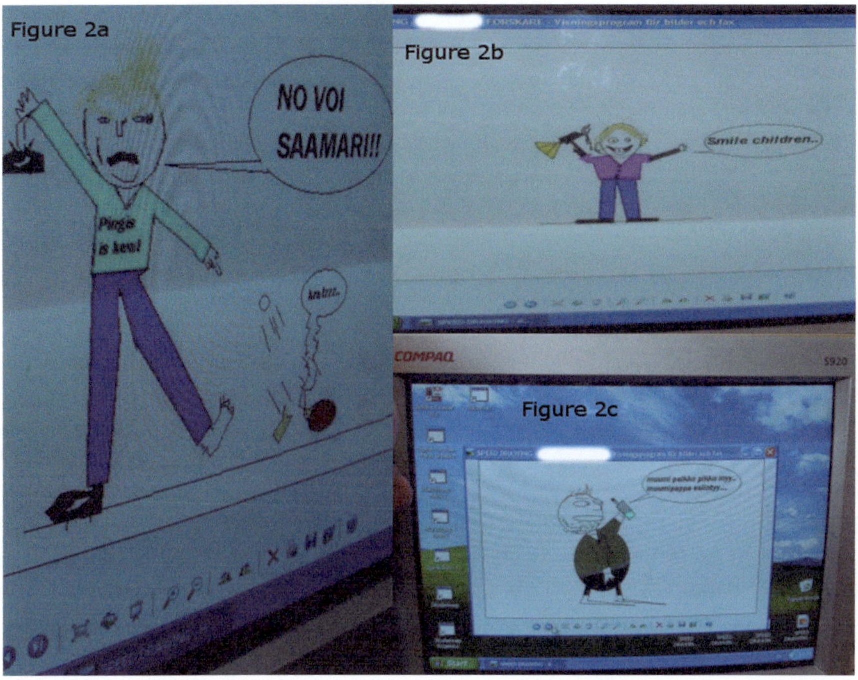

Fig. 13.2 **a**, **b**, **c** Windows office drawing program as a writing space

As the name "speed drawing" implies, the idea was to quickly create cartoon-like sketches of individuals in Class 5/6 C by using the Paintbrush for Windows program. The sketches, as seen above, were often accompanied by speech bubbles and other verbal commentaries that would imply something characteristic of the people depicted in them—or of particular social groups the people represented. For instance, in Fig. 13.2a, the slogan on Hans' t-shirt states "Pingis is kewl" [Swedish/Vernacular English for "Ping-pong is cool"], referring to a hobby of his that was known to all members of the class. Also, he is seen swearing "No voi saamari!!" [Oh damn!!] in Finnish, which was the linguistic variety he most often used in classroom interactions. The speed drawing in Fig. 13.2b is titled "Annaliina Researcher", referring to the Facebook profile name of the author of this chapter, and she is illustrated holding a video camera—as often was the case in the classroom during the ethnographic fieldwork, saying (in English variety, perhaps referring to her use of multiple linguistic varieties online): "Smile children…".

Figure 13.2c illustrates a speed drawing of one of the class teachers with an unshaven face, holding a half-empty bottle, singing a Finnish children's song with the lyrics "Muumi pappa Pikku Myy, Muumipeikko esiintyy…" [Moomin Pappa,

Little My, Moomin Troll perform again…]. Presumably, in a rather audacious mix of stereotypical elements this drawing indexes both the “Finnishness” of the teacher in general, but also the stereotypical drunken behaviour associated with certain social (male) groups in Finnish national culture. All in all, the image can be interpreted as resistance of adult authority, which is an important feature of adolescent peer culture. Studies within Sociology of childhood have also shown that the ability to make fun of adults is a way of becoming popular among peers (Corsaro 1997). Furthermore, the example illustrates one of many instances of members employing the Moomin characters in the classroom community, as the teachers often read Moomin stories out loud for the entire class, thus engaging them into this segment of Finnish (children’s) culture (see also Fig. 13.3).

In terms of languaging, Fig. 13.2a, b, c illustrates the ways in which August and Jonas engage in portraying other people’s identities in literacies that entail languaging in varieties that are seen as relevant for each of those individuals, whether they be Finnish, English or Swedish. This reinforces the heteroglossia taking place within the classroom community and highlights diversity, creativity and variability beyond formal educational practices. Furthermore, the participants’ engagement in this informal literacy practice is mediated and multimodal, as human-like sketches with emblematic material or discursive items are drawn and written into being with the help of a computer-based drawing program. As individuals-acting-with-mediational-means, the boys also contribute to a sense of class community, when representing other members, both students and adults, of the Class 5/6 C. Notable here is that the author, though not originally a “member” of the class, seems to have acquired enough legitimacy among the young people during the fieldwork to be included as a member of the community (see also Sect. 13.4.2). Moreover, using different linguistic and multimodal means that make the individuals depicted in speed drawings recognisable to both authors and viewers—the results of the speed drawing practice were often shared with class members in temporal spaces when teachers were out of sight—highlights aspects of “this is how we see each other’s identity positions”. Finally, as noted by e.g. Lotherington and Jenson (2011), multimodal engagement in literacies and learning supports collective authorship, as seen in the joint enterprise and shared agency which both August and Jonas contribute to in this practice.

Both literacy practices discussed thus far in this paper (Figs. 13.1 and 13.2) highlight different aspects of young people’s employing various linguistic and semiotic resources for meaning-making and social positioning when engaging in informal literacies of their own choice in institutional settings. Thus, it can be argued that in the social spaces of the class, the young people are not merely passive recipients of “education”. They engage in many activities which underline their agency as well as their social positionings beyond being “bilingual students”, which is the role attributed to them by the formal educational setting. Moreover, I note that both spatial and temporal aspects seem to affect the kinds of languaging, including literacies the participants are active agents in creating of—and that these literacies are not meant to be employed as a part of the formal "learning" or "teaching" activities taking place during the school days. Instead, they have the potential to contribute to identity positionings that highlight different aspects of a sense of belonging within the class community. The following examples that expand this theme originate from a literacy practice taking place outside the institutional setting.

13.4.2 Moving Beyond Physical Spaces: Identity Work and Informal Literacy Practices in Social Media

In this section, languaging and identity work are discussed as emerging in social media writing spaces in various discursive and intertextual functions. In Facebook, these discourses typically surface when users post something on their own or a friend's profile or "wall"; a status update, a photo, a link to a web site, or a combination of the above. The example below represents a profile picture update by Filippa, a member of Class 5/6 C. The status update function on Facebook can be considered a space for micro-blogging with a possibility to attach photos and other files, as well as tag people and add locations to the post (Barton and Lee 2013: 52). Moreover, the status updates appear also in a user's Facebook friends' news feed, which in turn invites other users to participate in dialogue by commenting on each other's status updates and other posts. In June 2010, Filippa posted a photo update on her profile. This picture is a collage of diverse Moomin[7] characters, to which Filippa tagged names and profiles of her class mates and teacher, as well as the name of the author of this chapter. In literacy spaces provided by Facebook, social tagging means labeling people in the picture with their name, or link to their profile, if they are among a user's friends. Tagging thus creates hypertextual links between user profiles and photos, videos and other updates. As a practice, it also positions users in relation to other users' aliases, people behind the aliases and semiotic materials created and available online. Let us now have a look at Filippa's post in Fig. 13.3 and some of the comments following it.

Figure 13.3 highlights Filippa's and other Class 5/6 C members' engagement in informal multilingual literacy practices in digital writing spaces. It entails a self-made collage of Moomin characters in various situations with different (English variety) descriptions highlighting their particular personality features such as "the Mystical", "the "Dancer", "the Shy one" as well as relations and groupings such as "Always together" and "The Fashion knowers". In the comment thread following the photo update, Filippa explicates the process of creating the collage, thus describing the actions of creating the entextualised photo update. Further on, both

[7]The Moomin characters were created by Tove Jansson, a Finnish author, cartoonist and artist. The characters have become emblematic for Finnish (children's) culture during the last few decades. Figure 13.3 is published with the permission of ©Moomin Characters™.

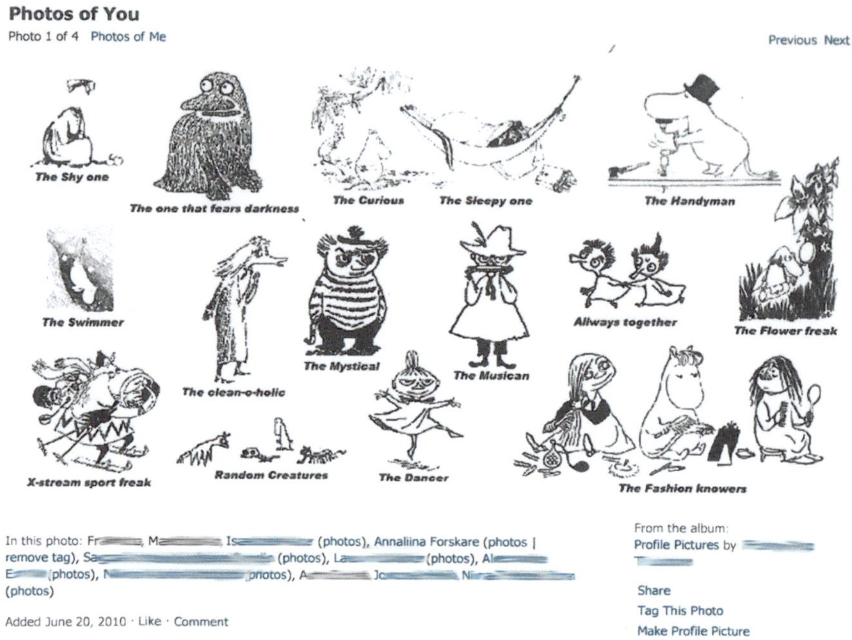

Fig. 13.3 Filippa's photo update "Moomin figures" with tags

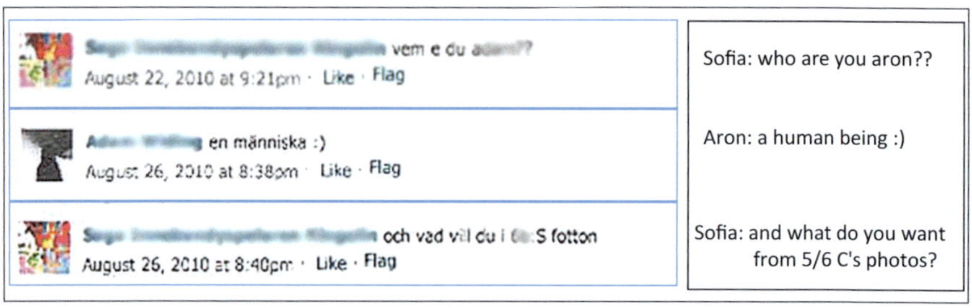

Fig. 13.4 Extract of discussion thread following Filippa's photo update (Swedish variety in original and my English translation)

characteristics of individuals depicted in the collage and their being and belonging are debated, in Swedish and Finnish varieties and through using a variety of so-called emoticons, in the discussion thread following the collage (cf. Figure 13.4). The layers of cultural knowledge associated with the interpretation of this activity have to do with (i) familiarity with the Moomin characters and the ways they were employed in story-telling, jokes and drawings by members of Class 5/6 C, (ii) having access to the English variety used in the descriptions and the other varieties employed in the discussion thread, (iii) being able to understand the connections between offline and online settings, emerging through the tagging of Class 5/6 C persons and their online profiles as well as (iv) the personality descriptions associated with the images and the people. The "success" of this post—and of Filippa's agentive actions—is thus dependent on her audience's access to specific linguistic features, but more importantly their ability to interpret the entextualised and resemiotised features of the collage and its connections with the world outside the virtual setting, referring to the class community. Due to spatial restrictions, the multilingual-multimodal comment thread will not be represented here as a whole, but aspects of members' communicative practices and agency emerging in and through this online writing space are discussed with the help of a few particular examples. As it appears, the entertainment value of Filippa's post is immediately appreciated by class mate Sofia, who we met in the first example. She responds to the post with "hahaahhahahah" in the first comment out of 44 emerging during the following 3,5 months, taking place mostly among members of Class 5/6 C.

On August 22, two months after Filippa's original photo update, Aron, a Facebook friend of hers—but not a member of Class 5/6 C community—writes "Where am I [in the collage]?" in the writing space, thus wondering why he is not tagged in the photo. This action prompts the update to appear on the news feed of everyone previously tagged in the photo, and a negotiation of belonging and group identity begins. Sofia is tagged in the collage as "always together" with Lina, another Class 5/6 C member. She asks Aron who he is and what he is doing in what is framed here as "Class 5/6 C's photos", thus questioning his being and belonging in this writing space.

Barton and Lee (2013: 23–24) note that in online writing spaces, people perceive and draw upon many different kinds of affordances in order to act according to their particular purposes—in this case portraying agency and group identities through social tagging of individuals from a class community in a collage and then negotiating belonging to that community linguistically and multimodally in the discussion thread. In the photo update and the discussion thread, the *chained* nature of languaging practices is prominent as the linguistic varieties of English, Swedish and Finnish, interplay in and between the update and comments (cf. Gynne and Bagga-Gupta 2013). However, language is here considered as only one of many resources people utilise in meaning-making that occurs in a multisemiotic manner. As seen in Figs. 13.3 and 13.4, so-called smileys and other paralinguistic means (such as Sofia's laughter-like "hahaahhahahah") carry different meanings. In this sense, the practices explored in the social networking site bear resemblance to the languaging practices in the "offline" writing spaces represented in Sect. 13.4.1, as in both, heteroglossia, texts, images and symbols are central elements in meaning-making and identity work.

In the present example, agency can be defined as the capacity to employ mediational means provided by writing spaces at a social networking site in order to create representations of group identity through signaling belonging and othering. When tagging members of a particular group of people and debating the meanings of those tags (or their non-existence), Filippa, Sofia and others also engage in identity work. Furthermore, tagging someone in online setting bears resemblance to "tagging" them in offline settings through writing their names and claiming they "were" there, such as in the literacy practice observed around the whiteboard writing space in Fig. 13.1. This entails similar functions in both spaces; claiming somebody's ownership or belonging to a particular space through writing their names and/or tagging them as well as positioning oneself as a person who can portray and position others (cf. Fig. 13.2).

Apart from agency, the data examples in Figs. 13.3 and 13.4 highlight the interconnectedness of online and offline settings in a number of ways. First, at least parts the community made up by "Class 5/6 C" in a school setting are re-established in an image tied to a literacy practice in a virtual writing space. Second, the social groupings, "belonging" and identity positions related to these become relevant as the users debate, "multilingually-multimodally", the image, the tags and their meanings in the discussion thread following the post. Third, the discussion following is open to all of Filippa's Facebook friends and possibly to friends of other tagged users, but the presence of an "outsider" (not a member of the presumed class community) in the interaction is met by those who perceive themselves as "insiders" or "legitimate members of Class 5/6 C" (cf. Lave and Wenger 1991) with suspicion. These indications accentuate both the ingroupness as well as othering of those outside the group. Finally, the social foundation as well as inconsequentiality of "being and belonging" becomes apparent when former members of the class, including the author of this chapter, are "allowed" to be tagged and their presence is not questioned by anyone (for further considerations concerning belonging and researcher role, see Bagga-Gupta et al. 2014, 2016; Gynne 2016).

13.5 Discussion and Concluding Remarks

This chapter has presented a variety of instances of identity work and "multilingual-multimodal" languaging emerging in writing spaces across the online-offline continuum. The leading question in the analysis has been to explore how so-called multilingual young people engage in languaging and informal literacy practices in writing spaces that provide different kinds of affordances for participation and identity work. The second key issue has been to examine in what ways individual and group identifications are performed, portrayed and negotiated in and through informal literacy practices. Finally, the study presented in the chapter has attempted to shed light on the ways in which the identity work contributes to creating a sense of (dis)engagement and belonging among the young people.

The empirical examples framed by the institutional educational setting as well as the writing spaces provided by the social networking site illustrate the flow and chained interconnectedness of different kinds of linguistic and multimodal resources in young people's languaging and agency. Furthermore, the affordances of distinctive kinds of discursive-technologies (Bagga-Gupta 2004, 2014; Barton and Lee 2013) become a central element in providing frameworks for meaning-making and identity work in literacy practices in all these spaces. The affordances of all the examined writing spaces: whiteboard, computerised drawing program and social media, offer different opportunities and constraints for the participants' languaging. For instance, the data illustrates many examples of chaining (see e.g. Gynne and Bagga-Gupta 2013; Humphries and MacDougall 2000) of linguistic, textual and other multimodal resources, which is to be considered a kind of multisemiotic languaging that seems to be a prerequisite for meaning-making in these spaces.

All the examined writing spaces can also be seen as dialogic spaces where dialogue and self- and other-expression take place in interaction between different tools and actors, and the spaces themselves. In the analysis of young people's informal literacy practices, it appears that participants employ different linguistic and semiotic repertoires that they are a part of in ways that are meaningful for those particular practices and writing spaces, as well as for themselves and each other as languagers. This embraces and extends the multidiscursivity and multivoicedness that are characteristic for heteroglossia (Bakhtin 1981). An important element here seems to be re-inventing and recycling of social, textual and linguistic materials from sources that originate from elsewhere, both culturally close and distant sources. Creating tags in offline writing spaces through claiming, in an emblematic phrasal sense, that "someone was here" is related to creating intertextual and interpersonal links between people and their social media profiles through tagging on Facebook—which is here considered an extension of entextualisation (cf. Kress and van Leeuwen 1996; Leppänen et al. 2013). Furthermore, recycling discursive materials from e.g. national gendered stereotypes and children's songs in "speed drawings" or cartoon images in social media writing spaces can be considered as agentive actions in which de- and recontextualisation of different cultural elements is at the core of the practice.

From identity work point of view, the examination of young people's engagements in languaging in different writing spaces (cf. Barton 2012) and reconceptualising identity as agency (van Lier 2008) entails also directing focus on relational aspects of identity work. Taking this perspective, the analyses of informal literacy practices in the classroom illustrate both conventional and creative solutions for portraying and negotiating identity positionings through agency. In writing spaces provided by the institutional educational setting, the students ascribe themselves and each other novel and recycled social positionings within the local classroom community. This occurs partly through insurgent agency, when young people engage in self-expression and creative collaborative languaging through occupying writing spaces habitually attributed to the teachers, and through employing linguistic and semiotic varieties that are not necessarily part of the formal institutional agenda of the educational setting. Furthermore, the practices of portraying identity-as-agency in the studied writing spaces are both individual and collaborative. This surfaces, among other things, in the ways in which interactions, agency and social positionings are emerging at the intersection of people, space, practice and technology both online and IRL. Young people who language on Facebook use various communicative resources in order to create boundaries and form alliances—in short, for crafting and contributing to identities and communities, imagined or other. Both reinforcement of local cultures emerging among peers and communities such as "Class 5/6 C", and contestation of being and belonging to them can be seen as common ways of enacting with the world.

Through the examination of agency and languaging in informal literacy practices in different kinds of writing spaces, the present study has highlighted the chained intertwinedness of the virtual and the physical in everyday life (cf. Gillen and Merchant 2013). Aspects of chaining, entextualisation and resemiotisation have been observed as emerging in spaces and practices across the offline-online continuum, and contributing to both individual and collective identity work.

Many of the elements central in young people's informal literacy practices both in and outside of classroom settings never truly enter the world of formal education. Students' experiences from diverse, e.g. digitally mediated cultural spaces are usually not recognized in the standardised formal learning settings, which continue to rely on standardised views of literacy ("bookish" literacies, cf. Bialostok 2014), and focus on assessment (cf. Gynne and Bagga-Gupta 2015). Previous scholars, e.g. Lotherington and Ronda (2011) have warned for students' "internalizing discourses that their extracurricular multimodal practices are not valid, relevant or valuable" (pp. 121–122). In conclusion, this study contributes to a strand of research that argues for the importance of bringing attention to young people's extra-curricular, heteroglossic and multisemiotic practices beyond formal educational goals. Future research prospects could benefit from its inclusive approach, and provide novel insights concerning how young people build up their life worlds through heteroglossic and multisemiotic languaging practices across virtual-IRL spaces.

Acknowledgements I would like to thank Associate Professor Tommaso M. Milani, University of the Witwatersrand, Johannesburg, and Professor Sirpa Leppänen, Jyväskylä University, for their critical feedback received to early drafts of this chapter. The insightful comments from the blind reviewers have also been greatly appreciated. Any remaining flaws are my own.

Appendix

Layout of the classroom spring term 2010.

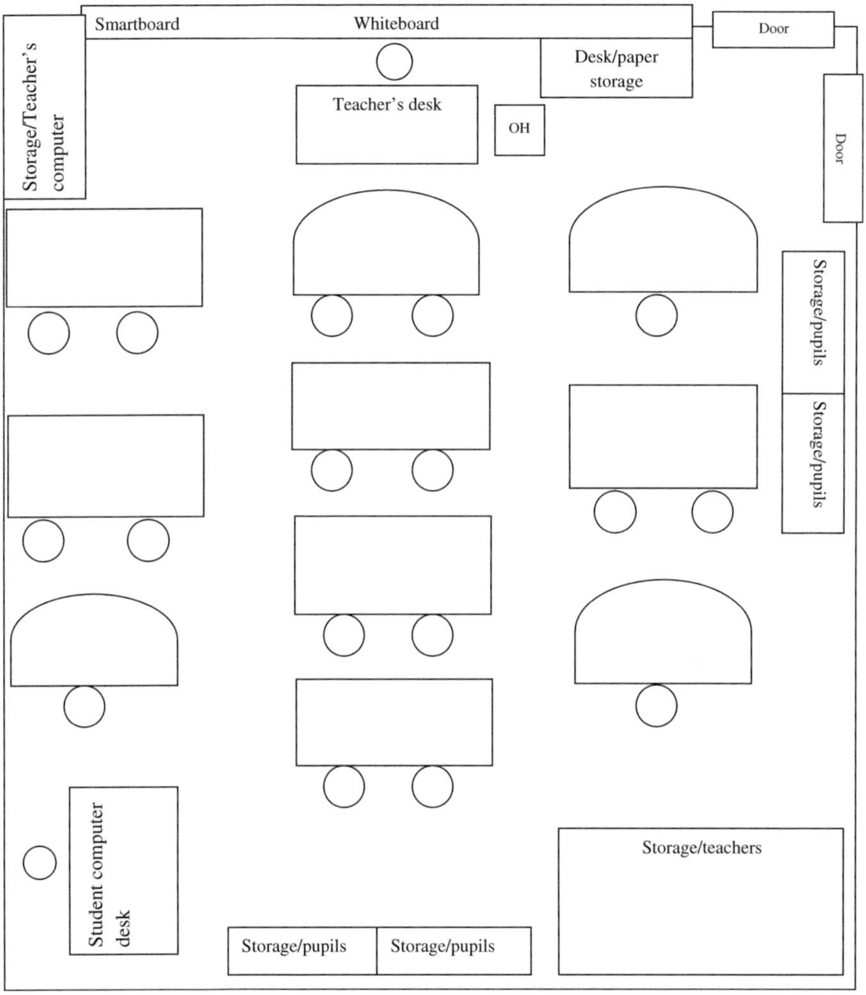

References

Agar, M. H. (1981). *The professional stranger: An informal introduction to ethnography*. New York: Academic Press.
Bagga-Gupta, S. (2004). Visually oriented language use. Discursive and technological resources in Swedish Deaf pedagogical arenas. In: M. V. Herreweghe & M. Vermeerbergen (Eds.), *Sociolinguistics in European Deaf Communities*: Vol. 10. The Sociolinguistics in Deaf Communities Series. (pp. 171–207). Washington, DC: Gallaudet University.
Bagga-Gupta, S. (2014). Performing and accounting language and identity: Agency *as* Actors-in-(inter)action-with-tools. In P. Deters, X. Gao, E. R. Miller, & G. Vitanova (Eds.), *Theorizing and analyzing agency in second language learning. Interdisciplinary approaches* (pp. 113–132). Bristol: Multilingual Matters.
Bagga-Gupta, S., Messina Dahlberg, G., & Gynne, A. (2016). Ethnography as fieldwork practice in and across physical-virtual spaces. Focusing current methodological practices. Paper at the 2016 conference for the American Association for Applied Linguistics (AAAL). April 9-12, 2016. Orlando, FL, USA.
Bakhtin, M. M. (1981). *The dialogic imagination: Four essays by M.M. Bakhtin* (M. Holquist ed., C. Emerson, & M. Holquist, Trans.). Austin: University of Texas Press.
Barton, D. (2007). *Literacy: An introduction to the ecology of written language*. Oxford: Wiley-Blackwell.
Barton, D. (2012). Participation, deliberate learning and discourses of learning online. *Language and Education, 26*(2), 139–150.
Barton, D., & Lee, C. (2013). *Language online: Investigating digital texts and practices*. New York: Routledge.
Bialostok, S. (2014). Metaphors that teachers live by: A Cultural Model of Literacy in the Era of New Literacies. *Language and Education, 28*(6), 501–520.
Björkvall, A., & Engblom, C. (2010). Young children's exploration of semiotic resources during unofficial computer activities in the classroom. *Journal of Early Childhood Literacy, 10*(3), 271–293.
Blommaert, J., & Rampton, B. (2011). Language and superdiversity. *Diversities 13*(2) UNESCO.
Boyd, D. (2008). *Taken out of context. American teen sociality in networked publics*. Berkeley, CA: University of California.
Bruce, B. C., & Bishop, A. P. (2008). New literacies and community inquiry. In J. Coiro et al. (Eds.), *Handbook of research on new literacies*. New York: Lawrence Erlbaum Associates.
Bucholtz, M., & Hall, K. (2005). Identity and interaction: A sociocultural linguistic approach. *Discourse Studies, 7*(4–5), 585–614.
Burnett, C. (2014). Investigating pupils' interactions around digital texts: A spatial perspective on the "classroom-ness" of digital literacy practices in schools. *Educational Review, 66*(2), 192–209.
Butler, J. (1990). *Gender trouble: Feminism and the subversion of identity*. New York: Routledge.
Cekaite, A., & Evaldsson, A.-C. (2008). Staging linguistic identities and negotiating monolingual norms in multiethnic school settings. *International Journal of Multilingualism, 5*(3), 177–196.
Chang, B. (2013). Voice of the voiceless? Multiethnic student voices in critical approaches to race, pedagogy, literacy and agency. *Linguistics and Education, 24*(3), 348–360.
Corsaro, W. (1997). *The Sociology of Childhood*. Thousand Oaks: Pine Forge Press.
Creese, A., Baraç, T., Bhatt, A., Blackledge, A., Hamid, S., & Wei, L. (2008). *Investigating Multilingualism in Complementary Schools in Four Communities* (final report). University of Birmingham. http://www.esrcsocietytoday.ac.uk/esrcinfocentre/viewawardpage.aspx?awardnumber=RES-000-23-1180. Accessed January 15, 2016.
Facebook. (2016). *About*. https://www.facebook.com/facebook?v=info. Accessed February 18, 2016.
García, O. (2009). *Bilingual education in the 21st century: A global perspective*. Malden, MA: Blackwell Publishing.

Gillen, J., & Merchant, G. (2013). From virtual histories to virtual literacies. In G. Merchant, J. Gillen, J. Marsh, & J. Davies (Eds.), *Virtual literacies: Interactive spaces for children and young people* (pp. 9–26). London: Routledge.

Gynne, A., & Bagga-Gupta, S. (2013). Young people's languaging and social positioning. *Chaining* in "bilingual" educational settings in Sweden. *Linguistics and Education, 24*(4), 479–496. doi:10.1016/j.linged.2013.06.002

Gynne, A., & Bagga-Gupta, S. (2015). Languaging in the 21st century: Exploring varieties and modalities in literacies inside and outside learning spaces. *Language and Education, 29*(6), 509–526. doi:10.1080/09500782.2015.1053812

Gynne, A., Bagga-Gupta, S., & Lainio, J. (2016). Practiced linguistic-cultural ideologies and educational policies. A case study of a "bilingual Sweden Finnish school". *Journal of Language, Identity and Education.15*(6), 329-343. doi: 10.1080/15348458.2016.1217160

Gynne, A. (2016). *Languaging and Social Positioning in Multilingual School Practices: Studies of Sweden Finnish Middle School Years*. (Doctoral Dissertations Mälardalen University 2015). Västerås, Sweden.

Humphries, T., & MacDougall, F. (2000). "Chaining" and other links: Making connections between American Sign Language and English in two types of school settings. *Visual Anthropology Review, 15*(2), 84–94.

Iedema, R. (2003). Multimodality, resemiotization: Extending the analysis of discourse as multi-semiotic practice. *Visual Communication, 2*(1), 29–57.

Ivkovic, D., & Lotherington, H. (2009). Multilingualism in the cyberspace: Conceptualizing the virtual linguistic landscape. *International Journal of Multilingualism, 6*(1), 17–36.

Kress, G. (2003). *Literacy in the new media age*. London: Routledge.

Kress, G., & van Leeuwen, T. (1996). *Reading images: The grammar of visual design*. Abingdon: Routledge.

Lankshear, C., & Knobel, M. (2006). *New literacies: Everyday practices and classroom learning* (2nd ed.). Berkshire: Open University Press.

Lave, J., & Wenger, E. (1991). *Situated learning: Legitimate peripheral participation*. Cambridge: Cambridge University Press.

Lee, C. (2011). Micro-blogging and status updates on Facebook. Texts and practices. In C. Thurlow & Mroczeck, K. (Eds.), *Digital discourse: Language in the new media.* Oxford: Oxford University Press.

Lefebvre, H. (1974). *The production of space* [La production de l'espace]. Oxford: Basil Blackwell.

Leppänen, S., Kytölä, S., Jousmäki, H., Peuronen, S., & Westinen, E. (2013). Entextualisation and resemiotisation as resources for (dis)identification in social media. *Tilburg Papers in Culture Studies 57.*

Linell, P. (2009). *Rethinking language, mind and world dialogically: Interactional and contextual theories of human sense-making*. Charlotte, NC: Information Age Publishing.

Livingstone, S. (2008). Taking risky opportunities in youthful content creation: Teenagers' use of social networking sites for intimacy, privacy and self-expression. *New Media Society, 10*(3), 393–411.

Lotherington, H., & Jenson, J. (2011). Teaching multimodal and digital literacy in L2 settings: New literacies, new basics, new pedagogies. *Annual Review of Applied Linguistics, 31,* 226–246.

Lotherington, H., & Ronda, N. S. (2011). Multimodal literacies and assessment: Uncharted challenges in the English classroom. In C. Leung & B. V. Street (Eds.), *English a changing medium for education*. Multilingual Matters: Clevedon.

Lytra, V. (2011). Negotiating language, culture and pupil agency in complementary school classrooms. *Linguistics and Education, 22*(1), 23–36.

Maybin, J. (2007). Literacy under and over the desk: Oppositions and heterogeneity. *Language and Education, 21*(6), 515–530.

Møller, J. S., & Jørgensen, J. N. (2009). From language to languaging: Changing relations between humans and linguistic features. *Acta Linguistica Hafniensia: International Journal of Linguistics, 41*(1), 143–166.
Pavlenko, A., & Blackledge, A. (Eds.). (2004). *Negotiation of identities in multilingual contexts*. Multilingual Matters: Clevedon.
Prinsloo, M., & Baynham, M. (Eds.). (2008). *Literacies, global and local*. Amsterdam: John Benjamins Publishing Company.
Säljö, R. (2000). *Lärande i praktiken – ett sociokulturellt perspektiv* [Learning in practice—A sociocultural perspective]. Stockholm: Prisma.
van Lier, L. (2008). *Agency in the classroom*. Unpublished paper available at http://www.dilit.it/allegati/LeoVanLierScrittaParte.pdf
Vygotsky, L. S. (1978). *Mind in society*. Harvard: Harvard University Press.
Vygotsky, L. S. (1986). *Thought and language*. Cambridge, MA: MIT Press.
Wertsch, J. V. (1991). *Voices of the mind: A sociocultural approach to mediated action*. Cambridge, MA: Harvard University Press.
Wertsch, J. V., Tulviste, P., & Hagstrom, F. (1993). A sociocultural approach to agency. In E. A. Forman, N. Minick, & C. A. Stone (Eds.), *Contexts for learning: Sociocultural dynamics in children's development*. New York, NY: Oxford University Press.
Wolcott, H. F. (2008). *Ethnography—A way of seeing*. Lanham, MD: Altamira Press.

Author Biography

Annaliina Gynne holds a Ph.D. in Education from the School of Education, Culture and Communication at Mälardalen University, Sweden. Her research interests include multilingual and multicultural education, languaging, literacies, learning and identities. In particular, her research has focused issues related to language and literacy practices as well as meaning making and identity work among multilingual young people in minority educational settings in Sweden.

Chapter 14
A Moment of Self-Revelation as a Turning Point in Understanding Language Learning

Elina Tapio

14.1 Introduction

Conflicting discourses characterise discussions on deafness and language learning. The history of deaf education—including the measures taken in relation to early language learning of deaf children—is characterised by the debate over which language, spoken or signed, should be provided for deaf children. In Finland, similarly to many other Western countries, several turns have occurred between favouring monolingual education—spoken language only—or bilingual education—signed and spoken language—(for more on the linguistic turns in deaf education, see Salmi 2010). One major turn took place in the 1970s, when both poor success of monolingual education and linguistic research on signed languages prepared the way for Finnish Sign Language (FinSL) to return to deaf schools after a period of *oralism*, which had begun in the late nineteenth century. Also the cultural-linguistic model of deafness, which had been introduced as an alternative to the medical perspective which sees deafness as a defect that should be cured, changed the intellectual and cultural climate in the 1970s (Padden and Humphries 1988; in Finland, Jokinen 1992, see also Bauman 2008). Consequently, in the 1980s and 1990s, deaf children were permitted to learn and to use FinSL, and hearing parents of deaf children were encouraged to learn and use FinSL. The use of FinSL was seen as the best way to achieve bilingualism in Finnish and FinSL.

However, the introduction of a new hearing aid, the cochlear implant, in the beginning of the 1990s led to a renewed emphasis on oral communication instead of signing. Medical authorities often discourage parents from using a sign language with children who have cochlear implants, claiming that the use of a sign language may disturb the development of a spoken language (Tapio and Takkinen 2012; Rainò 2012). The fact that no research exists that supports such statements

E. Tapio (✉)
Humak University of Applied Sciences, Helsinki, Finland
e-mail: elina.tapio@humak.fi

S. Bagga-Gupta et al. (eds.), *Identity Revisited and Reimagined*,
DOI 10.1007/978-3-319-58056-2_14

(see, e.g. Kirkehei, Myrhaug, Garm, Simonsen & Wie 2011; Marschark and Hauser 2012) has caused researchers to conclude that such persistent assumptions represent a "deep level of folk mythos" (Ladd 2003: 72), "systems of belief and practice that encourage the denial of observable facts" (Johnson 2006: 29) and crucial misunderstandings in relation to (signed) languages, language learning, deafness, and disability which have further strengthened the marginalisation of semiotic resources and practices used by sign language signers[1] in visually oriented communities (Tapio 2014). Similar shifts in the goals of language education have taken place elsewhere in Europe and America (Ladd 2003).[2]

Against this broader context, the aim of this study is to focus on the conflicting discourses in relation to the English language learning of deaf FinSL signers. Such discourses surfaced through an ethnographic study of English language in the everyday life of FinSL signers (Tapio 2013). The views that discount signed languages and other visual-embodied semiotic resources in visually oriented communities position deaf sign language signers as people who lack resources for learning English. This view can be seen in comments such as "It must be difficult to learn English when you don't hear it all the time", a typical comment that emerged in the ethnographic research (Tapio 2013). In other words, the English language learning of deaf people is often regarded as lacking auditive modes, yet as otherwise similar to the way hearing people learn English. Such a view can be identified as an authoritative discourse (Bakhtin 1981) that can have a negative effect on a learner's agency.

However, the above-mentioned views on deaf sign language signers and language learning are not the only prevalent understandings. Recent research on languaging and multimodal meaning making has brought to our attention the multiple and situated ways learners use semiotic resources for language learning (see, e.g. Dufva 2013; Kramsch 2002; van Lier 2002). Such research pays attention also to the visual and embodied resources involved in meaning making. This is in concordance with recent studies on the multimodal and multilingual practices that signers take with regard to languages (see, e.g. Bagga-Gupta 2010; Tapio 2013). Based on the empirical study of signed interaction in relation to English language (Tapio 2013), and a study on how deaf FinSL signers view themselves as language learners (Kelly, Dufva, & Tapio 2015), I have come to the conclusion that the mundane everyday actions of sign language signers are in conflict with the notion that they lack resources for English language learning. In other words,

[1]I have chosen to consistently use 'signer' when referring to people who participate in signing environments, for example at home or at school, and of whose historical body a sign language has become an integral part.

[2]In spring 2016, the global audience on the internet and the social media witnessed a heated discussion which began when the president of the Alexander Graham Bell Association for the Deaf and Hard of Hearing accused Nyle DiMarco, a famous deaf celebrity and activist promoting American Sign Language, of spreading myths about deafness. The open letter published by the association was opposed by a number of researchers and deaf people and highlighted research on the benefits of bilingualism in signed and spoken language.

while a learner of English might use diverse media and modes through which English emerges via embodied and visual resources, the dominant discourse positions the learner as struggling with limited resources when learning English.

The above-mentioned research (Tapio 2013), based on ethnographic material collected in 2004–2007, discussed how learners seemed to have adopted "the views of others" despite the fact that their everyday actions with English did not support such views. However, participation in the research activities seemed to trigger a change in how the research participants viewed themselves as English language users and learners. In this chapter, I will reanalyse one interview from the research material with a specific interest in examining the moment when a deaf FinSL signer becomes aware of her actions with English in relation to technology in particular. I will argue that the realisation triggers a change in the way the interviewee sees herself as an English language learner. I will do this by focusing on the clash between established views, authoritative discourses, and the reflection of everyday actions as it happens during the interview. The wider consequences of such a moment of realisation will also be considered, as the chapter discusses the way discourses and actions may transform into new discourses and practices when using nexus analysis as the research framework.

14.2 Nexus Analysis: Doing Research with the Research Participants

This chapter revisits and reanalyses an interview of a research participant, 'Hanna', who in 2007 participated in my ethnographic research on English language in the everyday life of FinSL signers (Tapio 2013). The study was conducted within the research framework of Mediated Discourse Analysis (MDA) and its practical research procedure, nexus analysis (Scollon and Scollon 2004). A nexus analysis connects two levels of discourse analysis—the micro-analysis of unfolding interaction and a broader analysis of social and power relationships—by examining social action from the viewpoint of *the historical body*: *the life experiences of an individual*, *the discourses in place*, and *the interaction order*. In this manner, a nexus analysis moves from describing *what* is happening to discussing *why* it is happening.

Nexus analysis has three main tasks: engaging the nexus of practice, navigating the nexus of practice, and changing the nexus of practice. The nexus of practice, "a network of linked practices", can refer to a group, a situation or a genre, and comes rather close to the term "community of practice" (Scollon 2001a: 150, 178). In the first phase of nexus analysis, *engaging the nexus of practice*, the analysis begins by placing the researcher within *a zone of identification* in relation to the community under scrutiny. The first stage of nexus analysis also concerns the discovery of the social actions and actors that are crucial to the social issue one has set out to investigate. Engaging with such actions through research is crucial for bringing about social change.

Scollon and Scollon (2004: 87) refer to the second phase of nexus analysis, *navigating the nexus of practice*, as a type of *mapping*. The goal is "to get a broader understanding of the ways that times and places prior to the social action (–) have brought their influence into the current situation and the ways in which this social action anticipates or presupposes outcomes". Navigating the nexus of practice is the main work of a nexus analysis. Scollon and Scollon (2004: 160–161) suggest that researchers using nexus analysis ask the following questions in order to guide that navigating procedure: (1) How do "the action-practice and mediational means you are studying come into the historical body (see Sect. 14.3) of each of the participants?"; (2) "How did these participants all come to be placed at this moment, in this way to enable or carry out this action?"; (3) "Is the action-practice habitual or innovative, intentional or accidental?"; and (4) "What discourses are transformed, resemiotized, or internalized in this action?" Another very important question is, "What types of discourses are present?" Such discourse types include talk, writing, signing, and gesturing, as well as signs, images, music and other aggregates present during the moment at which the social action occurs.

In nexus analysis, the researcher is part of the common activities of the nexus of practice. A nexus analysis not only positions the analyst within the nexus of practice, but brings the other participants into the nexus analysis. In other words, research is not conducted *on* the participants of the community of practice but *with* the participants (Cameron, Frazer, Harvey, Rampton, & Richardson 1993: 1–2). This leads inevitably to the third phase of nexus analysis, *changing the nexus of practice*. The crucial final question here is, "What actions can you take as a participant-analyst in this nexus of practice that will transform discourses and actions into new discourses and practices?" (Scollon and Scollon 2004: 178). Nexus analysis is motivated by an activist interest in promoting social change with respect to the issue the ethnographer sets out to investigate (Scollon 2002: 15).

One can view the third phase of the nexus analysis, *changing the nexus of practice*, as research activities occurring at the end of a nexus analysis, when enough material has been collected to gain a broad perspective of the research project, but also as occurring throughout the process (Scollon and Scollon 2004: 9–10). In other words, one may regard changing the nexus of practice as 'another analytical lens' through which to contemplate the role of the researcher inside the nexus of practice and the impact of the research on the research participants while conducting research through the phases of engaging and navigating. Scollon and Scollon describe how analysing change in the nexus of practice occurs through *re-engagement*, which can occur in practice in two ways: through direct actions motivated by the nexus analysis, or by bringing the analysis and understanding back into the semiotic ecosystem of the nexus of practice (Scollon and Scollon 2004: 177).

When examining the interplay of dominant discourses and an individual's view of oneself as a language learner, the concepts of historical body, voice and authoritative discourse become crucial and will be attended to in the following sections.

14.3 Historical Body: The Interplay Between Discourses as Social Structures and Actions of the Body

A 'historical body' means the history and the life experiences of an individual (Scollon and Scollon 2004: 13). Bourdieu refers to the same phenomenon as 'habitus'; however, Scollon and Scollon have chosen to use the term 'historical body,' a literal translation of *rekishi-teki-shintai*, originally from Kitaro Nishida (as cited in Scollon and Scollon 2004). The reason for choosing such a term comes from a need to employ a more concrete phrase to describe the interconnectedness of the psychological and social, and therefore to return "both social theory and activity theory to their materialist sources by disallowing any slippage of the term into super-organic categories such as frequently occurs with habitus" (Scollon and Scollon 2005: 108). This highlights one of the most crucial arguments Scollon and Scollon have propounded in their research: they believe that some psychological formations are internalised first as actions and later, in process, are externalised as discourse (Scollon 2001b; Scollon and Scollon 2009). This concurs with the contention of Bourdieu and Wertsch that real-time social action is rooted in the historical body, which is an aggregation of history, and that any action reproduces the identities of prior social actions (Scollon 2001b: 7) because "social identity is constructed through social and societal histories and internalized by the individual in habitus" (Norris 2005: 183) and is constructed, claimed, and contested in interaction (in-depth elaboration in Norris 2004, 2005, 2011).

Historical body has been further elaborated by Jones (2008) and Blommaert and Huang (2009). Jones (2008: 245) emphasises how the 'historical body' is "the storehouse of discourse sedimented in the history and memory of the individual and manifested in 'habitual' practices"; Blommaert and Huang (2009) describe the same as "an aggregate of discourse" and "repositories of histories of experience". In other words social structures are integrated into the historical body of the individual and manifested through mediated actions (through multimodal discourses, such as speech, gestures, and ways of being). According to Blommaert and Huang (2009), and also Jones (2008), the historical body as defined by Scollon is an *amendment* to the concept of habitus. The historical body links the discourse systems with actual, concrete actions of people. The historical body is "about becoming rather than being", dynamic, constantly interacting with its environment (Jones 2008: 247). Discourses as social structures in the world, integrated into the individual, are constantly being modified through interaction with the world. The concept of historical body emphasises the dialogical nature between discourses and actions. (Jones 2008: 247). Looking at the relationship between the actions people take and discourses is the key interest of MDA and nexus analysis. For example, by analysing anticipatory actions and precipitative actions, Jones (2008) sets out to understand sexual risk behaviour in situations where the safe sex discourse is or should be well-acquired. In other words, internalised discourse and habitual practice do not seem to meet. Jones' answer for this clash is found in the notion that discourses interact with a number of discourses and practices; the historical body is a dynamic system where several discourse trajectories meet. By understanding the complex linkages of the multiple discourse trajectories that are in play in one particular social action, one may grasp why an obvious, strong discourse—in Jones' example, safe sex and HIV prevention discourse—does not result in concrete actions. The link between prominent discourses and concrete actions seems to be missing.

14.4 Identity, Voice and Authoritative Discourse

This chapter draws on a sociocultural perspective on identity, according to which identities are neither unitary, static properties of individuals nor different phases in the evolution towards the "real" fixed self. Instead, identity is a social construction that can be negotiated and renegotiated (see, e.g. Giddens 1991; Pavlenko and Blackledge 2004). Identity is seen as the multiple ways in which people position themselves and are positioned in particular social, historical and cultural context. In other words, identity is a situated phenomenon (see, e.g. Davies and Harré 1990). This view on identity closely reflects the postmodern thinking that abandons the essentialist assumptions about the "natural" relationship between identity and nation, gender, or some other social category, but emphasises identity as fluid, ambivalent and dynamic over historical time and social space.

From the perspective of Critical Discourse Analysis (CDA) in particular, self-representations or identity positionings are constructed by drawing on the discourses that are socially available in a given situation (see, e.g. Fairclough 2003). The given socio-historical moment and the particular situation constrains or enables human action; in other words, people are positioned or position themselves in relation to the available social structures that exist. Researchers interested in how power operates within society in relation to language learning pay attention to taken-for-granted categories, such as race, gender and class, and how categorisation of individuals may impact language learner identities (Pennycook 2007: 39; Norton 2013: 11–13). The topic of the deaf as language users and learners triggers powerful discourses on (dis)ability, many of which can be seen as abnormalising the deaf as people who do not learn languages in "a normal way" but with limited resources that should be compensated for with special education measures (Tapio 2014; Tapio and Takkinen 2012).

The research on deaf identity, in general, views the deaf individual as struggling with the views of the surrounding community by emphasising the way deaf individuals construct their identities in the midst of strong, competing views on deafness, namely the medical view and the sociocultural view. Such studies have been criticised for being overly concerned with these two dualistic views on deafness and for not recognising the complex ways in which these discourses can also be seen as layered instead of "either/or", and that individuals draw not only on these discourses when constructing their identities but also construct and draw on both discourses (narratives) simultaneously, as well as other narratives (Luukkainen 2008). It is important to bear in mind that these two discourses and their existence are not to be taken for granted but are socially constructed and appropriated within particular relations of power (Norton 2013: 11).

In order to explore the identity work at play in situations where deaf language learners are refiguring the dominant discourses that they have adopted into their historical body, I will now turn to dialogism and two concepts originally Bakhtin's: multi-voicedness (polyphony) and authoritative discourse. Voice refers to the fact that the words we say are partly ours, partly someone else's. Further, the concept of multi-voicedness, on a practical level, means that we speak in combinations of words of others that are individually appropriated. Multi-voicedness can also be seen as a metaphor for having different perspectives (values, norms, etc.) present in the talk (Pietikäinen and Dufva 2006: 210). However, this does not mean that the individual is simply ventriloquating the voices of others, but the words of others are hybridised, appropriated by the individual in an individual manner (Bakhtin 1981: 304, see also Solomon 2012).

Drawing on dialogism and CDA, Pietikäinen and Dufva (2006) argue that identity must be understood as something which is both individual and social in nature. Their suggestion is to see identity as represented through a variety of voices and discourses, in other words, socially constructed and individually experienced. Yet some words resist the hybridising control and do not submit easily to such appropriation. Such authoritative discourse as "the word of a father, of adults and of teachers" (Bakhtin 1981: 294) and other generally acknowledged beliefs dominate and demand that we make them our own (Bakhtin 1981). The authoritative discourse thus has the power to be adapted as it is, taken for granted, leading to a hegemonic situation.

However, through reflexivity one can become aware of and acknowledge these authoritative discourses in such a way that the dominant discourses can be called into question and space for alternative identity positions may emerge. Such moments of emerging alternative visions can be called "ruptures of the taken-for-granted" (Holland, Lachicotte, Skinner, & Cain 1998: 141; Solomon 2012). Solomon in her study explored two women's accounts of themselves as successful mathematics students (a male-dominated field) and did so by analysing the multi-voicedness of their stories. Her point follows Bakhtin's argument on how the presence of multiple voices offers potential for new meanings as we self-author ourselves within new imagined spaces.

14.5 Everyday Actions as Alternative Discourses

As discussed earlier, the discourses that marginalise deaf people can be seen as authoritative discourses that draw on medical discourse which categorises deaf people as disabled. Similarly the discourse that positions the deaf learners of languages such as English as lacking the resources for language learning can be seen as an authoritative discourse that is strongly linked to other authoritative discourses, such as the compensatory agenda of deaf education in general (Bagga-Gupta 2010).

Scollon and Scollon (2004: 136) stress that when doing nexus analysis, an analyst should look for alternative discourses—should at least entertain those discourses—and should remain alert for discourses that are not presented explicitly but are instead silent. In my previous research on English in the everyday life of FinSL signers the goal was to examine the practices that FinSL signers apply to their use of English (Tapio 2013). First I mapped the focal social actions with English language through ethnographic fieldwork at a school, and then navigated through these social actions to see how they were interconnected with other social practices and discourses relating to the use of English by FinSL signers.

In the first phase of nexus analysis, engaging the nexus of practice, the research started to focus on the networking, technology, and media in the everyday life of FinSL signers. I found those to be the crucial scenes in which the participants used English. The data came from a focus group of eight 10- to 17-year-old FinSL signers and comprised interviews, photos, and video recordings inside and outside school, and a group interview. (See Tapio 2013 for more detailed description of data collection and analysis.)

My focus was, in particular, on how the participants managed mediational means in networking and online messaging, and how the participants dealt with English in a technological context, outside school. Through analysis of the data collected with the research participants, a wide variety of everyday actions with technology surfaced, including messaging and networking by the focus group participants. The data showed how English was present for the participants in an everyday technology context. However, a gap seemed to exist between the school English and everyday English. In most cases, the participants were unaware that they were using English frequently, or did not see everyday English as contributing to their formal English learning. It was also apparent that the participants were active in complex, multilingual, and multimodal networks, and actively managed the mediational means in such environments. Also, the hybrids of visual and embodied modes, such as fingerspelling English words, were resources that FinSL signers used in language learning. The concluding question of this research was: Are such resources recognised and actively used in formal education? Based on the research project, the everyday actions seemed to be in contrast with the discourse that emerged in the data. In other words, the discourse according to which deaf FinSL signers are excluded from the extensive English input because they lack the access to auditory modalities does not seem to be true in the lives of the people who participated in the research.

These finding echo with Bagga-Gupta's research in the Swedish context in which she studied everyday social practices, discourses about these practices, and policy documents (see, e.g. Bagga-Gupta 2004, 2010). The studies have shown a conflict between the ways visually-oriented communication is characterised by multimodal, multilingual meaning making and the discourses and conceptualisations of signers. In other words, while the empirically based analysis of interaction shows "the symbiotic relationship between different linguistic varieties, modalities and resources", the discourses around these arenas categorise the deaf in terms of hearing, and draw clear-cut boundaries between different language varieties and modalities (Bagga-Gupta 2012: 85).

14.6 Hanna's Case: An Individual and Conflicting Discourses

The aim of this chapter is to show through a case study of 'Hanna' how a research participant becomes aware of the conflict between a dominant, authoritative discourse—the perspective she has adopted from others that positions her as an English language learner who is struggling with limited resources to learn English—and the practices with English language in her everyday life. The moment of revelation, or the rupture that takes place during an interview, leads to a change in self-positioning. My aim is to examine what triggers such change on the personal level, and to argue that such moments of self-revelation offer possibilities for reverse discourses and new identity spaces to emerge. Finally, I will discuss the way the researcher can use nexus analysis to engage research participants in critical reflection of dominant discourses.

Hanna's interview is originally part of a larger, ethnographic study introduced earlier in this chapter (Tapio 2013). Figure 14.1 illustrates the data sets collected for the larger ethnographic study, and situates Hanna's interview in relation to other data sets collected within the project. As the figure shows, the interview I examine in this chapter was part of a complementary data set titled 'Hedgedog'. Hedgedog[3] was an intensive, two-week English course in summer 2007 which was launched for a small group of FinSL signers for a specific purpose: to re-engage with a nexus of practice in order to see whether another group of FinSL signers would confirm the observations on English language in the everyday life of FinSL signers that I had gained through the initial analysis of ethnographic data collected between 2004 and 2006. This applies to the data sets 'Beehive project' and 'Me & Languages,' as well as the interviews of the focus group in particular (Fig. 14.1). As explained earlier, the analyses of such data sets had brought to my attention how the FinSL signing participants of the study were actively using multimodal resources, such as visual and multilingual resources in online environments, when dealing with English language. Although an abundance of resources existed for language learning, the resources were often unrecognised by the research participants themselves.

For this reason, when designing the online course Hedgedog, my goal was to employ all the meaning making resources available when designing the online environment and teaching material, so that the activity would not depend only on linguistic resources. Another goal was to bring the participants together to discuss their past experiences of learning languages and their historical body in relation to English and English language learning. From the beginning, the important themes of the course were awareness and empowerment. The data from Hedgedog included

[3]As the teacher of the course, my aim was to communicate to the course participants that making mistakes is completely acceptable and mistakes can be used as a source for efficient language learning. For this reason, I named the course Hedgedog after my own mistake of calling a *hedgedog*, a mistake that had made me recognise the word *hedge* in *hedgehog*.

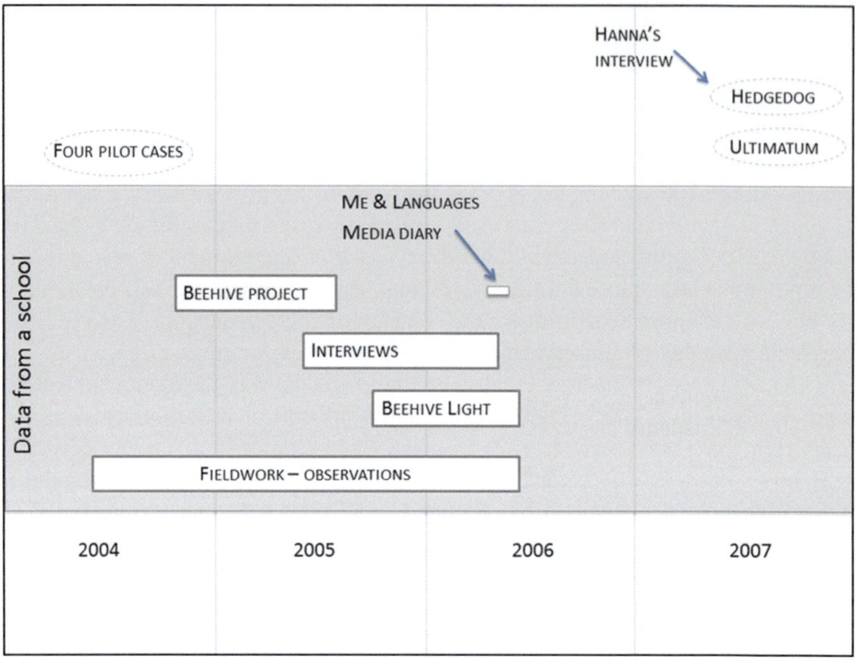

Fig. 14.1 Hanna's interview as part of a larger data archive

weblogs, Messenger conversations, emails, screenshots, screen videos, interviews, a group discussion, exercises, and forum conversations.

In this study, I reanalyse Hanna's interview using the analytical concepts of the historical body and authoritative discourse. (The earlier analysis of the data from Hedgedog including the analysis of Hanna's interview is presented in Tapio 2013, Chap. 10)[4]. Hanna is a deaf FinSL signer who at the time of the interview in 2007 was studying for the matriculation examination (equal to A levels in the British context). She was also planning on taking the English language examination in the near future. Her school background was in a special education primary school in Finland. The school she went to is one of three state schools for the hearing-impaired in Finland. The school is known for rigorously advocating for FinSL as the language of instruction for the deaf and hard-of-hearing pupils very early after the oralistic era. At the time of Hanna's elementary education at that

[4]The interview was done in FinSL and video recorded with a single camera. First, I recorded my simultaneous interpretation of the interview into spoken Finnish while watching the video recording. After that the spoken interpretation was transcribed into written Finnish, and the Finnish transcription was translated into written English. The final step for producing the transcription was to watch the original FinSL video and modify the English translation to be equivalent to the original FinSL signing. Hanna herself has read and commented on my translations, after which minor changes have been made both to the Finnish and English translations.

school, the school provided her with a signing environment. However, at the time of the interview, she was studying with hearing peers, integrated into mainstream education with two sign language interpreters. In English classes, the interpreters mediated spoken English through fingerspelling English words with the manual alphabet; however, most of the spoken English was mediated into FinSL. Hanna participated in classes either by writing on paper in English or signing in FinSL and fingerspelling English which again was translated into Finnish or English by the interpreter (see more detailed description of fingerspelling in Tapio 2013, Chap. 9).

Next, I will revisit one moment in Hanna's interview, a moment I would call a moment of epiphany or "a rupture" when Hanna realises the contradiction between the way she positions herself as an English language learner and the actions she takes with English. In the interview, Hanna tells how she is struggling with the language and she is rather frustrated with her "English skills". She explains how her feeling of inadequacy is caused by her being different from others, her being the only deaf student in the class. This causes situations where she feels misaligned with others. For example, writing her comments on paper when participating in group discussions is too slow for quick conversations, and she does not participate in the listening exercises which are emphasised as important for the hearing classmates. Also code-switching between languages and modes (e.g. English, FinSL, signing, writing, fingerspelling) makes her feel that "the brain freezes" and she does not know at all what to say and through which mode. The interviewer inquires about her spare time, curious to know whether she feels different with English language outside the classroom. Matter-of-factly Hanna explains how she does not watch movies or read any books, and that her use of English language through instant messengers is also very rare. She concludes that she uses English only at school or rarely with international friends.

Based on the observations of her online behaviour and how well she has managed the online environment during the Hedgedog course, the interviewer points out "Hey, the internet?", and again with certainty, she promptly answers "True, I use the computer almost every day". The interviewer is at that moment orienting towards the topic of different strategies of problem-solving when encountering English language outside formal spaces. In other words, the interviewer begins to direct the discussion towards the topic of how a visually oriented learner perceives written English and uses multimodal resources when languaging. However, Hanna's thoughts are now occupied by her own answer "True, I use the computer almost every day". While Hanna explains her surfing online to the interviewer, how she manages without using dictionaries, she slowly starts to realise that while explaining her strategies with respect to English language online, she is contradicting her previous comment "I only use English at school or just a bit with friends". While the interviewer is still orienting towards the topic of strategies and problem-solving, Hanna's confusion becomes more and more apparent in the way the interaction order changes. Until this point, Hanna has kept the floor during her turns which have been long and contained vivid self-narration with relatively fast signing speed. She has directed her gaze and comments to the video camera and answered back to the interviewer quickly, without hesitation, but now her eye gaze is either on the interviewer or roams about the room. She says (the length of pauses are in parentheses):

I don't notice it. (6.9)

It's true English is there almost all the time. (4.0)

Despite that I feel most of the hearing people pick up English language all the

time. But I feel, not me, not at all, because I don't hear anything.

But, true! There's the computer. But I don't notice that. (6.8)

The pauses are long, from four to nearly seven seconds in duration, during which she looks at the interviewer, eyes wide open, mouth open, then shrugs her shoulders and scratches her cheek. In other words, she expresses confusion and surprise with her embodied action and pauses in her talk (see Fig. 14.2, still images captured from the video). The interviewer, unfortunately, is still fixated on the topic of problem-solving yet slowly moves to align with Hanna. Hanna focuses on problem-solving strategies with the interviewer for a while and explains how she attends to the shapes of words instead of the sequence of letters when surfing online. However, when the interviewer ruminates on the topic, the surprised and confused expression stays on Hanna's face, showing how her thoughts are occupied with something else while simultaneously looking at the interviewer signing. After a while, Hanna moves away from the topic of problem-solving strategies by saying "It's also true that I played video games as a child", which expands her realisation of using English now to I have always used English.

At first, Hanna positions herself as a person who is not able to "pick up English all the time" as the hearing people do. This identity positioning can be seen as constructed by drawing on the discourses that have been available to her through "expert talk", as well as her personal experience in studying English at school among her peers where listening to English is emphasised as a way to learn English. However, her personal contacts with the people she has had since travelling abroad, as well as new technologies have enabled actions with English language outside school. When Hanna reflects on her everyday actions—the surfing of internet pages, messaging with friends via Windows Live Messenger and playing different video games—she makes the contradiction between her self-representation and

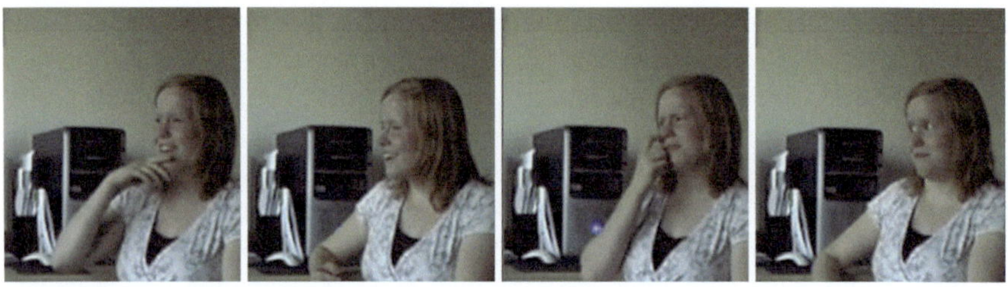

Fig. 14.2 The moment of rupture for the taken-for-granted: Hanna's expressions of confusion and surprise during the interview

everyday actions explicit. From the point of view of the historical body, the authoritative discourse of deaf people having limited resources in English language learning has been integrated into the historical body of Hanna, and is manifested in her narration during the interview (Blommaert and Huang 2009; Scollon and Scollon 2004). However, as mentioned, the historical body is constantly being modified through the dialogue between discourses and actions (Jones 2008: 247). The alternative discourse which sees deaf people as having multiple, multimodal resources for learning English is already evidenced by Hanna's habitual practices with English language (Jones 2008: 245), and during the interview the practices are externalised as discourse (Scollon 2001b or Scollon and Scollon 2009). Hanna identifies her "embodied knowledge" (Blommaert and Huang 2009) in relation to English language use, and in this way goes beyond the practices promoted and recognised institutionally. In the beginning of the interview, reading books and using dictionaries are recognised by Hanna as actions related to English language learning, while playing video games becomes recognised as such only after her active reflection later in the interview.

The interview alone, I suggest, would not have triggered such reflection. Hanna's participation in research activities opened space for "a rupture of the taken-for-granted" to take place during the interview. Participation in the Hedgedog course had given Hanna an experience of direct access to the interaction occurring. In particular, she had access to English language produced by other participants in the online course. Hanna did not have access to such interaction when studying English in mainstream education with two sign language interpreters. She stated that seeing other people "making mistakes, using Finnish when not remembering the right English words" encouraged her to use English more freely. Long, Vignare, Rappold and Mallory (2007) and Tapio (2013) report similar positive experiences of online language learning among deaf and hard-of-hearing learners of English language. After the interview, Hanna actually wanted to discuss her ideas with another participant of the course, Jesse, who also is a deaf FinSL signer. Consequently, I arranged a meeting between myself, Hanna, and Jesse to discuss the experiences gained during the course. One of the themes of our discussion, indeed, was how the powerful, authoritative discourse that presents deaf people as lacking access to (spoken) languages has made Hanna "blind" to all the English around her. During the process of participating in the research, Hanna recognised the constraints of the dominant discourses she has adopted, and began to question them based on her own individual experience.

The concept of voice and the idea of identity being represented through a variety of voices is useful when examining the way a language learner positions oneself. Some voices may be dominant for a while until "pushed aside" by a competing voice in the community of voices within a person (see, e.g. Hermans 2002). Critical studies on multilingualism and identity have explored similar cases in which individuals appropriate and re-evaluate identity positions that are either imposed or assumed of them, leading to the negotiating of identities (Pavlenko and Blackledge 2004, drawing on positioning theory by Davies and Harré 1990).

However, in Hanna's case we see something else happening. There are no alternative voices on offer to Hanna as a deaf signer, she has many multimodal, multilingual practices that she can draw on when using English. Instead, the authoritative discourse has been powerful enough to be taken for granted by Hanna, yet the rupture of the taken-for-granted takes place during the interview and the authoritative discourse submits to individual appropriation (Bakhtin 1981; Pietikäinen and Dufva 2006; Solomon 2012). This rupture of the taken-for-granted, or moment of epiphany, becomes a crucial point which opens up new space for the identity positions of a capable learner of English.

14.7 Conclusion: Navigating the Nexus of Practice with the Research Participants

The critical research paradigm has produced research on identity construction which focuses on, for example, the strategies of resistance in contexts where marginalised groups develop resistant discourses against powerful, discriminatory discourses. Critical studies on multilingualism and identity explore cases in which individuals or groups of people are negotiating their language identities. Such negotiation of identities, or resistance to assumed and imposed identities can emerge, according to Pavlenko and Blackledge (2004), through any type of discursive practices, not just through conversational interaction. I take this to mean all multimodal actions of meaning making, which deserve much more attention than we researchers have previously given. MDA and nexus analysis encourage us be alert to discourses that are embedded into built environments, objects and the historical bodies of participants. I followed this advice in my earlier research in showing the contradiction between the dominant discourses and the actions with English language by FinSL signing research participants. In other words, the discourses of the analyst—my interactions with the research practices and my characterisations of the research I was engaged with—*represented and produced* alternative discourses for the dominant discourse that positions deaf signers as lacking resources for English language learning. In this study which reanalysed an interview done in 2007, however, it is not only the researcher who is navigating the discourses crucial for the social issue of deaf signers as English language learners. One could say that the research participant, Hanna, begins to navigate the nexus of practice by mapping the crucial actions in relation to English language learning, and moreover, by forming a broader understanding of the practices and discourses linked to her language learner identity.

When reflecting on nexus analysis as a research approach that can contribute to promoting social change by transforming discourse and actions into new discourses and practices, I argue for the importance of merging research activities with the activities of the research participants. This study suggests that an efficient way to promote change is to invite the research participants to participate in research activities beyond the data collection, in other words, to participate also in the multimodal analysis of the discourses that are prominent in their everyday actions.

There are various marginalised groups that are confronted with strong hegemonic discourses that position them as non-competent participants in relation to different activities in today's society. Hanna's case offers an example of how alternative identity positions may be triggered by reflection on rather mundane actions. My suggestion is to promote research among marginalised groups with a conscious focus on the link (sometimes invisible) between actions and prominent, authoritative discourses. Firstly, such research may provide us with new knowledge that questions the previous understandings or myths in relation to such marginalised groups (similar to cases presented in Sect. 14.5) and, secondly, such research can trigger the rearrangement of the discourses in the historical bodies of the research participants.

14.8 Afterword: Meeting with Hanna Seven Years Later

I met Hanna again in 2014 in order to discuss the analysis on the Hedgedog online project and her interview. She also watched and commented on the clip of the video recorded interview, as well as commented on my analysis of the interview. The discussion (2014) was captured with by video camera as it is very difficult to make notes when engaged in signed interaction. The interview in 2014 has not been further analysed.

After watching the clip of the interview I reanalysed in this chapter, Hanna spontaneously told me how she remembers the particular moment in the interview when her view of herself as a non-competent English language learner was challenged by the interviewer. She situated the interview and the Hedgedog course in her past, in a particular phase in her life trajectory. As she was now familiar with CDA, ethnographic research on multilingual identities, as well as multimodality in language learning, she saw "Hanna in the past" considering herself as a non-competent English language users and learner linked to the context she was in 2007: she was the only deaf student integrated in mainstream education which foregrounded the limitations of her English language skills. She remembered how participating in the research—the Hedgedog course and the interview—changed her view of herself as a language learner. In her opinion, the support from the researcher, who acknowledged her resources for language learning, played an important role in the shift. In our discussion (2014) she was rather amused when noticing what a difference there is between the time of the first interview and the way she sees herself now. She no longer feels she lacks anything as a language learner; quite the contrary, she sees herself as a very competent multilingual person who not only uses several languages daily, but also masters a range of repertoires in different modal and linguistic varieties.

References

Bagga-Gupta, S. (2004). Visually oriented language use: Discursive and technological resources in Swedish deaf pedagogical arenas. In M. V. Herreweghe & M. Vermeerbergen (Eds.), *To the lexicon and beyond: sociolinguistics in European deaf communities* (pp. 171–207). Washington, D.C.: Gallaudet University Press.

Bagga-Gupta, S. (2010). Creating and (re)negotiating boundaries: representations as mediation in visually oriented multilingual Swedish school settings. *Language, Culture and Curriculum, 23* (3), 251–276.

Bagga-Gupta, S. (2012). Privileging identity positions and multimodal communication in textual practices: Intersectionality and the (re)negotiating of boundaries. In A. Pitkänen-Huhta & L. Holm (Eds.), *Literacy practices in transition: Perspectives from the Nordic countries* (pp. 75–100). Bristol: Multilingual Matters.

Bakhtin, M. (1981). Discourse in the novel. In M. Holquist (Ed.), *The dialogic imagination: four essays* (pp. 269–422). Austin, Texas: University of Texas Press.

Bauman, H. L. (Ed.). (2008). *Open your eyes: Deaf studies talking*. Minneapolis, MN: University of Minnesota Press.

Blommaert, J., & Huang, A. (2009). Historical bodies and historical space. *Journal of Applied Linguistics, 6*(3), 267–282.

Cameron, D., Frazer, E., Harvey, P., Rampton, B., & Richardson, K. (1993). Ethics, advocacy and empowerment: Issues of method in researching language. *Language & Communication*. doi:10.1016/0271-5309(93)90001-4

Davies, B., & Harré, R. (1990). Positioning: The discursive production of selves. *Journal for the Theory of Social Behaviour., 20*(1), 43–63.

Dufva, H. (2013). Language learning as dialogue and participation. In E. Christiansen, L. Kuure, A. Mørch, & B. Lindström (Eds.), *Problem-based learning for the 21st century* (pp. 51–72). Aalborg: Aalborg University Press.

Fairclough, N. (2003). *Analyzing discourse: Textual analysis for social research*. London: Routledge.

Giddens, A. (1991). *Modernity and self-identity: self and society in the late modern age*. Cambridge: Polity.

Hermans, H. J. M. (2002). The dialogical self as a society of mind. *Theory & Psychology, 12*(2), 147–160.

Holland, D., Lachicotte, W., Jr., Skinner, D., & Cain, C. (1998). *Identity and agency in cultural worlds*. Cambridge, Massachusetts: Harvard University Press.

Johnson, R. E. (2006). Cultural constructs that impede discussion about variability in speech-based educational models for deaf children with cochlear implants. *Perspectiva, 24,* 29–80.

Jokinen, M. (1992). *Kuuroutta koskevia näkemyksiä peruskoulun kuulovammaisten opetussuunnitelman perusteissa 1987* [Views on deafness in the Foundations of the comprehensive school curriculum for hearing-impaired 1987]. Helsinki: Kuurojen liitto.

Jones, R. H. (2008). Good sex and bad karma: Discourse and the historical body. In V. K. Bhatia, J. Flowerdew, & R. H. Jones (Eds.), *Advances in discourse studies* (pp. 245–257). London: Routledge.

Kelly, R., Dufva, H., & Tapio, E. (2015). Many languages, many modalities: Finnish Sign Language signers as learners of English. In J. Jakonen, J. Jalkanen, T. Paakkinen, & M. Suni (Eds.), *Kielen oppimisen virtauksia. Flows of language learning* (pp. 113–125). Jyväskylä: Publications de l'association Finlandaise de linguistique appliquée (AFinLA) 73.

Kirkehei, I., Myrhaug, H.T., Garm, N., Simonsen, E., & Wie, O.B. (2011). Kommunikasjonsformer for barn med cochleaimplantat [Communication modes for children with cochlear implant]. (Rapport nr. 15–2011). Oslo, Nasjonalt kunnskpassenter for helsetjenesten.

Kramsch, C. (Ed.), (2002). *Language acquisition and language socialization: Ecological perspectives*. London: Continuum.

Ladd, P. (2003). *Understanding deaf culture: In search of deafhood*. Clevedon: Multilingual Matters Ltd.

Long, G., Vignare, K., Rappold, R., & Mallory, J. (2007). Access to communication for deaf, hard-of-hearing and ESL students in blended learning courses. *The international review of research in open and distributed learning, 8*(3). http://www.irrodl.org/index.php/irrodl/article/view/423/933. Accessed April 4, 2016.

Luukkainen, M. (2008). *Viitotut elämät: Kuurojen nuorten aikuisten kokemuksia viittomakielisestä elämästä Suomessa* [Signed lives. Experiences of deaf young adults on life as sign language users in Finland.] Helsinki: The Service Foundation for the Deaf.

Marschark, M., & Hauser, P. C. (2012). *How deaf children learn—what parents and teachers need to know*. Oxford: Oxford University Press.

Norris, S. (2004). *Analyzing multimodal interaction: A methodological framework*. London: Taylor & Francis Group.

Norris, S. (2005). Habitus, social identity, the perception of male domination—and agency? In S. Norris & R. H. Jones (Eds.), *Discourse in action: Introducing mediated discourse analysis* (pp. 183–196). London: Routledge.

Norris, S. (2011). *Identity in (inter)action: Introducing multimodal (inter)action analysis*. Berlin: De Gruyter Mouton.

Norton, B. (2013). *Identity and language learning. Extending the conversation* (2nd ed.). Bristol: Multilingual Matters.

Padden, C., & Humphries, T. (1988). *Deaf in America: Voices from a culture*. London: Harvard University Press.

Pavlenko, A., & Blackledge, A. (Eds.). (2004). *Negotiation of identities in multilingual contexts*. Clevedon: Multilingual Matters Ltd.

Pennycook, A. (2007). *Global Englishes and transcultural flows*. London: Routledge.

Pietikäinen, S., & Dufva, H. (2006). Voices in discourses: Dialogism, Critical discourse analysis and ethnic identity. *Journal of Sociolinguistics, 10*(2), 205–224.

Rainò, P. (2012). *Sisäkorvaistutteen saaneiden kuurojen lasten ja nuorten kielivalinnoista ja tulkkauspalvelujen tarpeesta* [Language choices and the need for interpreting services for deaf children and young people with cochlear implants]. Helsinki: HUMAK University of Applied Sciences.

Salmi, E. (2010). *Linguistic turns in teaching of the deaf in Finland*. Helsinki: HUMAK University of Applied Sciences.

Scollon, R. (2001a). Action and text: towards an integrated understanding of the place of text in social (inter)action, mediated discourse analysis and the problem of social action. In R. Wodak & M. Meyer (Eds.), *Methods in critical discourse analysis* (pp. 139–183). London: Sage.

Scollon, R. (2001b). *Mediated discourse: The nexus of practice*. London: Routledge.

Scollon, R. (2002). Intercultural communication as nexus analysis. *Logos and Language: Journal of General Linguistics and Language Theory, 3*(2), 1–17.

Scollon, R., & Scollon, S. W. (2004). *Nexus analysis—Discourse and the emerging internet*. New York, NY: Routledge.

Scollon, R., & Scollon, S. W. (2005). Lighting the stove: why habitus isn't enough for critical discourse analysis. In R. Wodak (Ed.), *New agenda in (critical) discourse analysis: Theory, methodology and interdisciplinarity* (pp. 101–169). Philadelphia, PA: John Benjamins Publishin Company.

Scollon, R., & Scollon, S. W. (2009). *Breakthrough into action. Text & Talk, 29*(3), 277–294.

Solomon, Y. (2012). Finding a voice? Narrating the female self in mathematics. *Educational Studies in Mathematics, 80*(1–2), 171–183.

Tapio, E. (2013). *A nexus analysis of English in the everyday life of FinSL signers—A multimodal view on interaction* (Doctoral dissertation). Finland: University of Oulu.

Tapio, E. (2014). The marginalisation of finely tuned semiotic practices and misunderstandings in relation to (signed) languages and deafness. *Multimodal Communication, 3*(2), 131–142.

Tapio, E., & Takkinen, R. (2012). When one of your languages is not recognized as a language at all. In J. Blommaert, S. Leppänen, P. Pahta, & T. Virkkula (Eds.), *Dangerous multilingualism—Northern perspectives on order, purity and normality* (pp. 284–308). Basingstoke: Palgrave Macmillan.

van Lier, L. (2002). An ecological-semiotic perspective on language and linguistics. In C. J. Kramsch (Ed.), *Language acquisition and language socialization: ecological perspectives* (pp. 140–164). London: Continuum.

Author Biography

Elina Tapio is principal lecture at the Humak University of Applied Sciences, Finland. She is doing ethnographic research on signed interaction with a particular interest on space, multimodality, and multilingualism within the framework of Mediated Discourse Analysis.

Erratum to: Identity Revisited and Reimagined

Sangeeta Bagga-Gupta, Aase Lyngvær Hansen and Julie Feilberg

Erratum to: S. Bagga-Gupta et al. (eds.), *Identity Revisited and Reimagined*, DOI 10.1007/978-3-319-58056-2

In the original version of the book, the belated corrections to update editor affiliation in copyright page as "Sangeeta Bagga-Gupta, School of Education and Communication, Jönköping University, Jönköping, Sweden" and to include abstracts for all chapters in online version have to be updated. The erratum book has been updated with the changes.

The updated online version of this book can be found at
http://dx.doi.org/10.1007/978-3-319-58056-2

S. Bagga-Gupta et al. (eds.), *Identity Revisited and Reimagined*,
DOI 10.1007/978-3-319-58056-2_15

Afterword
Cultural Experience, Identities and Diversification in the Hands of Researchers

Roger Säljö
University of Gothenburg, Gothenburg, Sweden

Introduction

This volume invites the reader to share research and reflections on identity and identity formation in a multitude of settings in contemporary society—in schools, professional settings, political processes, interviews, in collaborations in virtual spaces and in other conversational contexts that together form what we refer to as society. What we learn is that if we avoid assuming that identity is a given essence of a person or a group, we will see how identities are shaped, performed, negotiated, contested and accomplished in interactional settings. Thus, what to many will appear as a stable core of a person or a group—identity—turns out to be flexible, dynamic, situated, attributed and continuously talked into being. Such a perspective simultaneously has a meta-message; it forces us to consider seriously, even reconsider and unlearn, some of the assumptions on which social science research traditions have been built. Let me begin by briefly revisiting some of the ideals of social inquiry that we will be wise to reconsider in order to advance our understanding of the questions we need to ask about our own time and its challenges. As is pointed out repeatedly in the contributions to this book, there are "tellings" about society, some of which exercise considerable power in institutions, that turn out to be far from obvious or innocent.

In the wake of the enlightenment and the French revolution, the kinds of inquiry we now understand as social science emerged. Even though philosophers and scholars of various backgrounds had taken an interest in human conduct and life conditions since the ancient Greeks through inquiries into areas such as moral philosophy and various branches of theology, it was during the late 18th and the 19th century that the ideas of an empirical social science in the modern sense were shaped and institutionalized as disciplines. An important intellectual driving force that paved the way for social inquiry was the emergence of positivism. Through the writings of Comte (1830–1842) and others, the ideas of a scientific approach to

S. Bagga-Gupta et al. (eds.), *Identity Revisited and Reimagined*,
DOI 10.1007/978-3-319-58056-2

studying society, in order to uncover the laws that regulated social life, were articulated and spread across the world. The spirit of this epistemology pulled in the direction of limiting scholarly attention to what is directly observable to the senses, and to seeking explanations in terms of cause and effect in the mechanical sense. An important imperative, with almost moral underpinnings, was the idea that the attempts to achieve maturity as a science must be grounded in seeking methodological inspiration from the more advanced sciences, where methods and observations had resulted in mathematical modelling and successful prediction. Following in the footsteps of these maxims, it was assumed, the various social (and human) sciences would soon place themselves among the mature disciplines, and, as a consequence, they would provide valuable insights into how to predict human behaviour and how to organize society through the scientific principles of social engineering.

Although these ideals of going beyond metaphysics and speculation, and turn to data and observation, have been of great service to social research by sharpening our understandings of what it means to generate and analyse data, the limitations of the strong versions of the positivist programme soon became obvious. Max Weber, Georg Simmel and many other late 19th and early 20th century scholars, including leading natural scientists, pointed to the limitations of staying within such a narrow paradigmatic worldview. The price paid for this would be to leave many important social issues outside the realm of scientific inquiry, and, at worst, going down this road would risk making method into ontology. And this, to a large extent, is what happened in many corners of the behavioural sciences, for instance when behaviourism stepped in and rapidly excluded from what could be studied issues of culture, values, minds and the role of collective action in the lives of humans.

During the 21st century we have seen a systematic and dedicated battle against many of the legacies of positivism that continue to exercise influence inside and outside research. A range of alternative philosophical perspectives and epistemologies has entered the stage with the explicit ambition of broadening the role of research by expanding the domains in which systematic exploration and analysis of social action may take place. In the case of empirical social science research, one of the most influential early proponents of an alternative agenda appeared within the intellectual framework of the so-called Chicago school of sociology (Bulmer 1984). In view of the important issues of contemporary society that the authors of the present volume address when exploring issues of identities in various settings, the tensions in social inquiry—theoretical as well as methodological—that the leading scholars in the Chicago school experienced almost a century ago are worth returning to. By learning from them we need not fear that the edifice of social research is crumbling when we adopt methods and research approaches that are adapted to studying processes of diversification and identity transformation; on the contrary, we will be sensitized to what we take for granted or do not yet see.

What the members of the Chicago school—inspired by scholars such as the pragmatist John Dewey and the founders of symbolic interactionism George Herbert Mead and Herbert Blumer—encountered as they set about their research on social life were the consequences of a radical restructuring of life conditions of large groups of people in the wake of industrialization. The unequal distribution of wealth created conditions, where in a short time enormous fortunes were built up by successful industrialists, while their workers lived in poverty with miserable and insecure working conditions, poor housing and health care, and lack of other physical and social resources. The schooling offered to large proportions of the children, especially those of migrants, was limited and low in quality, and in most cases whatever was offered in terms of education was not relevant to the needs of children who, in many cases, did not even speak the majority language. This apparent mismatch between the agenda of schools and the backgrounds, interests and needs of children in urban environments triggered Dewey (1902, 1966) to explore the possibilities of replacing the abstract and teacher-centered traditions of communication in classrooms with something different; a democratic and more participatory role for children where what was going on in class would be consequential for their lives.

To make a long and interesting story short, what the members of the Chicago school experienced were the consequences of social diversity brought about by migration and urbanization, and they realized that urban sociology, and social research more generally, would have to adopt different methodological and theoretical premises if they were to have anything interesting to say. Large-scale surveys based on the language and ideals of mainstream society were simply no longer alone producing the data that would provide insights into the dynamics of urban life and the conditions of the homeless, the immigrants, the elderly, those suffering the consequences of alcoholism, or, more generally, those who were marginalized or considered deviant in an increasingly diverse society.

Several important theoretical and methodological advances followed from these ambitions to design research that would illuminate the conditions of living and working in complex societies. At the theoretical level, one of the avenues followed was to study communities rather than societies (or even cities). Society, following this logic, is an abstraction; communities are the contexts in which people develop their worldviews, identities, values and practices. Communities are organic and offer interactional settings where—as the editors of this volume put it in their preface—people and institutions are shaped by the "living and daily doings" of its members. The other side of this coin, with a profound impact on social research that is still visible, is of course the development of research methods that followed from this recognition of the challenges introduced by social complexity. Approaches to data generation such as ethnographies, participant observation, research interviewing and several others emerged as responses to the needs of analysing how members of communities went about their daily lives and how they produced social order through interaction. This interest in how to properly do qualitative research is still a matter of debate, quite often with the ideals of quantification, prediction and (statistical) generalization launched by positivism, hovering in the background as preferences irrespective of what the research questions are.

The Challenges of Studying Complex Societies

The metaphor of the traditional and functionalist perspective of social science is of studying society as a machine with clearly separate elements (i.e. individuals) that add up to the collective (i.e. institutions and society). Ideally, this machine should operate with as little friction as possible, and any dysfunctional unit should be immediately attended to and corrected, preferably before the dysfunction appears. And the role of research is to detect deviance and suggest methods that institutions may use in order to bring the person back on track. If this naïve functionalism did not hold water as a figure of thought a century ago, as the efforts of the members of the Chicago school have taught us, it is even less relevant today in a world of globalization, migration, virtualization and diversification. Hopefully, we will soon see the end of the paralyzing powers of neoliberalism and its offspring in terms of new public management, simplistic performance measurements and an economistic ideology, where all features of human life have been reduced to ideas of individuals maximizing their personal gains in all walks of life. The limiting perspectives following this ideology have reduced social research to studying the kinds of indicators that inform ready-made and reified conceptions of society and social change—who fits in, and who does not.

There are several features of the arguments and the results presented in this volume that I think have to be taken seriously if social sciences are to play a significant and emancipatory function in our time. I will limit myself to commenting on three points. One of these concerns accepting diversity and diversification as productive base lines of social inquiry, which is a point made very clearly in the first chapter by the editors and in the first section of this volume, and it reappears as a matter attended to in all sections. This is a challenge for most areas and disciplines, since they on many occasions build on, even sanction, stereotypes and hegemonic conceptions of people and social practices. In my own research area, it is fascinating to observe how a very narrow, and Eurocentric, perspective on human development for a long time dominated theoretical perspectives. Intellectual development, for instance, was construed as a capacity for increasingly abstract forms of thinking, and the implication was that reasoning in terms of abstract logic should be the target for the mature mind (and a guide for educational practices). Looking at how tests in developmental research were designed, we see how this ideal materialized in scholarly practices of designing experiments and empirical research that privileged abstraction at the expense of more contextual modes of reasoning (cf, e.g., Grossen 1988). The famous, and much debated, study by Harvard psychologist Gilligan (1982) in an interesting manner raised the question if a dominant, and very Western, perspective on moral development was biased in terms of gender. One of Gilligan's points, illustrated through empirical observations, is that women and men seemed to relate differently to moral dilemmas used in standardized psychological tests. In brief, men seemed to follow the expected abstract logic when providing responses, while women were more contextual in their reasoning, sometimes to the extent that they would not accept the premises on which the dilemmas were formulated by the test designers. A similar example of a massive exercise of hegemonic research practices may be found in cross-cultural research on human development. As many studies have shown, the assumptions regarding cognitive, social and other forms of development result in research designs and practices that end up portraying non-Western populations as less well performing and less advanced (for critical discussion of such normativity, see Dasen 1972; Gay and Cole 1967; Greenfield 1976). A critical intellectual issue is, as is pointed out in many of the chapters of this volume, that there is a long tradition in research and theorizing of making assumptions about the universality of human development and life in general. Even when acknowledging differences between groups in terms of how societies are organized and lives are lived, the differences between societies and cultures are not given full attention, since we are not able to fully cope with the problem that even our epistemologies differ as the authors of this volume remind us of. We will never be able to critically scrutinize how identities emerge, are remade and performed, unless we are willing to acknowledge that they are embedded in societal and institutional practices and assumptions of what it means to grow up or to act in specific settings as is illustrated in the contributions to this volume analysing virtual as well as physical encounters.

A second important lesson to be learned from the contributions to the book is the necessity of analysing processes of social change, and to do this by linking the individual and the collective level, which is a topic explored in several chapters. Societies are constantly coming into being; they are never finished or in an end-state. A corollary of this assumption is that we have to continue producing insights that demonstrate how social practices, identities, values and so on are shaped through interactional and institutional processes, and how they are transformed. Interactional practices and joint-activities make up the glue that simultaneously creates continuity and transformation of the ways in which we lead our lives. Such a focus on studying dynamics and change will serve as an important antidote to the problems of essentialism and reification of human identities, values, language practices and capacities pointed to by many of the authors in this volume (cf. Hasnain et al. 2013). It is also precisely in this domain that we must unlearn some of the legacies of the cultural history of social science research. As Linell and Mäkitalo (2017) point out, there is an unrecognized assumption in many approaches to social inquiry that society is made up of individuals, and that collective practices are accessible by attending to indicators of individual performance. Or, in other words, the method determines ontology by assuming that individuals are real while collective practices such as interaction and collective action are epiphenomenal.

As a third point, and most importantly, there is a meta-message in the research reported in this volume, which I hope we all take seriously. As scholars we are dependent on language and categorizations when we attempt "to sort things out" (Bowker and Star 2000). The world cannot be studied and conceptualized in all its complexity, and reduction of complexity is a *sine qua non* for scholarly work. A corollary of this is that as researchers we have to be cautious in our claims and sensitive to the categories and explanations we rely on in our work, and that we perhaps endorse outside academia as well. Analytical frameworks never tell the full story; they are always partial, and what we claim to find is relative to our conceptualizations and methodological procedures. In this sense, research is a moral enterprise where we have to exercise epistemic responsibility. Our categories, and the claims they produce, may be recycled by politicians, policy-makers and the general public as rhetorical resources in arguments and debates that are consequential for our perceptions of society, our views of others and for decision-making. Categories are not merely abstract terms, they are enacted in social discourse between people, in media and in professional discourse within institutions, and in this sense they contribute to producing social reality—they are part of our procedures for "worldmaking" as Goodman (1978) put it a long time ago. An important ambition of the work presented in this volume is the attempt to question essentialist and reified categories about how human interaction, identities and relationships are conceived in scholarly work across a range of societal practices. The outcome of such endeavours is a richer and more fine-grained understanding of what it means to live and develop in a complex society. At present, when populist ideologies and narrow-minded accounts of cultural traits and ethnic identities proliferate around the world, we urgently need to be sensitized to our biases and blind spots. Currently we see how a wealth of prejudices, unfounded arguments and nationalist claims are allowed to play an increasing role in the public sphere, and they feed directly into aggressive policies against minorities and spur ethno-political tensions in many parts and regions the world (cf. Wertsch, 2017; Garagozov, 2017). Counteracting these trends must be a prominent mission for contemporary social science.

References

Bowker, G., & Star, S. L. (2000). *Sorting things out. Classification and its consequences*. Cambridge, MA: The MIT Press.

Bulmer, M. (1984). *The Chicago school of sociology. Institutionalization, diversity and the rise of sociological research*. Chicago, IL: Chicago University Press.

Comte, A. (1830–1842). *Cours de philosophie positive. 1re et 2e leçon* [Course on positive philosophy. 1st and 2nd lecture]. Retrieved November 23, 2014, http://classiques.uqac.ca/classiques/Comte_auguste/cours_philo_positive/cours_philo_positive.html

Dasen, P. (1972). Cross-cultural Piagetian research. *Journal of Cross-Cultural Psychology, 3*(1), 23–40. doi:10.1177/002202217200300102

Dewey, J. (1902). *The child and the curriculum*. Chicago: The University of Chicago Press.

Dewey, J. (1966). *Democracy and education*. New York, NY: The Free Press.

Garagozov, R. R. (2017). Collective memory in dynamics of ethnopolitical mobilization: The Karabakh conflict. In Å. Mäkitalo, P. Linell, & R. Säljö (Eds.), *Memory practices and learning. Interactional, institutional, and sociocultural perspectives* (pp. 249–275). Charlotte, NC: Information Age Publishing

Gay, J., & Cole, M. (1967). *The new mathematics and an old culture: A study of learning among the Kpelle of Liberia*. New York, NY: Holt, Rinehart & Winston.

Gilligan, C. (1982). *In a different voice. Psychological theory and women's development*. Cambridge, MA: Harvard University Press.

Goodman, N. (1978). *Ways of worldmaking*. Indianapolis, IN: Hackett Publishing.

Greenfield, P. M. (1976). Cross-cultural research and Piagetian theory: Paradox and progress. In K. F. Riegel & J. A. Meacham (Eds.), *The developing individual in a changing world* (Vol. 1, pp. 322–333). The Hague: Mouton.

Grossen, M. (1988). *L'intersubjectivité en situation de test* [Intersubjectivity in test situations]. Fribourg, Switzerland: Editions Delval.

Hasnain, S. I., Bagga-Gupta, S., & Mohan, S. (Eds.). (2013). *Alternative voices: (Re)searching language, culture, identity...* Cambridge, England: Cambridge Scholars Publishing.

Linell, P., & Mäkitalo, Å. (2017). Memory practices writ large and small. In Å. Mäkitalo, P. Linell, & R. Säljö (Eds.), *Memory practices and learning. Interactional, institutional, and sociocultural perspectives* (pp. 383–401). Charlotte, NC: Information Age Publishing.

Wertsch, J. V. (2017). Narrative tools, truth, and fast thinking in national memory. A mnemonic standoff between Russia and the West over Ukraine. In Å. Mäkitalo, P. Linell, & R. Säljö (Eds.). *Memory practices and learning. Interactional, institutional, and sociocultural perspectives* (pp. 233–248). Charlotte, NC: Information Age Publishing.

MIX
Papier aus verantwortungsvollen Quellen
Paper from responsible sources
FSC® C105338

If you have any concerns about our products,
you can contact us on
ProductSafety@springernature.com

In case Publisher is established outside the EU,
the EU authorized representative is:
Springer Nature Customer Service Center GmbH
Europaplatz 3, 69115 Heidelberg, Germany

Printed by Libri Plureos GmbH
in Hamburg, Germany